Clinical Skills for Student Nurses
Theory, Practice and Reflection

Edited by

Robin Richardson

reflectpress.co.uk

First published in 2008

ISBN: 978 1 906052 04 1

British Library Cataloguing in Publication Data
A catalogue record for this book is available from the British Library

The authors and publisher have made every attempt to ensure the content of this book is up-to-date and accurate. However, health care knowledge and information is changing all the time so the reader is advised to double-check any information in this text on drug usage, treatment procedures, the use of equipment, etc. to confirm that it complies with the latest safety recommendations, standards of practice and legislation, as well as local Trust policies and procedures. Students are advised to check with their tutor and/or mentor before carrying out the procedures in this textbook.

Production project management by Deer Park Productions
Cover and text designed by Oxmed
Printed and bound by Bell & Bain Ltd, Glasgow
Distributed by BEBC, Albion Close, Parkstone, Poole, Dorset BH12 3LL
Published by Reflect Press Ltd
11 Attwyll Avenue
Exeter
Devon, EX2 5HN
UK
01392 204400

reflectpress.co.uk

Contents

PART 4 Medicine Management

Introduction

The Faculty of Health, within the University of Central Lancashire, is committed to the teaching of clinical skills to its health care students within safe, controlled, simulated clinical environments. My team of academic staff contributes a great deal of practice-based teaching expertise to many vocational curricula, particularly within the Department of Nursing.

We have written this book, predominantly, for pre-registration student nurses, who are either in their common foundation programme or in the adult branch. Other students of health care disciplines may also find certain sections of use.

The origins of this book go back, if I may be so bold, to the nineteenth century when, in 1860, Florence Nightingale founded the first training school for nurses at St Thomas' Hospital in London. She did this because she believed that nursing should have its own theoretical basis and that nurses should be formally trained (Peate, 2006). At the same time, she published her book *Notes on nursing – what it is and what it is not* and it is from this that I now quote:

> It [nursing] has been limited to signify little more than the administration of medicines and the application of poultices. It ought to signify the proper use of fresh air, warmth, cleanliness, quiet, and the proper selection and administration of diet – all at the least expense of vital power to the patient. (Nightingale, 1860, p.2)

Nightingale's view of nursing as a practical discipline seems to be just as valid 147 years later. For example, how often do we read media stories regarding cleanliness in hospitals and horror stories around hospital-acquired infections such as MRSA?

However, much has occurred since 1860 to turn nursing into an academic-based profession, distinct from medicine and other professions allied to it. In 1984 the United Kingdom Central Council for Nursing, Midwifery and Health Visiting (UKCC) set up a project to consider the reform of nurse education. This radical change to the education of nurses took place in the form of Project 2000 (UKCC, 1986). The implementation of this initiative in 1989 in England and Wales and 1992 in Scotland heralded the move of all pre-registration nursing programmes into the higher education setting. Student nurses were given full supernumerary status in clinical areas, as well as an academic award attached to their professional qualification. However, because the new pre-registration curricula placed greater emphasis on the theoretical underpinnings of the discipline, they were soon being criticised for being too theoretical. Indeed, research conducted by the National Board for Nursing and Midwifery Scotland in 1996 highlighted that graduates of the new Project 2000 programmes were lacking in clinical skills when compared with their traditionally trained counterparts (NBS, 1998).

The most popular view at the time of this overall 'de-skilling' of the nursing fraternity was that the new curricula, steeped as they were in the theoretical underpinnings of the profession, were producing qualified nurses with all the knowledge, but lacking in the practical, psychomotor skills.

This leads us to the notion of 'practical' or 'clinical' skills and their perceived value to the nursing profession. The whole discourse around skills was taken up by Corbett (1998) who makes an interesting differentiation between psychomotor (or practical) skills and what he terms 'skilled clinical knowledge'. Practical skills are able to be objectified and qualified in terms of performance ability and could thus be taught to and performed by health care assistants without them having to know the theory that underpins skills such as, for example, giving a patient a bed-bath. In contrast, skilled clinical knowledge is experiential in nature, formed through reflection on clinical experience in a variety of learning environments over a period of time, involving the development of mastery and intuitive practice. Such higher order skills are not easily taught in a classroom setting, or even in a clinical environment. However, if the emphasis within nurse education is now to promote cognitive skills such as critical thinking, reflection and problem-solving, alongside the nursing theory and practical skills, surely we are helping you, our students, to begin to develop this skilled clinical knowledge which sets nurses apart from health care assistants.

In 1999 the then regulatory body for nursing, the UKCC, published a review of pre-registration nurse education, based on the Peach Report, entitled *Fitness for practice*. This report highlighted the necessity for twenty-first-century nurses to be 'knowledgeable doers', critical thinkers, problem-solvers and reflective practitioners (UKCC, 1999). It also recommended that the balance between theory and practice in educational programmes should be restored, by introducing practice skills and clinical placements early in the curriculum. The recommendations of this report were incorporated into the government White Paper *Making a difference* (Department of Health, 1999), which also emphasised the importance of clinical skill acquisition in students of health care professions. This was almost a 'U-turn' with respect to the initial ethos of Project 2000 with its emphasis on theory. But can practice be separated from theory? Much is made of the so called 'theory–practice gap' in nursing. This is generally referred to as the situation in which students of nursing are taught one thing in university and experience something quite different in practice. However, I would argue that practice drives theory and vice versa, thus practice can never be separated from theory.

Skills development was also highlighted in another government paper of 2001, which provided a strategic framework for the continuing professional development of all NHS staff (Department of Health, 2001). This has led to the recently published NHS careers ladder, which has linked salary to the skills of the individual, rather than length of service (Department of Health, 2005).

Thus, having experimented with the theorisation of nursing within the higher education setting, practical nursing skills are once again high on the NHS agenda. More and more clinical skills teaching is being introduced as part of the 'Making a Difference' curricula throughout the UK. Simulation in a controlled environment (such as a skills laboratory) is being recommended for the teaching of clinical skills in order to allow students to acquire confidence prior to practising their skills on real people. More recently, the Nursing and Midwifery Council have introduced the Essential Skills Clusters (NMC, 2007), which stipulate what a nurse should be able to do, both on entry to the branch programme and on registration. These will be informing your own nurse education programme, wherever you are doing it within the United Kingdom. The NMC document segregates clinical nursing skills into five distinct 'clusters', namely:

❏ care, compassion and communication;

❏ organisational aspects of care;

❏ infection prevention and control;

❏ nutrition and fluid management;

❏ medicines management.

It is on these skills clusters that the sections of this book have been based, with infection control and prevention issues incorporated into all sections. Incidentally, have you noticed how these skills clusters are not a million miles away from Florence Nightingale's nursing ethos?

Therefore, clinical nursing skills appear to be defined in some quarters as the psychomotor 'tasks' associated with physical care, and by others as a much more complex entity, involving cognition, critical thinking and mastery. We believe that the latter definition is true of the professional nurse in the twenty-first century, which is why the skills in this book are not simply presented as 'how to' checklists but as part of clinical scenarios that have a patient at their centre. Each section relates to a particular patient and the skills attached to that patient's nursing care. Underpinning knowledge is also presented, so you will not only know what to do, but why you are doing it.

Additionally, interspersed within the sections are various exercises. Some of these are designed to test your knowledge and comprehension while others are reflective exercises. These reflective exercises will help you to consider your own position within the care you are delivering. They will help you to examine your own feelings, attitudes and prejudices, as well as those of others. This, we hope, will help you to develop critical thinking skills, as well as making you a more caring and compassionate nurse.

Remember, it is a privilege to be a nurse and to help and be with your patients (and their families) at some of the most difficult times in their lives. At all times, treat them as you would wish to be treated yourself. Good luck with your nurse education programme and in your future careers.

In the preparation of this book, my team and I are indebted to our colleagues within the Nursing Department at UCLan for their support and assistance, as well as their stoical determination to provide high-quality nurse education to the many students who pass through our doors.

I would also like to thank our clinical colleagues who do such a good job of mentoring our student nurses during their clinical placements. You are vital to all our success. I would particularly like to thank Dr Jenny Wilson and Katie Swarbrick, Consultant Nurse at Lancashire Teaching Hospitals NHS Trust, for their expertise and advice on early warning scoring.

Robin Richardson
MA, BSc (Hons), RGN, RNT

References

Corbett, K. (1998) 'The captive market in nurse education and the displacement of nursing knowledge'. *Journal of Advanced Nursing*, 28(3): 524–31

Department of Health (1999) *Making a difference: strengthening the nursing, midwifery and health visiting contribution to health and healthcare*. London: HMSO

Department of Health (2001) *Working together, learning together: a framework for lifelong learning for the NHS*. London: HMSO

Department of Health (2005) *Agenda for Change: NHS terms and conditions of service handbook*. London: HMSO

National Board for Nursing, Midwifery and Health Visiting for Scotland (1998) *Information base on arrangements which support the development of clinical practice in pre-registration nursing programmes in Scotland*. Edinburgh: NBS

Nightingale, F. (1860) *Notes on nursing: what it is, and what it is not*. Edinburgh: Churchill Livingstone

Nursing and Midwifery Council (2007) *Essential skills clusters for pre-registration nursing programmes*. London: NMC

Peate, I. (2006) *Becoming a nurse in the 21st century*. Chichester: Wiley

United Kingdom Central Council for Nursing, Midwifery and Health Visiting (1986) *Project 2000: A new preparation for practice*. London: UKCC

United Kingdom Central Council for Nursing, Midwifery and Health Visiting (1999) *Fitness for practice: the UKCC Commission for Nursing and Midwifery Education*. London: UKCC

Acknowledgements

The editor, authors and publisher would like to thank the following people and organisations for permission to reproduce their material in this book.

The Nursing and Midwifery Council for permission to reproduce the Essential Skills Clusters for Pre-registration Nursing.

Dementia Care Australia Pty Ltd – Abbey, J., De Bellis, A., Piller, N., Esterman, A., Giles, L., Parker, D. and Lowcay, B., funded by the JH & JD Gunn Medical Research Foundation 1998 – 2002 for the Abbey Pain Scale.

The World Health Organisation for the WHO Pain Relief Ladder and the Handwashing Guidelines.

Professor Ernst for the data used in the examples of complementary medicine used for pain control. This comes from Ernst, E., Stevinson, C., Pittler, M.H. and White, A.R. (2001) *The desktop guide to complementary and alternative medicine*. Edinburgh: Mosby.

University Hospitals of Morecombe Bay NHS Trust for the Early Warning Score chart.

Sue Anderson, Lecturer in Nursing at UCLan for her contribution to Chapter 9.

The Resuscitation Council UK for the Adult Basic Life Support Algorithm and the Advanced Life Support Algorithm.

Every attempt has been made to seek permission for copyright material used in this book. However, if we have inadvertently used copyright material without permission/acknowledgement we apologise and we will make the necessary correction at the first opportunity.

Author Biographies

Robin Richardson

Robin Richardson is principal lecturer and divisional leader of the Practice Learning Division at UCLan. Robin's nursing career began in the 1980s at the Royal Infirmary of Edinburgh. On qualifying, he worked in London for several hospitals, including the Royal Free Hospital, and St Mary's, Paddington. Robin specialised in vascular surgical nursing and went on to be a Nurse Practitioner. During the latter part of his clinical career Robin began working as an associate lecturer at Thames Valley University, eventually taking up a permanent lecturer post there. He came to UCLan in 2003 as a Senior Lecturer in the Foundation Studies Division.

The Practice Learning Division is a comparatively recent addition to the Department of Nursing divisional structure at UCLan. The Division believes that clinical skills are fundamentally important in nursing and staff are committed to the promotion and teaching of them. The Faculty of Health has excellent practical teaching facilities in the form of a suite of purpose-built skills laboratories. These not only benefit students of nursing, but also those studying paramedic practice, operating department practice, midwifery, physiotherapy and sports therapy.

Paul Cairns

Paul Cairns is a Clinical Skills Lecturer at UCLan. He embarked on his career in Nursing in 1987. Throughout the following years he has gained a vast array of knowledge and skills in both medical and surgical environments. Since 1995 he has practised within a variety of senior positions in renal medicine, including transplantation and dialysis (acute and chronic). Paul's underpinning knowledge base has been enhanced through the completion of specialist renal education at diploma and degree level. Subsequently, he relocated from London to Blackpool in 1999 and was the unit manager for a locally based haemodialysis service until he joined the teaching staff at UCLan in 2004.

Julie Cummings

Julie Cummings is a Senior Lecturer. As the representative of the Practice Learning Division within Children's Nursing, Julie participates in the teaching, learning and assessment of student nurses on both pre- and post-registration courses. Julie is the module leader for the pre-registration module developing skills and competences in children's nursing and the post-registration enhanced seamless care module. She is currently course leader for the foundation degree – child health and social care pathway.

Prior to joining the Practice Learning team Julie practised as a children's community nurse and was the team leader for the hospital at home children's nursing team at Burnley. Before working in a community setting she worked in children's medical and surgical/orthopaedic nursing.

Julie has a particular interest in the nursing of children with chronic and complex needs, in particular cystic fibrosis, and she has published on the subject. Julie is also interested in inter- and intra-disciplinary team working and protecting and safeguarding children.

Simon Dykes

Simon Dykes is a Lecturer and joined the Practice Learning Division in July 2006 to pursue a career within the higher education setting. He is developing paramedic education and practice as part of his role within the university. This will involve participation within the BSc Paramedic Practice programme and the Graduate Certificate in Emergency and Unscheduled Care.

Before joining the university Simon served with the North West Regional Ambulance Service NHS Trust and this enabled him to develop a strong clinical pre-hospital care portfolio. He gained the Institute of Health and Care Development (IHCD) Paramedic qualification in 1995 and further advanced his career with the ambulance service with the attainment of the IHCD tutor award in 1999. Simon's main function with the service took the form of Clinical Paramedic Tutor and he became heavily involved with the appraisal, traditional training and re-accreditation of clinical staff. Simon also gained a Certificate in Education and BA (Hons) in Education and these qualifications have further augmented his teaching practice.

Alison Eddleston

Alison Eddleston is Senior Lecturer in the Critical Care Division at UCLan. She is course leader for the University Certificate in Critical Care Skills and the University Advanced Certificate in the Care and

Management of the Highly Dependent Patient. Her areas of academic interest include curriculum development for the teaching of clinical skills and practice development.

Alison has extensive clinical intensive care experience and maintains her competency by holding an honorary contract with East Lancashire Hospitals NHS Trust. She is an active member of the British Association of Critical Care Nurses, serving on the North West regional committee. She is also a clinical link lecturer for both intensive care and high dependency specialities at East Lancashire Hospitals NHS Trust and Southport and Ormskirk NHS Trust.

Renette Ellson

Renette Ellson is a Senior Lecturer in the Practice Learning Division at UCLan. Renette completed her training at the Blackburn School of Nursing and acquired a staff nurse post on a two-year rotational contract in the Surgical Unit at Blackburn Royal Infirmary. This enabled her to gain experience in ear, nose and throat, urology, and general surgery. She was then employed for many years on one general surgical ward that specialised in both vascular and colorectal surgery.

Renette has long been interested in nurse education. She attained the ENB 998 in 1993 and regularly adopted the role of student nurse mentor. She has also worked as a night nurse practitioner where her remit included managerial tasks, responding to emergency situations, performing extended roles and teaching those roles to qualified night staff. Her experiences since this post have included surgical assessment, respiratory medicine and surgical high dependency.

Renette has a law degree and a Post Graduate Certificate in Education. She has been employed at UCLan since September 2004 and is currently studying for a Masters in Medical Law and Ethics.

Tony Heyward

Tony Heyward is a Senior Lecturer in the Practice Learning Division at UCLan. Being a representative of the Practice Learning Division within the Mental Health team, Tony teaches on pre-registration modules and on some of the post-registration courses including BSc Community Mental Health Nursing and Return to Practice. Tony is Course Leader for the University Advanced Certificate Caring for People with Dementing Illness, and module leader for Older People's Mental Health: Assessment and Interventions.

Tony has had a lot of experience of working with older people with mental health problems in a variety of clinical settings. Before taking up this teaching post he was a Practice Development Advisor for older people in Burnley, employed by Lancashire Care Mental Health Trust.

Tony has a particular interest in promoting a positive attitude to nursing older people and the promotion of 'person-centred care'. He has clinical links with Older People (Mental Health) Services and the Community Mental Health Teams (Working Age) in Burnley. He has recently completed his MA in Gerontology at Salford University.

Elizabeth Hickson

Elizabeth (Lizi) Hickson is a Lecturer in the Practice Learning Division at UCLan. She has recently been working for UCLan on a part-time secondment. This has allowed her to work operationally on front-line emergency vehicles and her duties also involved assessing and supporting staff in their development. In September 2007 she joined UCLan on a full-time basis and this allowed Lizi to focus on the developing future of the pre-hospital health care provider. She is the module leader for the Managing Trauma and Environmental Emergencies module and she also teaches on many of the modules on the Paramedic Practice BSc (Hons) programme. Lizi is currently studying for a BA (Hons) in Education.

Lizi began her career with North West Regional Ambulance Service NHS Trust in January 2000. She progressed to registered HPC Paramedic status in 2003 and gained her IHCD Tutor certificate in 2005. Since becoming a paramedic she has completed her Certificate in Education as well as becoming an ASA Decontamination Provider and a Pre-hospital Paediatric Life Support Provider. She is registered with the British Paramedic Association.

Ivan McGlen

Ivan McGlen is a Lecturer in the Adult (Pre-registration) Division at UCLan. He is currently course leader for the DipHE in nursing (pre-registration) adult branch. Ivan is also module leader for NU2001 and has other teaching commitments in various other modules. He has clinical link responsibilities within the Wigan and Leigh area. His present area of academic/scholarly interest is in the field of risk in clinical practice.

Ivan commenced his nursing career in 1986 and qualified as a Registered General Nurse at the South West Durham School of Nursing based at Bishop Auckland General Hospital, County Durham. In 1991 he qualified as a Registered Midwife at the Liverpool School of Midwifery based at the Liverpool Maternity Hospital. His clinical background is in the fields of midwifery and accident and emergency care, working most recently within the Accident and Emergency Department of the Royal Liverpool University Hospital.

Sam Pollitt

Sam Pollitt is a Senior Lecturer in the Practice Learning Division at UCLan. Prior to coming into higher education, Sam qualified as a RGN in 1991 and worked in a variety of clinical settings specialising in Acute Medicine and Elderly Care. Previous roles in education include a period of time as a Research Fellow in the Department of Nursing, during which time she achieved a Masters by Research degree in nutrition, and a Senior Lecturer within the Foundation Studies Division.

Sam's current role demonstrates her commitment to teaching clinical skills to pre-registration student nurses. She is module leader for a pre-registration adult branch module that reflects her research interests in the subject of nutrition. Sam also has an interest in problem-based learning and is a member of the SONIC Project group.

Sue Quayle

Sue Quayle is a Clinical Skills Lecturer in the Practice Learning Division at UCLan. Sue teaches clinical skills within the university and also co-ordinates mandatory basic life support. She has Link Lecturer responsibilities in Leigh and Adlington.

Sue trained in London and has a clinical background in emergency nursing. She has worked in Australia and New Zealand for many years and was involved working in both management and teaching while she was there.

Sue has recently completed an MBA. She also holds a Postgraduate Certificate in Emergency Nursing. Her special interests lie in the acquisition of clinical skills in the curriculum.

Susan Ramsdale

Susan Ramsdale is a Senior Lecturer in the Practice Learning Division. Susan is Course Leader for the MSc Advanced Skills and Practice in Primary

Care Mental Health and is also the module leader for subjects ranging from stress management to teaching the management of violence and aggression. She also teaches on the pre-registration nursing course and is the Link Lecturer for the Wigan and Leigh area (mental health). Within the Practice Learning Division she contributes to the teaching of basic life support, manual handling and breakaway techniques. Her current research focus is on the involvement of service users in education.

Susan qualified as a Registered Nurse (Mental Health) in 1996 and worked as a staff nurse and then team leader on acute in-patient wards in Chorley, Preston and Blackburn until 1999. In 1999 she became part of the team that set up the new Crisis Response Team in Blackburn, which was a joint venture between Blackburn, Hyndburn and Ribble Valley NHS Trust and Blackburn with Darwen Social Services. In 2003 she was briefly part of the team setting up the new crisis service in Chorley and South Ribble before moving into the world of academia in September 2003.

Paul Tipping

Paul Tipping is a Senior Lecturer in the Practice Learning Division at UCLan. His clinical background is in accident and emergency care. Paul recently left clinical practice where he was a charge nurse responsible for the education and training of staff in a busy department. Since joining the university as a senior lecturer he has been heavily involved in pre-registration training of both nurses and paramedics. However, Paul also maintains his high level of clinical skills by retaining strong links with clinical practice.

Angela Wilton

As Clinical Skills Lecturer Angela Wilton works within the Practice Learning Division team delivering high quality and enjoyable learning experiences for both pre- and post-registration nurse students. She also delivers clinical skills teaching across departments when required.

With dual qualifications in adult and paediatric nursing, Angela's clinical background is in adult and paediatric accident and emergency departments across London, as well as a short stint on a renal ward at Great Ormond Street and then a number of years as a school nurse in Lambeth. Returning north to Preston in 2001 resulted in her working at UCLan as the Senior Clinical Skills Technician. While in this post Angela developed a passion for clinical skills teaching and 2005 saw her move into an academic post within the newly formed Practice Learning Division.

Apart from clinical skills, Angela's main academic interests include the provision of separate facilities for children in A&E and pain assessment in children. She recently completed her BSc in Nursing Studies and is currently studying for a post graduate teaching qualification.

Part
1
COMMUNICATION

This part includes the following chapters:

Scenario: George Clarke

George Clarke is 72 years old and lives at home with his wife Mary and their 32-year-old son Max. George was diagnosed with Alzheimer's disease six months ago. This manifests itself in some minor memory difficulties around the home and disorientation when George is away from his home. He stopped driving three months ago following advice from his GP. Other than this, George has been relatively healthy with no hospital admissions in the last ten years. However, he did have to attend accident and emergency last month when he accidentally walked into a door because he wasn't wearing his glasses. He does take four lots of medication, one each for his Alzheimer's and arthritis and two for his blood pressure. His wife tends to all the household chores and finances, and she has to supervise George with his medication but, other than that, he is normally relatively independent.

Recently, George has started to experience some abdominal discomfort. This is exacerbating his memory problems and he is becoming a little agitated. After a visit to his GP, George is admitted to the medical assessment unit at his local general hospital.

Following admission, George is examined by a doctor and assessed by his named nurse. Bloods are taken and investigations are ordered to try to ascertain the cause of George's pain. George is kept nil by mouth and an intravenous infusion is commenced. Shortly after admission a pain assessment is performed and it is clear to see that George's pain is increasing and that it is radiating into his back. In view of the findings following the doctor's examination, his blood results and the fact that he has been on long-term non-steroidal anti-inflammatory drugs for his arthritis, the doctors decide that he needs an urgent laparotomy for a suspected perforated duodenal ulcer.

His operation goes as planned, with the provisional diagnosis proving to be correct. Post-operatively he is transferred to a surgical ward as his problems are no longer medical in nature and the surgical ward is much more experienced in dealing with his present needs. He makes an uneventful post-operative recovery apart from the fact that he is a little more confused than normal for the first 24 hours or so. However, in view of his age and his complex needs, it is felt that he would benefit from a spell of rehabilitation and he is therefore transferred to a rehabilitation ward in a nearby local community hospital seven days after his operation. Following a spell of rehabilitation he is discharged home (14 days after his admission) with a care package.

INTERPERSONAL SKILLS

Tony Heyward and Susan Ramsdale

This chapter includes three sections. The first section looks at verbal and non-verbal communication skills. The second section focuses on dementia and the skills needed when communicating with patients with this condition. The third section discusses the interpersonal skills needed to deal with aggressive and violent patients. Together these three sections cover key Nursing and Midwifery Council (NMC) Essential Skills Clusters (ESCs) in 'Care, Compassion and Communication' and in 'Organisational Aspects of Care', including the following.

Patients/clients can trust a newly registered nurse to:

Section 1	Provide care based on the highest standards, knowledge and competence.
Section 2	Engage them as partners in care. Should they be unable to meet their own needs then the nurse will ensure that these are addressed in accordance with the known wishes of the patient/client or in their best interests.
Section 3	Treat them with dignity and respect them as individuals.
Section 5	Provide care that is delivered in a warm, sensitive and compassionate way.
Section 6	Listen, and provide information that is clear, accurate and meaningful at a level at which the patient/client can understand.
Section 19	Work to resolve conflict and maintain a safe environment.

Communication skills

Introduction

This first section will raise your awareness of the skills we use when talking and interacting with patients. Activities will be suggested so that you can practise these skills with friends and colleagues, and assess and evaluate how effective your communication skills are, either in or away from the clinical environment. The section will provide you with an opportunity to develop interpersonal skills for health and social care practice, enabling you to engage, develop, maintain and disengage from therapeutic relationships through the appropriate use of communication skills.

Throughout the section you will be asked to consider how you communicate now, what influences your interaction with people, when you find it easy to communicate with others and when you find it difficult. For example, when you are out with friends or family 'chatting' is easy. You have lots of things in common and, when you are in an environment that is relaxed, you can chat freely. However, what about when you have to hand over in the clinical environment? How does it feel when you are feeding back information to other nurses about patients that you have cared for that morning or afternoon? Are you 'chatting' freely? If not, why do you think this is? What is making it difficult to communicate?

The handover situation can be anxiety-provoking as we feel that we are being watched, scrutinised and assessed. However, it is important that what we have to say is accurate and is being heard by others. Sometimes, if we are anxious, we may try to rush what we have to say or become 'tongue-tied' and get our words mixed up. Of course, this is a feeling any one of us can experience and it is perfectly normal for people to become anxious in certain situations. We all adapt our interpersonal skills depending upon the situation and environment. However, we still want our communications to be effective so, by being aware of how we adapt, we can take control of how effective our communication is.

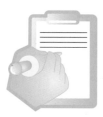

Activity 1.

Think about situations in clinical practice that cause you to feel anxious – for example, feeling that you are being watched and assessed. List these situations on a piece of paper and consider what may be causing your anxiety in each one. Then score the situations out of 10, with 10 being the most anxiety-provoking and 1 being the least. You could do this with other students and see if there are any similarities. Use the exercise to discuss the ways in which each of you deals with anxiety-provoking situations and share ideas for ways to combat the anxiety. If you are doing this exercise on your own, consider what causes you to feel anxious in the worst of the situations and how this is different in the situations you scored 1–3. Is there anything you can learn from the least scored situations that you can practise in the higher scored ones? Try to adopt these coping strategies when you next face a situation that causes you anxiety.

Communicating with George Clarke

The scenario for this part of the book describes George Clarke's admission to hospital in order to assess his condition, pain level and general health. During George's stay in hospital he will require a skilled approach and your understanding that the Alzheimer's disease may affect his well-being and influence how he responds to nurses and doctors. If George does experience periods of confusion it is important that you can adapt the way you communicate with him, to ensure that he understands what is happening to him and so that he can be involved in the decisions being made about him.

Communicating with people with dementia can be very challenging, and I would like you to consider George and his situation throughout this chapter. Ask yourself how George would be best dealt with using your interpersonal skills, and bear in mind that, if your interaction with him is poor, he is likely to feel isolated and afraid. Later in this chapter I will discuss dementia and the associated communication issues in more detail.

Effective non-verbal skills

What are non-verbal skills? Can we really control them so that they say what we want them to say? Non-verbal skills, sometimes referred to as 'body language', are the ways we communicate to each other through the use of our bodies. Our body language may include our posture and the way we stand for example, or the way we 'fidget', which may indicate that we are bored or anxious or even in a rush. Often, in lectures, the lecturer may observe that students are getting bored, distracted or even tired. No one has told the lecturer that this is happening but, through observing the students' body language, they realise that maybe students should take a break or even engage in some group work to change the way the lecture is being delivered. Next time you are in a lecture, take a look around (don't let this interfere with your learning) and try to spot which students have become bored, tired or distracted in some way. The gestures we make are referred to as 'cues', and it is these that we use to communicate with each other.

Non-verbal cues

Some basic body language cues are the same world-wide. For example, if someone is smiling it can indicate that they are happy or pleased.

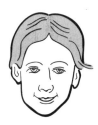

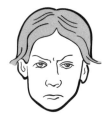

When they are sad or angry they frown and/or their mouth is slightly turned down at the corners.

Nodding the head is generally known as 'yes', while shaking the head indicates 'no'. These are gestures that we can easily control and use to reinforce what we are saying to someone, though we usually do them without thinking about the gesture. It is also the case that often, when people read the body language of another person, they do it without thinking about it. We know that a person is saying 'yes' by nodding the head but we don't need to make a conscious effort to think about the gesture; we just acknowledge it as everyday communication. However, when we are trying to communicate with someone who speaks a different language to us, on holiday for example, we rely much more consciously on these non-verbal cues.

We also use more complicated non-verbal gestures where the meaning is not as obvious as nodding or shaking the head. For example, it is suggested that if we avoid looking someone in the eye, we have something to hide or we may not be telling the truth. Another example is that when we position our bodies at an angle away from the person close by, we are indicating that we don't want to be with that person or we are trying to ignore them. Again these cues can be picked up and reacted to by the other person, sometimes consciously and sometimes unconsciously.

Our gestures or cues will also change with how well we know someone. For example, we may feel very comfortable standing close to a family member or good friend but, with a stranger, we will distance ourselves by moving away to a more comfortable position.

Adapting our body language

It is possible to consciously adapt our body posture so that we can use our bodies to reinforce what we are saying and to support positive and effective communication. For example, when we are assessing a patient we can position ourselves so that we are facing them and so that we can make eye contact easily. The patient then knows that we are interested and listening to them. Egan (1990) suggests that, with practice, we can use our bodies as a vehicle to communication. It takes time and practice to achieve this and it is something that we need to constantly re-evaluate during communication. Therefore, when you have begun to assess your patient, you may have positioned yourself so that you are facing them, but you will need to consider what your body language is communicating to the patient from time to time during the assessment as well. So, for example, if you find that you have started to turn away from the patient, you can make a conscious effort to bring yourself back to face them again.

A patient like George needs to feel that he has your full attention and that you are interested in and value his input. You can meet George's needs very effectively by learning to adapt your body language and use non-verbal cues. You also need to actively consider the non-verbal cues that George uses to communicate his needs. What is his body language telling you about the way he feels?

Effective listening skills

Earlier in the chapter I talked about the fact that sometimes, during a lecture, the lecturer might notice that students have stopped listening and may need to give them a break or an alternative activity in order to regain their attention. The lecturer has picked up on the non-verbal cues that tell him that the students have stopped listening to what he is saying. Your body language can indicate that you are not listening to someone or not interested in what they have got to say. This can be quite distressing, particularly for our patients as they depend upon us to listen to them and then act on what they have said when they are not in a position to take any action themselves. The promised action might be as simple as refilling a jug of water, which may seem a minor issue to the nurse but, for the person waiting for fresh water, it is very significant. Now imagine if the patient had asked you to convey an important message to the ward sister, charge nurse or the consultant in charge of their medical treatment, or if they were telling you about an allergy that they have. How do you think they would feel if your body language made it clear that you were not listening to them? If a patient believes that their nurse is not listening to them then they will start to lose confidence in the service that the nurse provides and in the nurse's ability and willingness to do what they have promised to do.

From the patient's point of view it is important to remember that emotions such as anxiety and embarrassment can prevent people from listening effectively. It is well known that someone may go to see their GP but will forget what the doctor has said to them just a few minutes after the appointment. Our patients may experience the same thing when we are talking to them, so it always worth considering this when giving instructions to your patients.

Listening to George

Our patient George is constantly looking for reassurance, sometimes so much so that this irritates the nursing staff on the ward. Nursing staff are busy and will rush past George promising to be back in 'two minutes' but, of course, they don't always come back. On more than one occasion he is asked to 'go back to his bed and stay there, someone will come to him' but, unfortunately, he forgets that it is only five minutes since he last asked a member of staff the question he has just asked again. George will often ask for his wife because he is worried or afraid and, because he is not sure who people are, he wants someone familiar to be with him. However, again, he will often receive a 'brush off' from some nurses and this leads to George becoming angry (which often accompanies feelings of being afraid).

Reflection

Consider a time when you felt you weren't being listened to. Reflect on this.

❏ What did it feel like and what emotions did you experience?

❏ How did you know that the person wasn't listening to you?

❏ How important was it that you were listened to?

❏ Would you want to talk to that person again?

Is there a time you can think of when you didn't listen to someone? How did your own body language indicate that you were not listening?

Indicating that you are listening

How do we indicate that we are listening to someone? Firstly, it is very important to remember to look at the person talking to you. Consider your body posture and your non-verbal cues – what are they saying to the person you are listening to? You may have heard a parent say to their child, 'look at me when I am talking to you' because they want to know that they have the full attention of the child. Face the person with your whole body and stop and make time for them – don't look back over your shoulder as you are leaving the room. However, be aware that facing someone with your whole body can be intimidating, so it is important that you have a relaxed posture to covey the message that you are listening to them in an interested and friendly manner.

Make sure you have an open posture – i.e. make sure your arms are not folded and your legs are not crossed. Try to relax and lean forward slightly if you are sitting down, but not too far as this may intimidate the person talking to you and invade their personal space. Subtle gestures can also indicate that you are listening to someone. These can include nodding slowly to the person as they speak to you and tilting your head to one side can show that you are interested in what they are saying. Responding verbally will acknowledge that you have listened to what they are saying and using phrases such as 'I see' will indicate that you have understood them.

Eye contact

Eye contact is important when communicating and is particularly so when you are listening to someone. However, be careful not to let the eye contact become a stare, so that the person you are talking to has to look away to break the contact. Eye contact should be more of a gaze that will occasionally move away and then come back to eye-to-eye contact. Maintaining direct eye contact for too long can become intimidating or even start to indicate anger. This will make the person you are listening to uncomfortable and they will start to show their discomfort non-verbally, by fidgeting or moving away. If you do observe the person starting to fidget or move away, check your own body posture and become conscious of what you are communicating with your body. Correct your body posture and reduce your eye contact and see if that has an effect upon the person talking to you.

Conscious control of body language

Obviously, indicating that you are listening to someone needs to be done extremely discreetly. Of course, as we become interested in the person talking to us our body posture will usually adjust unconsciously and this will indicate our interest. On the other hand, if we are becoming embarrassed or bored by what is being said to us, we will unconsciously move into a body position that indicates this. What is important is that you are actively aware of how you react and use body language when you are listening to someone. You need to learn to consciously control your body language and this can take a lot of practice and effort.

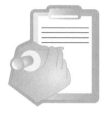

Activity 2.

Spend some time one day observing the body language of people around you – this might be when you are with your family and friends, or when you are out supermarket shopping for example, or on the bus. Consider what those around you are indicating through their body language and what they are saying verbally. Is what they are saying verbally coinciding with their body language? Discuss your own body language with friends and colleagues and see if they can help you to practise adapting your non-verbal communication.

Effective verbal skills

Speech is a very complicated area of communication and the way we speak can be influenced by many external triggers such as fear or anxiety, for example. An awareness of these triggers can help us to control our speech and therefore make it more effective. It is very important that your verbal communication is effective because, as a nurse, what you say can and will matter to individuals and groups – your patients, their families and your colleagues. The way you communicate verbally will also influence the response you get from those listening to you.

Making sure you are understood

Choosing the right words

It is vital that we are understood when we speak to each other and that we choose to use the right words for the context. Sometimes it is easy to use language that confuses others. This can be quite common among doctors and nurses when talking to a patient about their illness. It is easy to slip into using medical jargon which can leave the patient confused and lost.

Choosing the right speed

The speed at which we speak can vary and be affected by emotions such as anxiety, fear, excitement or embarrassment. In these situations speech speed tends to increase and rapid speech can cause difficulties for the listener. Slow speech can also be a response to an emotional state; it may indicate depression or feeling low. It may also indicate a shyness or lack of confidence or even someone being defensive. You will need to become aware of the ways in which your emotions can affect your speech as this will help you to control the speed at which you talk.

Choosing the right tone and pitch

The tone and pitch of our voices can also be influenced by our emotions. Of course, it is also important that we are aware of the tone of voice used by someone who is telling us how he or she is feeling as this can indicate their emotions. Some of the emotions that can influence tone of voice include anger, sadness, joy or confusion. Often we are unaware of the tone of our voice. Has anyone ever said to you 'there's no need to shout' when you weren't aware that you had raised your voice?

It is possible to deliberately adapt your tone and pitch for certain situations. For example, if we are being sympathetic with someone we will use a softer tone. We can change the tone we use to try and calm a situation if we are faced with an aggressive patient or, in the case of our scenario patient George, when he is becoming confused and anxious he is likely to respond better if you use a calm tone of voice. On the other hand, shouting at people can exacerbate certain situations and fuel anger in others, particularly with people who are already anxious such as, for example, those in accident and emergency (A&E) waiting rooms.

The pitch of our voices is part of our intonation – the way we use our voices to convey meaning. Pitch is usually described as high or low and, again, can influence how people listen to us. When we are anxious this can tighten our voice boxes, which will have an effect upon the pitch of our voice, making it sound higher. One way of dealing with this is to have a drink of water to moisten our throat and relax our voice box. Also, the pitch of our patients' voices can indicate their emotional state. A flat low pitch, for example, can be an indicator of depression or someone feeling 'fed-up'.

Our patient George can sense when people are frustrated with him from the tone and pitch of their voices, though he doesn't always understand why this is the case. He sometimes believes that some of the nurses on the ward treat him like a child when they speak to him in a short, sharp tone of voice.

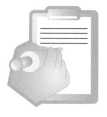

Activity 3.

Think about a time when you have been faced with someone who is getting angry with you, in a work situation, perhaps, or with family or friends. Consider the tone and pitch of voices used – your own and that of others around you. What was keeping the anger going? How could the situation have been calmed? (Consider the information you have been reading in this section.)

Summary

This section has given you an introduction to the ways in which we use our whole body to communicate and not just our voices. We are constantly communicating and our communication is being interpreted by others all the time, some of it consciously and some of it subconsciously. In nursing it is important that you communicate as effectively as possible, verbally and non-verbally, to maintain your professional image and to effectively care for your patients. To achieve this, you can learn to adapt and control your verbal and non-verbal communication by being aware of the ways in which your emotions affect the way you communicate, and by being aware of the effect this has on others. This understanding will also help you to interpret the verbal and non-verbal cues that your patients are sending you, via their body language and their verbal communication. Interpreting these cues will help you understand the feelings and emotions that lie behind what your patients are saying to you.

Dementia and interpersonal skills

Introduction

There are more and more people experiencing dementia and they frequently find themselves being admitted to hospital. In a lot of hospitals today the majority of beds will be occupied by people who are over the age of 65 (Department of Health, 2001) and, as a person becomes older, there is an increase in the possibility that they will experience dementia. However, this does not mean that all older people will experience dementia. Also, as with George's situation, the dementia is not always the primary reason for admission to hospital, but it can have a huge impact on how the person is cared for and on the way in which the patient adjusts to being in hospital. Hopefully, this section of the chapter will encourage you to read more about dementia and about how to care for the person experiencing the disease. It can be very challenging communicating with this client group but it also has its rewards.

Understanding dementia

Dementia is often misunderstood. Dementia is not a disease or illness in itself. It is, in fact, a broad term that is used to describe a range of signs and symptoms that are involved in a progressive decline in a person's mental abilities. This decline is the result of damage caused by specific brain diseases or by a trauma within the brain such as a stroke. Whatever the cause of a person's dementia the end result is the same and this is the death of brain cells (neurons). Unfortunately, brain cells do not reproduce themselves, so once they are gone they are gone for good. Dementia therefore affects memory, thinking and reasoning. It is a progressive illness and the person deteriorates over time.

Dementia is usually associated with old age, but it is possible to experience dementia at younger ages, i.e. in people in their thirties, forties or fifties. The prevalence of dementia in people over 65 is approximately 5 per cent, increasing to 20 per cent of the population over 80 years of age. The prevalence of dementia in people between the ages of 60 and 65 years of age is 1 per cent. The Department of Health estimates that there are 17,000 people under the age of 65 with a diagnosis of dementia.

Diagnosing dementia

Dementia is an umbrella term. In the same way as 'heart disease' can mean a variety of heart problems such as, for example, angina, so there are different types of dementia – for example, Alzheimer's disease or Lewy-body dementia. Alzheimer's disease is the most common type of dementia, vascular dementia is the second most common and Lewy-body dementia is the third. It is important to point out that, while no two people diagnosed with dementia will be the same, many types of dementia do follow a similar pattern. Some or all of the following signs and symptoms may be present:

❏ short-term memory loss;

❏ disorientation;

❏ loss of problem-solving skills;

❏ loss of independence;

❏ loss of the ability to care for own personal hygiene;

❏ loss of control over bodily functions.

It is also important to remember that certain treatable conditions can present symptoms similar to those of dementia, and they should be considered when diagnosing dementia and treated as appropriate. These conditions include:

❏ depression;

❏ delirium (caused by physical illness);

❏ alcohol dementia;

❏ vitamin deficiency;

❏ brain tumours;

❏ thyroid problems;

❏ neurosyphillis;

❏ poor diet with reduced fluid intake;

❏ endocrine disturbances such as diabetes or thyrotoxicosis;

❏ cerebral hypoxia caused by anaemia, pneumonia or transient ischaemic attacks.

Also remember that some drugs can also cause symptoms similar to dementia if not managed effectively.

People who are confused can also present similar symptoms to those of dementia. Even something as simple as dehydration, malnutrition or a chest infection may cause someone to appear confused. The main difference between confusion and dementia is that in dementia, people continue to experience memory problems and also have thinking and communication difficulties over an extended period. Confusion is usually short-lived, perhaps present for two to three weeks, and you can expect to see your patient make a good recovery. However, with dementia, the memory, thinking and communicating difficulties will have been present for at least six months.

Caring for dementia patients

All of our patients should be treated with respect and dignity and it is no different for people with dementia. However, their care needs can be very different from those of other patients. People with dementia can feel more afraid than most people because of their short-term memory difficulties. Also, their ability to fully assimilate new information regarding their surroundings or treatments may be impaired. So you may find that you are repeating yourself when it comes to giving information, which may be frustrating for you, but the person with dementia will think that this is the first time you have told them. It is easy to believe that someone is doing this 'on purpose' but be assured they are not.

Being in new surroundings can be unsettling for someone with dementia, and sometimes this can manifest itself in behaviours that can be difficult to understand and manage. These behaviours can include:

❏ aggression (physical and verbal);

❏ wandering;

❏ uninhibited behaviour;

❏ repetitive questioning;

❏ suspicion;

❏ pacing;

❏ lethargy.

Try to understand the behaviour more fully and ask yourself: Who is this behaviour causing a problem for? Would it be possible to accept the behaviour rather than try to change it or stop it? Consider possible causes for the behaviour. Quite often the patient is trying to communicate something. It is important that you go at the patient's pace and that you respect them as adults. Don't infantilise them (treat them as young children) and allow them freedom of choice whenever possible. If you are developing a care plan that focuses on the challenging behaviour then involve carers and relatives in the planning. They will help to give you a bigger picture of what the patient is like and what, if anything, will distress them.

Caring for George

In our scenario George was only diagnosed with dementia six months ago. However, the new surroundings and being in hospital could still cause him anxiety. George would benefit from having familiar things around him, so you could ask his wife if there is anything that she could bring in for George such as, for example, family photographs. Obviously, though, the ward will have to be able to safely accommodate whatever is brought in for him.

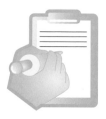

Activity 4.

Imagine that you are in a busy marketplace in a foreign country. You don't know how you got there or even where you are and you don't understand the language being used there. You try to speak to people who are going past, to try to find out some information about what has happened to you. However, they don't understand what you are saying to them. They just speak to you, give you a sympathetic look and walk on. As the people walk away you shout to them or try to grab them to stop them from leaving you, but they seem to brush you aside so they can get on with their day. They haven't got time for you. The marketplace is big, busy, noisy and frightening.

Think how you would feel in this situation. Who would you want with you, to help you or even just to share this experience with you? How would you like to be treated by the people around you? What would you need to help you feel better?

Communicating with a dementia patient

Communication can be problematic for patients with dementia and this can be for a variety of reasons:

- ❑ **Receptive aphasia** – where the person has difficulty interpreting the spoken word. Detailed information can become a jumble of sounds for them, but their understanding of non-verbal communication may be reasonable.

- ❑ **Expressive dysphasia** – where a person may understand what you say to them but they cannot find the words to reply.

- ❑ **Apraxia** – where a person is unable to follow a command to carry out purposeful movement.

It is important to remember that so-called 'problem behaviours' may actually result from not being able to communicate effectively.

You may have decided that the person you would want with you in the situation described in Activity 4 is your partner or a parent – someone who will help you and support you. It can be the same for patients with dementia. They become afraid and anxious, they want reassurance from staff that are busy and speak in a language they don't fully understand, and the staff don't seem to understand what they are saying to them. They may ask you where their partner or even a parent is and you may need to be very tactful when you respond. Telling them that their mother or father is dead can be extremely distressing for the patient.

Finally, it is important that the patient with dementia is seen as a person with all the components that each of us has: personality, past, present, social life, family or significant others, likes and dislikes, and a need for privacy and dignity. If we try to compromise in any of these areas by restricting the person or forcing them to do something they don't want to do, we start to make caring for people with dementia difficult for ourselves and extremely uncomfortable for our patients.

Dealing with aggression and violence

Introduction

When you work in health care you will meet people who are acting in a violent or aggressive way. This may be directed towards you or at someone nearby. It can become frightening if it is not managed successfully. The terms 'violence' and 'aggression' are sometimes confused or thought to mean the same thing, but there is a difference. Look at the following definitions and try to remember when you have seen examples of each – perhaps in real life or even on your favourite television show. Aggression has been described as 'a disposition to inflict harm. This may be verbally expressed in threats to harm people or objects, or result in actual harm.' Violence has been described as, 'acts in which there is use of force to attempt to inflict personal harm' (Wright, *et al.*, 2002). There are many things that can trigger violent or aggressive acts, some of which may be out of your control. Other factors, if you are aware of them, you can do something about in order to reduce the possibility of a situation escalating.

Factors causing violence and/or aggression

It has been said that there are some personality types that have a tendency towards aggression. This may be a combination of genetic factors and/or childhood environmental factors. This is hard to deal with because if you don't know much about the person, you are unlikely to be aware of this risk. However, sometimes it is easier to predict violence.

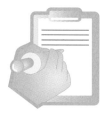

Activity 5.

Imagine that you are working in the local Accident and Emergency department late on a Saturday night. A man has been there for over two hours. He has been drinking and looks as though he has been in a fight prior to arriving. He is pacing up and down the waiting room and his voice is getting louder. Do you think there is a chance that he could become violent? Usually after an episode of violence or aggression it is easy to identify why it happened or what contributed to it. What do you think could contribute to this man becoming violent?

Factors contributing to aggression can relate to the environment. For example, noise and lighting are known to aggravate situations and changes in climate can affect some people (Blackburn, 1993). People don't like their personal space being invaded and boredom or lack of structured activity can also create aggression. People also tend to become very frustrated, which can lead to anger when they feel ignored or treated disrespectfully. Alcohol and substance misuse can also increase the risk of violence. Can you see now why the man in A&E might have become increasingly aggressive?

It is not just people in overtly stressful situations that can become aggressive. Consider our scenario patient George. He could be feeling very frightened and confused. He doesn't know the staff and they are always busy. They don't know much about him and communication is quite difficult. Can you see how George might react by becoming aggressive? What do you think that you could do to help him to remain calm?

Identifying anger, aggression and violence

People tend to display anger quite quickly so knowing what to look for can help you to stop anger growing into aggression and possibly violence. Garnham (2001) identifies some bodily reactions that indicate anger:

❑ stammering, twitching, refusal of eye contact, pacing, nonchalance;

❑ tremor, staring, clenched fists, shifting body weight;

❑ excessive swearing, spitting marring speech, exaggerated gestures;

❑ rapid movements, increased volume, poking;

❑ hitting self, grimacing, turning sideways, puffing out chest, refusal to listen;

❑ refusal to speak, defensive posturing, leaning forward, jerky movements, tearfulness;

❑ banging furniture, grinding teeth, increased voice pitch, provocative speech, inciting violence, dipping head, rapid speech;

❑ excessive sarcasm, standing too close, inappropriate laughter, pointed hand movements, stamping;

❑ wavering voice, insulting, rocking, rising to full height, screaming.

Think back to a situation involving anger or aggression. Can you visualise the situation escalating. Do you recognise any of these reactions? What can you do to try to manage this situation?

Core interpersonal skills required to prevent and manage aggression

According to Leadbetter and Patterson (1995) there are four core skills required to prevent and manage aggression:

1 empathy;

2 respect;

3 genuineness;

4 integrity.

By being empathic you show that you understand another person's point of view, their feelings, and can convey an accurate understanding of their situation. It does not mean that you have to agree with everything they say or do. Respect means respect for that person's individuality – not classing them as part of a group but showing an interest in them and what they are involved in. It is easy to dismiss people by considering them as part of a group with no individual ideas or needs. To display genuineness you need to be yourself. Often people hide behind the mask of 'professionalism', which often restricts their responses to stereotypical phrases which don't really mean much. Try to respond in an open, spontaneous and personal manner, which will show warmth and understanding. Lastly there is the need for integrity, which means you need to be aware of your own competence, responsibility and fairness. Be mindful of any biases that you may hold and try to assess the situation fairly.

De-escalation

If a situation involving aggression does arise then this needs to be addressed immediately. The term that is used to describe the calming down of such situations is 'de-escalation'. This term covers many aspects of the process of calming someone down and maintaining a safe environment but the main focus throughout is on communication. If you are confronted with someone who is being aggressive your body language and verbal communication are both extremely important. You need to be aware of your posture and eye contact. What you don't want to do is aggravate the situation by adopting an aggressive stance and shouting or talking over the other person. This would look more like an argument than a negotiation.

It might be difficult but try to appear calm, self-controlled and confident, while also showing respect for the other person's point of view. Easy? Think about situations in which you have been involved, or witnessed, where de-escalation has worked. What did the person do to calm things down? It isn't about agreeing with everything and promising the earth. It is about establishing a rapport based on co-operation and negotiating realistic options rather than issuing threats. Remember what we said earlier about respect and empathy? You can display these by asking open questions and showing concern and attentiveness through your verbal and non-verbal responses. Listen carefully and avoid coming across in a patronising or dismissive way.

If you are in a situation where there are patients, visitors and/or other staff around, you must also be mindful of their safety and enlist the help of other staff to make the environment safe. Clear communication and confidence in delivering brief assertive instructions are essential skills.

Following an aggressive or violent incident it is good practice to take some time out and allow those involved the chance to express their feelings about the situation. This also gives the opportunity to discuss how the matter was handled and enables both good practice and areas needing development to be identified.

Finally, managing aggression is a skill that requires you to examine how you use your basic interpersonal skills in day-to-day situations so that you are sure that your attitude, posture, tone and body language work with you rather than against you. It is important to remember that the most important aspects of managing violence and aggression are communication with and observation of your patient. Most violent incidents are predictable and preventable. If you use your interpersonal skills well and are approachable and understanding then you will have the opportunity to develop your skills in de-escalation and aggression management.

References and further reading

Bhaduri, R. (ed.) (2002) *Caring with confidence: a handbook for training in dementia care for nursing and care assistants in continuing care homes.* Cheshire: JRW Group

Blackburn, R. (1993) *The psychology of criminal conduct: theory, research and practice.* New York: Wiley & Sons

Burnard, P. (1992) *Know yourself! Self-awareness activities for nurses.* London: Scutari Press

Department of Health (2001) *National service framework for older people.* London: Department of Health

Egan, G. (1990) *The skilled helper: a systematic approach to effective helping,* 4th edn. Belmont, CA: Wadsworth

Garnham, G. (2001) 'Understanding and dealing with anger, aggression and violence'. *Nursing Standard,* 16(6): 37–41

Hartley, P. (1999) *Interpersonal skills,* 2nd edn. London: Routledge

Innes, A. (2000) *Person centred dementia care: an introductory course.* Bradford: Anchor Trust.

Kitwood, T. (1997) *Dementia reconsidered: the person comes first.* Buckinghamshire: Open University Press

Leadbetter, D. and Patterson, B. (1995) 'De-escalating aggressive behaviour', in Kidd, B. and Stark, C. (eds), *Management of violence and aggression in health care.* London: Gaskell/Royal College of Psychiatrists

Mason,T. and Chandley, M. (1999) *Managing violence and aggression: a manual for nurses and health care workers.* Edinburgh: Churchill Livingstone

Pease, A. (1988) *Body language: how to read thoughts by their gestures.* London: Sheldon Press

Thompson, N. (2002) *People skills,* 2nd edn. London: Palgrave

Wright, S., Gray, R., Parkes, J. and Gournay, K. (2002) *The recognition, prevention and therapeutic management of violence in acute in-patient psychiatry: a literature review and evidence based recommendations for good practice.* London: UKCC

Chapter 2

ASSESSMENT OF PATIENTS

Renette Ellson

Throughout this chapter reference will be made to the Nursing and Midwifery Council (NMC) Essential Skills Clusters (ESCs). Patient assessment and its subsequent nursing interventions are extremely important aspects of nursing care and as such the NMC has identified several subsections within two of the Essential Skills Clusters titled 'Care, Compassion and Communication' and 'Organisational Aspects of Care' that relate to these necessary skills.

Patients/clients can trust a newly registered nurse to:

Section 2   Engage them as partners in care. Should they be unable to meet their own needs then the nurse will ensure that these are addressed in accordance with the known wishes of the patient/client or in their best interests.

Section 3   Treat them with dignity and respect them as individuals.

Section 6   Listen, and provide information that is clear, accurate and meaningful.

Section 7   Protect and treat as confidential all information relating to themselves and their care.

Section 8   Ensure that their consent will be sought prior to care or treatment being given and that their rights will be respected.

Section 9   Make a holistic and systematic assessment of their needs and develop a comprehensive plan of nursing care that is in their best interests and which promotes their health and well-being and minimises the risk of harm.

Section 10   Deliver and evaluate care against the comprehensive assessment and care plan.

Introduction

Nursing can be described as a process. When this process was initially identified, Yura and Walsh (1978) showed that it is a four-stage cycle. The cycle begins with assessment, then a plan of care is devised, the care is implemented and then an evaluation of that care completes the cycle. Then the cycle begins again (see Figure 1).

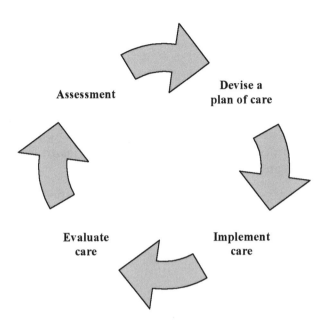

Figure 1
The nursing process

How does the nursing process relate to the NMC's Essential Skills Clusters?

It is quite clear to see that the NMC has related ESC numbers 9 and 10 directly to the nursing process. Essential Skills Cluster 9 highlights that patients/clients can trust a newly registered nurse to 'make a holistic and systematic assessment of their needs and develop a comprehensive plan of nursing care that is in their best interests and which promotes their health and well-being and minimises the risk of harm' (NMC, 2006, p.9). Essential Skills Cluster 10 then goes on to say that the registered nurse should then 'deliver and evaluate care against the comprehensive assessment and care plan' (NMC, 2006, p.10).

What is assessment?

The first stage in the nursing cycle is assessment. Everyone is different and people differ in many ways – age, sex, physical form, ethnicity, religion, the job they do, their home life and background, etc. – and all of these different factors can influence and affect their health and the care you give them. Therefore nursing assessment is about identifying which of these factors are important in relation to a particular patient's health and care. So, the purpose of the nursing assessment is to find out about your patient in relation to:

❏ their physical needs;

❏ their psychological needs;

❏ their spiritual needs;

❏ their sociological needs.

By asking questions in relation to the above headings, usually on admission, the nurse can identify the patient's health care problems. These problems can be further divided into:

❏ actual problems – problems and needs that the patient actually has at the time; and

❏ potential problems – these are problems and needs that may arise as a result of the patient's condition or predicament.

How do we assess patients?

There are a great many different things you could find out about patients so how do we know which of these things are important in relation to nursing care and, therefore, which factors we should assess? Luckily, several academics have developed nursing frameworks and models in order to assist the nurse with the practice of nursing assessment. Nursing models have been in existence since the 1960s and many different terms, such as 'models', 'frameworks' and 'theories', have evolved and have been used freely to refer to the same thing. However, this is not without its problems and many academics, such as Fawcett (1989) and Fitzpatrick and Whall (1989), have attempted to differentiate between the different terms. I will not go into these issues and problems here but I do advise you to carry out further reading on the development of nursing models, frameworks and theories (see the list of References and Further Reading at the end of the chapter).

It is, however, important that you understand the principles underlying nursing models. The models take all of the important factors that a nurse needs to consider when assessing a patient and organise them into a number of broad concepts. These concepts are based on the model author's beliefs about nursing and their nursing philosophy. Different academics have different beliefs and nursing philosophies and so they have come up with different nursing models. For the purpose of this section, we have selected Roper, Logan and Tierney's Model of Living

(1980) (Roper *et al.*, 2000) as this is the main model utilised by the author in her experience and it also appears to be the most widely-used model in the nursing profession.

Roper, Logan and Tierney's Model of Living (1980)

The Model of Living identifies five concepts (though many of them interrelate – see Figure 2):

1. the activities of living;

2. lifespan;

3. dependence/independence;

4. factors influencing the activities of living; and

5. individuality in living.

(Holland *et al.*, 2004)

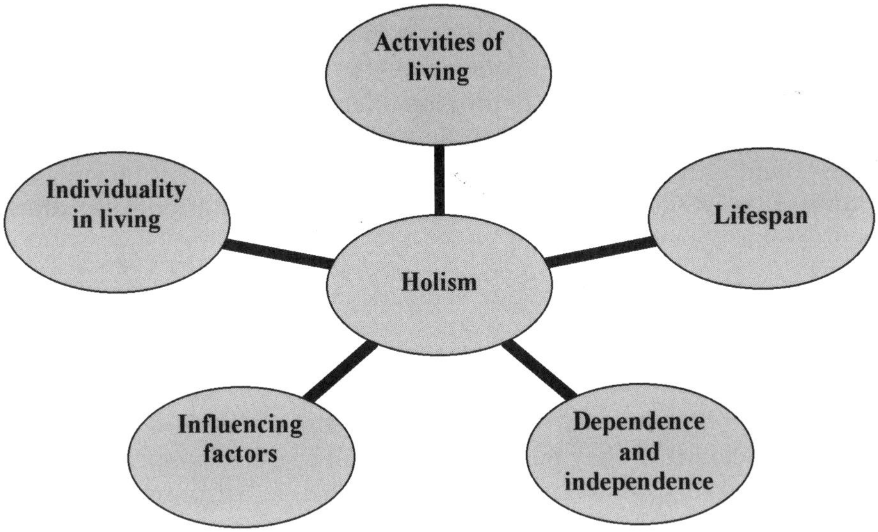

Figure 2
The Roper, Logan and Tierney Model of Living

The activities of living

The activities of living include:

❑ sleeping;

❑ dying;

❏ personal cleansing and dressing;

❏ elimination;

❏ eating and drinking;

❏ communication;

❏ work and play;

❏ maintaining a safe environment;

❏ controlling body temperature;

❏ mobilisation;

❏ breathing;

❏ expressing sexuality.

As healthy individuals we often go about daily life without even considering these activities because many of them just 'happen', we do not generally have any problems with them and, as such, we take them for granted. However, because many of these activities interrelate or are dependent upon each other, when someone becomes ill it is often the case that several of these activities are affected. Each of these activities will be explained in more depth and advice will be given on how to assess them effectively in the section on patient assessment on page 33. However, as an illustration, here is an example of the interrelationships between the activities of living.

See this chapter, page 33.

Breathing

A patient who has a problem with breathing may find that this affects sleeping as they may find it difficult to get to sleep or be too frightened to go to sleep (see Figure 3). This, in turn, involves the issue of dying and the fear of dying may also be present when the patient is awake as they are not able breathe properly. Personal cleansing and dressing will be affected as they won't be able to carry this out effectively if their breathing is impaired. This may also be the case with eating and drinking, communication, work and play, mobilisation and expressing sexuality and the actual procedures

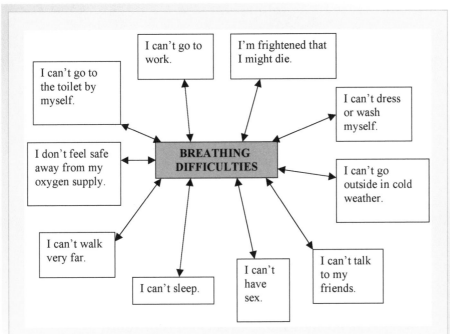

Figure 3 Activities of living interrelationships

involved in elimination (getting to the toilet, etc.). Maintaining a safe environment is affected as the individual's oxygen requirements will be compromised and controlling body temperature may be affected due to a potential risk of infection and the need to have a warm, well ventilated environment (which also ties in with maintaining a safe environment).

Reflection

Reflect on your own illnesses and identify times when some of your activities of living were compromised and why and how they were compromised.

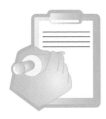

Activity 1.

1.   There are only twelve activities of living and now that you have read them you may think that they will be quite easy to remember. See how many you can actually remember without looking back at them.

Some tips to aid your memory

If you got them all then that's excellent but, just in case you didn't and you found them somewhat difficult to remember, I would suggest that you consider one of the following mnemonics:

❑ **SDP** (Social Democratic Party), **EEC** (European Economic Communities), **WMC** (Working Men's Club) and **MBE** (Member of the British Empire).

❑ 'Mastering Essential Skills Clusters Ensures the Patient's Well-Being is Maintained and Excellent Care is Delivered.'

❑ 'Mastering Essential Skills Clusters Ensures Excellent Care Delivery While Making Patients Better.'

Alternatively, you may find it easier to develop your own way of remembering.

2.   Try the last exercise with the aid of one of these mnemonics and see if it makes it easier for you to remember them. Consider the activities of living and try to identify any medical or surgical conditions which may affect these activities.

3.   Consider our scenario patient George. Which of his activities of living might be affected by his health problems and why? Discuss your findings with fellow students.

Lifespan and dependence/independence

From a legal viewpoint our lifespan may either begin at conception or when the foetus is potentially viable outside of the mother's womb, either prior to birth or, alternatively, at birth. The need for nursing or medical intervention may arise at any of these stages but, as this is a rather in-depth legal and ethical argument, we shall assume for the purpose of this book that our lifespan begins at birth.

From birth we continue to develop and, as a rule, we become more and more independent. However, in all sorts of ways we are actually still dependent upon others in order to achieve the activities of living. For example, a toddler may be able to feed himself/herself but would he/she be able to cook the food, or go out and buy the food or be able to earn the money to pay for the food? From childhood we develop into teenagers and then into adults where hopefully our dependence upon others is minimal. However, as we become older people, unfortunately, our independence may progressively diminish and, again, for whatever reason, we may develop a reliance on others in order to achieve the activities.

However, irrespective of what is classed as the 'norm', when a person develops an illness their independence may become threatened on either a short- or long-term basis. It is at this stage that the important skill of assessment is needed. Ultimately, the ideal care plan will allow as much independence as possible for the individual but, at the same time, it will highlight which activities need assistance or support and at what level this assistance or support needs to be.

Furthermore, following the cyclical stages of the nursing process ensures that the level of assistance or support continues to be provided at the right level for the individual until their optimal level of independence is achieved. Indeed, good nursing is very much like good parenting where independence is promoted, limitations are recognised and assistance is given as and when physical or emotional safety is compromised.

Reflection

Reflect upon your own stages of life and identify times when you were dependent upon others. Discuss your findings with fellow students.

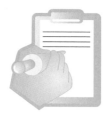

Activity 2.

Consider our scenario patient George. How might he be dependent upon his wife or other family members? Discuss your findings with fellow students.

Factors influencing the activities of living

The Roper, Logan and Tierney model (1980) has been criticised in the past. One of the criticisms is that there is an emphasis on 'the physical aspects of patient care' (Minshull *et al.*, 1986, and Walsh, 1989, as cited in Bellman, 1996, p.129). However, in agreement with Bellman (1996, p.129), one would also argue that this problem has been exacerbated by an 'inappropriate introduction and implementation of the model in practice'.

Indeed, personal observations of certain individuals utilising the model have highlighted what can only be classed as a naivety in its use, with several practitioners being unaware of the many complexities that the model can address. In some instances, this ignorance may also be due to time constraints and the need, on the nurse's part, to prioritise what he or she perceives as being the most important needs for the patient. However, in order to achieve the ESC 9, patients/clients should be considered holistically, taking every issue into account, irrelevant of whether we, as nurses, feel they are particularly important or not. Therefore, it is imperative that practitioners consider all the factors that influence the activities of living.

To keep the model as simplistic as possible, Roper *et al.*, (2000) identified five main factors that may influence the activities of living (see Figure 4). These are biological, psychological, socio-cultural, environmental and politico-economic factors, and quite often they interrelate with each other.

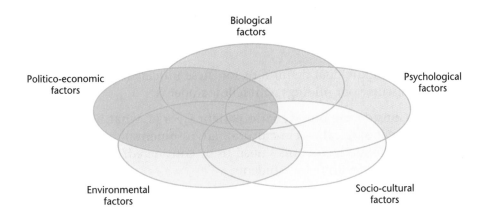

Biological
factors

Politico-economic
factors

Psychological
factors

Environmental
factors

Socio-cultural
factors

Figure 4
Factors that
influence the
activities of living

The interrelationship between the factors that influence the activities of living

A patient may be admitted following a diagnosis of breast cancer. The biological factor is the structure of the breast and the invading cancer while the psychological factor is how the patient may respond to the cancer and the threat to her life and her womanhood, and the changes that may be necessary to her body image. The socio-cultural factors may interrelate with the psychological factors as her beliefs about the illness will need to be addressed as well as any religious issues that need to be considered with regard to her treatment. The environmental factors may include the woman's lifestyle in general. Have any of her lifestyle practices predisposed her to the illness and can they be modified? Furthermore, her home environment can be considered in order to prepare her for her eventual discharge, which will ultimately depend upon the success of her treatment. The politico-economic factors will consider the woman's rights to treatment and care, present and continuing, with particular reference being paid, in this instance, to the NHS Cancer Plan (2000).

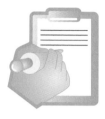

Activity 3.

1. Find individual definitions for these influencing factors and discuss your findings with fellow students.

2. Considering our scenario patient George, what biological, psychological, socio-cultural, environmental and politico-economic factors may need to be considered? Discuss your findings with fellow students.

Individuality in living

This is the final concept of Roper *et al.*'s model and, hopefully, the explanations of the first four concepts, the nursing process and the NMC's ESC 9 has provided you with enough information in order to understand what this concept is about. In short, it is about treating the patient/client as an individual and planning their care appropriately, according to their own specific needs.

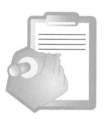

Activity 4.

1. When next in clinical practice consider two different patients/clients and compare and contrast their needs. Are they the same? If not, why?

2. Think about our scenario patient George. What individual specific needs do you think he might have? Discuss your thoughts with fellow students.

Reflection

Think about yourself. What individual needs do you have? Think about a close friend or relative – what individual needs do they have? Are your needs the same as your friend's or relative's?

Patient assessment

As nurses are the ones who usually have the most contact with patients, it is true to say that the patients are more likely to develop a closer relationship with the nursing staff than any other members of the multidisciplinary team. It is therefore imperative that updated and accurate nursing records are maintained throughout the patient's hospital stay as these are a potential source of essential information (Sturdy and Carpenter, 1995). Indeed, effective documentation not only helps to reveal nursing care to others (Lawler, 1991, as cited in Heartfield, 1996) but, if it is accurate, complete and up to date, it is also a vital component of high-quality care (Moores, 1996). Records should be completed clearly and logically and not be open to interpretation. Ideally they should also be free from error. However, should any errors occur, they should be highlighted appropriately. More information about this aspect can be found in the NMC's (2004c) *Guidelines for records and record keeping* available at **www.nmc-uk.org/aDisplayDocument.aspx?DocumentID=223**, and the NMC's (2006) *A to Z on record keeping* is also very useful and is available at **www.nmc-uk.org/aDisplayDocument.aspx?DocumentID=1587**.

The admission procedure and care planning

Admitting and planning the care of our patients are fundamental aspects of our nursing role. The two procedures interrelate as the admission procedure, if performed comprehensively, can very much inform the process of care planning. The nurse's interviewing skills are especially important and must include many of the therapeutic communication techniques. Asking the right type of questions at the right time is very important. In some instances basic 'yes' or 'no' questions will suffice but quite often 'open-ended' questions, which allow the patient to expand on an issue, are required in order to perform an in-depth assessment.

All hospitals have an admission process with specific documents that need to be completed in order to collect objective and subjective data. Generally, the most important document is known as the 'Nursing Kardex'. Because many of the sections within this document relate directly or indirectly to the activities of living, the nurse is given the ideal opportunity to ask vital questions that can provide valuable information about the patient. This valuable information can then identify and generate a number of problems and needs, thus providing a collection of attainable goals and, therefore, a solid basis to ensure that the care plan produced is indeed individual and, as the NMC (among others) advocate, holistic.

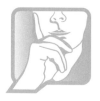

Reflection

Research the difference between objective data and subjective data. Think about the last time that you were ill and try to identify what objective and subjective data may have been collected had you been admitted to hospital with this illness.

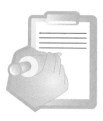

Activity 5.

1.   Think about our scenario patient George. What type of objective and subjective data may be collected for him?

2.   When next in clinical practice, ask your mentor about the Nursing Kardex that is used on his/her ward. Ask if you can have a copy so that you can familiarise yourself with the different sections on the form. If the form is difficult to understand or follow then ask your mentor if he/she would kindly explain those issues to you in more depth.

The Nursing Kardex

Not all hospitals will use the exact same Kardex, but generally they will be quite similar. Furthermore, there may be variations between wards and departments within the same hospital. This is because in some instances, such as, for example, in surgical day case units where the patient is likely to be discharged home on the same day following a very minor procedure, the process of performing an in-depth admission assessment would be quite futile and a waste of resources. However, for patients who are likely to have a lengthy hospital stay, the Kardex is likely to include the following sections. (Questions that may be asked are highlighted within each section but it must be remembered that these lists of questions are not exhaustive. They provide basic guidelines that I feel will give a good introduction to the assessment process.)

Name, address, telephone number, hospital number and date of birth of the patient

Obviously, we need to know who our patient is, but we also need to ask them how they would like to be addressed as this may not necessarily be the same as their proper name, or they may have a preference as to whether we call them by their first name or surname. Collectively, all the information in this section should ensure that the correct medical records, which could provide vital information for that individual patient's future management, are easily located. Knowledge of where they live may also need to be considered when arranging the patient's discharge. For example, you will need to know their address when arranging for a district nurse to visit the patient or when you are dealing with social services. There may also be environmental issues that need to be considered such as, for example, access to their house, the overall condition of the house and the location of the house for arranging transport for any subsequent appointments, etc.

Next-of-kin information

This is important for various reasons. The next of kin may be the only source of information if the patient is incapable of providing the necessary information themselves. They may also be an added source of information, especially if they live with the patient and have witnessed the events prior to admission. They may know of any previous illnesses and how the patient has coped in general with the activities of living. They may know of the patient's prior wishes with regard to treatment and/or of any living wills, should the need arise, although, of course, the decision about consenting to treatment rests with the patient if they are capable of making it. In times of stress the next of kin may also be a source of help with the situation.

Activity 6.

Consider our scenario patient George. How important is his wife's role likely to be during George's admission and hospital stay? Discuss your thoughts with fellow students.

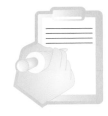

The person to contact in any emergency

This may be someone different from the next of kin though, generally, they are the same person. However, if, for example, the patient is elderly and they have an elderly spouse, that spouse may be hard of hearing or have other communication problems. The spouse may also be suffering from an illness, they may find it difficult to cope with the issue of an emergency situation or it simply may just be that they don't have transport. In this situation the person given to contact in an emergency may be their son or daughter or other close relative or friend.

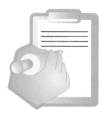

Activity 7.

1. Imagine that you are elderly, frail and have no transport of your own. Your spouse or partner has been admitted to hospital with a serious illness leaving you at home alone. The telephone rings and you are informed that your partner has taken a turn for the worse and you are asked to go to the hospital immediately. How do you think you would feel and how might you react? Discuss your thoughts with other students.

2. Now imagine that it was George's wife who had been admitted to hospital. What issues might arise if he was listed as the person to contact in an emergency in his wife's notes? Discuss your thoughts with fellow students.

Any known allergies?

It is imperative that you document any known allergies as the possibility of an allergic reaction on its own, never mind on top of an existing illness, could have fatal consequences. Even if the patient is unsure, it is better to document it just in case. It is also vital that you document the information that there are no known allergies as this demonstrates that the issue has been addressed and, should an allergic reaction subsequently occur, the patient is unlikely to be able to prove negligence.

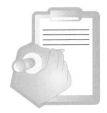

Activity 8.

1. In some instances people have an illness or problem but they do not realise that that this is actually an allergy. Therefore, when asking about this issue, it is important that you do not just ask 'do you have any allergies?' You need to expand on the question by giving some examples of allergies. When you have some free time, go to the library or read your nursing textbooks and identify the different types of allergies.

2. Think about our scenario patient George. How might you ascertain if he has any allergies? Consider the different types of sources of information that you may have. Discuss your thoughts with fellow students.

Reflection

Do you, or anyone that you know, have an allergy? If so, have you suffered or have you witnessed someone else suffering from an allergic reaction? How did you feel at the time? How serious do you think that failing to find out about someone's allergies could be?

Past medical history

A patient's past medical history is extremely important as previous illnesses may have implications for the patient's present admission and/or treatment. Ascertaining these facts may help with reaching a diagnosis and they will also help with the formulation of the care plan as certain illnesses may be long-term or still be apparent and, as such, these may also need to be considered when planning that individual's care.

Present medications

Knowledge of a patient's medications may help with a diagnosis and treatment. For example, if a patient is admitted with **haematemesis** (vomiting blood), then it may be that a particular medication is causing this. Furthermore, if a patient is on one form of medication, then it may be contra-indicative to prescribe certain other medications that may be needed in order to treat their present illness. Moreover, it is extremely important that patients are able to continue on their present medication regime to prevent any exacerbation of the condition for which those medications were prescribed in the first place.

Observations on admission

There are numerous nursing observations that can be recorded upon admission but, as a general rule, the most usual ones are temperature, pulse, respirations, oxygen saturations and blood pressure. The patient's weight should also be recorded. Depending upon the patient's condition or symptoms other observations may be performed such as, for example, blood sugar levels in diabetic patients. There are also different samples that may need to be collected. Routinely, a nurse would collect a urine sample for a urinalysis that checks for any abnormalities in the urine (see Chapter 21, page 463). Other samples may include a stool sample, a wound swab or swabs for methicillin-resistant staphylococcus aureus (MRSA). Samples that are usually collected by the doctor (though more and more nurses are now doing this) are blood samples for various laboratory tests. The most usual blood tests are for urea and electrolytes and for a full blood count (FBC).

See Chapter 21, page 463.

It is often said that observations on admission provide a baseline for the patient's normal range of observations. However, this is not necessarily the case as a patient who is admitted as an emergency may be in pain or shock, for example, and these conditions are likely to affect that person's normal range. In these instances the observations may actually help with the diagnosis of the patient's condition. Having knowledge of the normal ranges for observations and the potential causes of any deviations is therefore imperative and these issues will be discussed in Part 5 on Care Management.

Communication needs

As mentioned in Chapter 1, communication is a vital component in all nursing care and procedures. Identifying any problems with the patient's communication abilities is extremely important as this allows the nurse to solve these problems, if possible, or to find aids to try and improve the situation. Questions to consider include the following.

❑ Does the patient have any hearing difficulties?

❑ Do they have a hearing aid? Have they brought it with them?

❑ Do they have problems with their eyesight?

❑ Do they wear glasses? Have they brought them with them?

❑ Do they speak and understand English adequately? If not, why not?

❑ Do they understand another language? If so, which?

Asking these questions can help to ensure that all forms of communication are maintained to a high standard. Even basic things like filling in a menu can cause problems if the person filling it in can't read because they have no glasses or don't understand English. Furthermore, personal items like glasses and hearing aids sometimes go missing and documenting these items in the Kardex can help to ascertain whether or not they were in the patient's possession upon admission.

Activity 9.

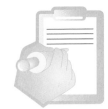

1.   When next in clinical practice ask your mentor if you can accompany him/her or another nurse on a doctor's ward round. Listen carefully and see if you can understand everything that is being said.

2.   Think about George from our scenario. Can you identify any particular communication problems that he might have both before admission and during his hospital stay? Discuss your thoughts with fellow students.

Reflection

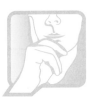

Following the last exercise, try to imagine how the patients feel when they are listening to the doctors talking about them and their condition. Think about your own communication abilities. Do you have any problems? Have you ever been on holiday and had problems understanding the locals? Discuss your thoughts with other students.

Other valuables

For legal reasons it is important to make a note of what valuables the patient has with them upon admission. In some instances patients bring large amounts of money or expensive valuables with them as they don't want to leave them at home. In such cases, it is often Trust policy to have them checked, documented and locked away safely. Alternatively, if possible, the patient may be asked to send certain items home with their next of kin but, again, it is important to document this.

Religious practices

Documenting a patient's religion helps to ensure that some of their socio-cultural needs are addressed. Offering the patient the option of prayer can help them on a psychological basis. This may even be the case for those who do not normally practise their religion as many people turn to religion in times of need. For those who practise regularly, denying them the facility to maintain their practice may be extremely detrimental to their well-being.

See Chapter 14, page 276.

Furthermore, a person's religion can affect that person's treatment and care in many ways. For example, some treatments (and, in some cases, life-saving treatments) may be refused on religious grounds. However irrational this refusal may seem to us, the legal rules of consent mean that the patient's wishes and autonomy must be adhered to (see Chapter 14, page 276). With regard to the patient's care, there may be certain issues that need to be considered where their diet or hygiene needs are concerned. Developing a sound knowledge of cultural aspects is extremely important and further reading on this topic is strongly advised.

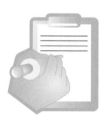

Activity 10.

1.   When next in clinical practice ask your mentor what facilities there are to cater for people's religious beliefs.

2.   Think about our scenario patient George. How might you be able to address his religious needs?

Reflection

If you are religious, how would you feel if your opportunity to worship was taken away from you? If you are not religious, has there ever been an occasion in your life where you have turned to worship in one form or another? If you are happy to do so then discuss your feelings with fellow students.

Admission notes

The admission notes section of the Kardex allows the nurse to record a history of the symptoms and/or events that have led up to the patient's admission. Again this is very important as it can help with a diagnosis and with identifying that particular person's present needs. Questions including the following:

❏ What specific symptoms has the patient been suffering from? Ask how often the symptoms have occurred, when they have occurred, where they have occurred and if anything particular brought the symptoms on.

See Chapter 4, page 92.

❏ Have they been in pain and, if so, assess this pain (see Chapter 4, page 92).

❏ Have they had any similar problems in the past?

❏ What exactly have they done in order to address their problems prior to admission?

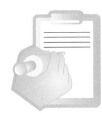

Activity 11.

1. When next in clinical practice, have a look at a selection of different admission notes for different illnesses. Try to relate these notes to the specific illness that the individual patient is suffering from by identifying typical symptoms.

2. Think about our scenario patient George. Given that he has pain in his abdomen, what type of questions might you ask him or his wife? Discuss your thoughts with fellow students.

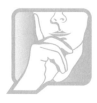

Reflection

Have you ever been to your GP with an illness? How did he or she ascertain what was wrong with you? Have you ever suffered from an illness that was similar in its symptoms to someone else's but your actual diagnosis was different?

Sleep

When a patient comes into hospital it is important that they are able to get their rest and that we try to keep their sleeping pattern as normal as possible. Different people use different methods in order to aid their sleep and a person who is admitted to hospital should be allowed to use these methods during their hospital stay. Questions to consider include the following.

❑ What time do they normally go to bed?

❑ How many pillows do they normally use?

❑ How many hours do they normally sleep?

❑ Is their sleep normally interrupted? If so, why?

❑ Are they a light sleeper? If so, you may consider putting them in a bed that is in a quieter spot of the ward or in a side room.

❑ Do they take any night sedation? If so, what? (This can be especially important as a withdrawal of certain medications can cause confusion in some patients.)

❑ Has their present illness affected their sleep and, if so, how?

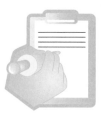

Activity 12.

1. When next in clinical practice, observe a selection of patients and make a note of their differences where sleeping is concerned. Do they all have the same amount of pillows? Do they all have the same number of blankets? Do they all stay awake during the day or do they have a sleep at some time? Do they all go to bed at the same time?

2. Think about our scenario patient George. Can you identify any particular sleep problems that he might have both before admission and during his hospital stay? Discuss your thoughts with fellow students.

Reflection

Think about your own sleep pattern and ask yourself the questions highlighted above. Would there be any particular problems that you might encounter should you be admitted to hospital? Discuss your thoughts with fellow students.

Personal cleansing and dressing

Ask questions about the patient's normal cleansing and dressing regime because replicating this in hospital, if at all possible, would be the best thing for your patient's well-being. Questions to consider include the following:

❏ How often do they have a wash, bath or shower?

❏ How often do they wash their hair?

❏ Do they have any problems or difficulties in performing these tasks independently?

❏ Do they use any particular toiletries?

❏ Do they have any problems with their skin, feet, hands, nails or teeth?

❏ Do they have any medications or treatment regimes for these problems?

Maintaining a high standard of hygiene while in hospital is imperative on health and safety grounds. However, a potential conflict with this principle could be the issue of patient autonomy. Some patients may, for whatever reason, be a little less meticulous than others where their hygiene standards are concerned or they may have their own specific reasons for not wanting to wash or bathe. In this instance it is important to ascertain these reasons and try to address them if possible. It may be that a compromise can be achieved. However, should a patient continue to refuse to wash, the nurse has very little option but to abide by that patient's wishes, provided of course that all the legal requirements for the ability to consent are present. Trying to achieve a happy medium can be difficult but any deviation in standards that result in a potential danger to the patient and/or others should be addressed and on these grounds the nurse's actions may be justified. Of course it is quite often the case that tactfully explaining the issues and discussing your concerns with the patient are likely to help gain their co-operation. On occasions it may be that the patient is embarrassed about being washed by the nursing staff so another option may be to involve the relatives with that side of their care. Hopefully, this dilemma may not present itself that often and, in most instances, it will be possible to adhere to the patient's normal regime.

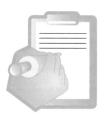

Activity 13.

1. When next in clinical practice make a note of the patients that need assistance with their hygiene needs. Try to ascertain why this is. Observe how this might change as their condition changes.

2. Think about our scenario patient George. Can you identify any particular needs that he may have where hygiene is concerned? Research the requirements for valid consent. How might George's situation differ from your own? Discuss your thoughts with fellow students.

Reflection

Think about your own hygiene standards. What is the 'norm' for you? Has there ever been a time when you were not as clean as you would have liked to be such as, for example, after playing sport or during an illness/injury of your own? How did you feel at that time? How did you feel once you had showered or bathed?

Elimination

Elimination is mainly concerned with the urinary and bowel function of the patient (though perspiration may also be considered). Again, ascertaining their normal and continual functions is important. Questions on this aspect need to be more in-depth when the patient's present condition relates to the process of elimination. Otherwise, ascertaining a 'norm' for the patient should suffice. Questions to consider include the following.

❏ How often do they urinate and have their bowels opened?

❏ Has this changed since they became ill?

❏ Does their urine and faeces look or smell any different? For example, are they constipated, have they had diarrhoea, is there any blood in their urine or faeces, is their urine or faeces a different colour?

❏ Have they had or do they presently have any bladder or bowel problems? Asking a question like this helps to avoid being too direct about issues that may be embarrassing but not necessarily a problem to the patient and, therefore, something that they do not particularly want to disclose such as, for example, stress incontinence.

❏ If there is a problem highlighted, how is it managed and has anything been done about it? This may then allow the patient to disclose whether they have a colostomy or urostomy.

❏ Do they have any pain when urinating or defecating?

❏ Do they have any urinary urgency, frequency or retention?

❏ Do they have any mobility problems or difficulties when going to the toilet?

In some instances, elimination may be affected by the patient's condition or illness at a later date, and it may also be affected by the fact that they have been admitted to hospital and are in unfamiliar surroundings, so continual assessment of this activity is imperative. Asking questions on this aspect can be embarrassing for both the patient and the nurse so a professional attitude is essential. Equally, the care of patients during this activity can be embarrassing for the patient so maintaining privacy and dignity throughout is also essential.

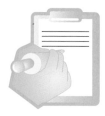

Activity 14.

1.   When next in clinical practice, assess a selection of different patients with regard to their elimination needs. How do they differ and why?

2.   Think about our scenario patient George. Can you identify any particular elimination needs or problems that he may have? Discuss your thoughts with fellow students.

Reflection

Has there ever been a time in your life where you have had problems with your elimination such as, for example, while on holiday or before an exam or interview? How did you feel about it? Did you find it easy to talk to other people about it? How would you feel if you had to have your bowels opened on a commode at the side of a hospital bed with only a set of curtains between you and the outside world? If you are happy to do so then discuss your thoughts with other students.

Eating and drinking

See Chapter 10, page 216.

Many patients are either admitted with, or subsequently suffer from, malnutrition following an admission to hospital (the causes and consequences of this will be discussed in Chapter 10, page 216). In view of this, it is extremely important that we as nurses are aware of the need for a well-balanced diet for our patients. In some instances it may be the patient's lack of education about nutrition that causes or predisposes them to the possibility of malnutrition. Therefore, asking the right questions in this section can provide the first step to re-educating that individual. Questions to consider include the following:

❑ How good is their appetite?

❑ Has their appetite changed since they became ill?

❑ Have they suffered from any nausea or vomiting recently?

❑ Do they have any problems eating and drinking such as, for example, problems with swallowing?

❑ If they wear dentures, do they fit properly?

❑ How many meals do they eat each day?

❑ What kind of diet do they eat? Is it well balanced?

❑ Are they diabetic and eat a sugar-free diet?

❑ Do they follow any other type of diet through choice or illness such as, for example, a low sodium diet, a low fat diet or a low protein diet?

❑ Are they allergic to any food?

❑ Is there any particular food that makes their present illness worse, or that they dislike or that doesn't agree with them?

❑ Do they have any religious beliefs that we need to cater for where their diet is concerned?

❑ Do they have any difficulties at home in preparing their food?

❑ Do they have any financial difficulties that prevent them from buying nutritious food?

❑ Do they have any problems getting to the shops to buy their food?

❑ Have they lost or gained any weight recently?

❑ Are they likely to need any help with filling in the diet sheet? If so, what kind of help do they need?

❑ Are they able to feed themselves? If not, why not?

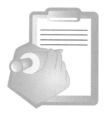

Activity 15.

1. When you are next in placement, have a look at the food menu and see if it is self-explanatory. Are there any symbols that denote the type of food on the menu? If so, do you understand them?

2. Think about our scenario patient George. Can you identify any particular eating and drinking needs or problems that he may have? Discuss your thoughts with fellow students.

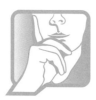

Reflection

Has there ever been a time where you have been invited to someone's house for lunch, dinner or tea and they have given you food that you didn't like? What did you do? Have you ever been to a restaurant and ordered something without really knowing what it was and, when the food was served, it looked and tasted awful? What did you do?

Mobilisation

Ascertaining a patient's normal mobility is extremely important. In many instances this activity overlaps with others such as, for example, their ability to feed themselves, their ability to wash and dress themselves and their ability to tend to their own toileting needs. With this in mind, it can be seen that a reduction or impairment in the ability to mobilise can quite often be the root cause of many other problems. Also, many problems in mobility can be transient and caused by the person's present state of health or injury.

However, for many people, the problems may be long term and relate to the actual ageing process, for example arthritis, or they may be caused by previous illness or surgery, for example following an amputation of a limb. Mobility problems may also be due to the person's social or economic status. For example, problems may be caused by where they live or their access (or lack of it) to funds in order to improve their mobility by, for example, installing a stair lift. Questions to consider include the following.

- ❏ Do they have any problems with any of their limbs? If so, what problems do they have?

- ❏ Do they suffer from any illnesses that affect their mobility such as, for example, osteoporosis or multiple sclerosis?

- ❏ Do they have any mobility aids and, if so, what are they?

- ❏ How far can they walk independently?

- ❏ Do they have any pain when mobilising?

- ❏ Do they take any medications to ease the pain and, if so, what medication do they take?

- ❏ Are there any aspects at home that affect their mobility such as, for example, steps or stairs?

- ❏ Could modifications at home improve the issue?

Please note that other questions about mobility could also be included when considering other activities of living.

From an assessment point of view, it is important that the person's normal abilities are ascertained and the care planned for them will return that person to as close to their normal abilities as possible. However, as mentioned, it may also be possible to improve their abilities through the use of aids or adaptations, and other members of the multidisciplinary team such as, for example, physiotherapists and occupational therapists may also be able to help to improve a patient's mobility.

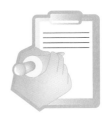

Activity 16.

1. When next in clinical practice have a look at all the mobility aids that are available in the placement area. Ask your mentor if you can spend some time in either or both the physiotherapy department and the occupational health department to see what they can provide for patients.

2. Think about our scenario patient George. Can you identify any potential or actual needs or problems that he may have with mobility? Discuss your thoughts with fellow students.

Reflection

Have you ever suffered from an injury that has affected your mobility such as, for example, a fracture or a sprain? How did you cope at the time? Did your dependence upon other people increase and, if so, how did you feel about this?

Breathing

The ability to breathe is vital to life and is quite often performed effortlessly. However, any difficulty in this ability (**dyspnoea**) can be very frightening for the individual concerned. Breathing can change throughout our lives, with the demands on our breathing fluctuating depending upon the activity that we are performing at any given time. For example, during exercise an individual's breathing demands will increase, and this is also the case when an individual's adrenalin rises. Illness and disease may also affect an individual's breathing demands, especially when those illnesses or diseases directly affect the lungs such as, for example, asthma, chronic obstructive pulmonary disease (COPD), pneumonia and lung cancer. Communicating with a patient who is suffering from dyspnoea requires more skill as it is important to phrase questions that allow for straightforward answers, which will therefore minimise the breathing demands for that individual (and this applies throughout the admission procedure). In some instances, involving relatives or carers can assist the process. Questions to consider include the following.

❑ Have they had any difficulties with their breathing such as, for example, dyspnoea, coughing or wheezing?

❑ If they have a cough, is it productive? If so, what colour is the sputum? Is there any blood in the sputum (haemoptysis)?

❑ Has this changed since becoming ill?

❑ Do they have any long-standing problems with their breathing such as, for example, asthma or COPD?

❑ Do they take any medication to help with their breathing?

❑ Does their ability to breathe affect any other activities?

❑ Do they smoke? If so, how many a day?

❑ Would they consider smoking cessation?

Social circumstances

The patient's social circumstances are very important as they will help to formulate the plan for discharge. As discussed in Chapter 3, page 65, many people are readmitted to hospital due to problems with their previous discharge. Unfortunately, in some instances, the individual may have been diagnosed as being terminally ill and their wishes are that they return home to die. Therefore ensuring adequate support on discharge is vital and the only way that this can be achieved is by ascertaining the individual's present circumstances. Other issues that may need to be addressed include the aspects of work and play. For some people an admission to hospital may affect their finances as they may not be entitled to their normal income while absent from work, and this may add to their anxieties and fears. It may be that they are concerned about the care of a pet or relative while they are in hospital. Issues surrounding the activity of 'expressing sexuality' may be a potential problem depending on the cause of admission. For example, their illness may affect their ability to perform sexual intercourse on discharge, or their treatment may have had an effect on their body image. These concerns may also be addressed in other areas of the care-planning process or alongside the health education needs before or upon discharge. Questions to consider include the following.

See Chapter 3, page 65.

❑ Do they live alone?

❑ Do they have any family who live locally?

❑ How do they generally manage at home?

❑ Is there anyone who helps them with shopping, cleaning or general care?

❑ What type of house do they live in?

❑ Do they have any features that may cause mobility problems such as, for example, steps or stairs?

❑ Are their bathroom and bedroom upstairs?

❑ Do they have any mobility aids at home? If so, what are they?

❑ Do they have any emotional or financial concerns about their hospital admission?

❑ Do they envisage any problems on discharge?

Please note that the needs and coping abilities of relatives and carers should also be taken into consideration.

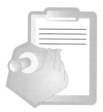

Activity 17.

1. Think about an elderly relative. If they were admitted to hospital and needed time to convalesce on their discharge, what aspects of their home life may impede this? What resources might be available to assist this process?

2. Think about our scenario patient George. What specific questions may need to be asked? How would these differ if it was George's wife who had been admitted to hospital?

3. When next in clinical practice, ask your mentor for another Kardex. Then, using role play, ask a fellow student/colleague to imagine that they are the patient in our scenario or ask a patient if you can go through the assessment process with them. If these options are not possible, imagine that you are that patient yourself and try to complete the admission form. What questions might you ask this patient or his wife in order to perform an in-depth admission assessment? You may find it useful to refer back to the information already given in this chapter. Following this exercise, ask your mentor if you can observe him or her performing the task for real. When you feel confident enough, ask your mentor if you can actually do an admission assessment yourself with supervision.

Care planning

Performing the admission assessment is the first step towards formulating your patient's care plan. Care plans are made up of problems and needs and, for each of these problems or needs, a goal is set in order to address the problem or meet the need. Goals must be realistic and attainable and must describe exactly what needs to be done in order to achieve them. Furthermore, the process must involve the patient as we cannot make assumptions about what that patient's problems or needs are. However, in some instances, due to our knowledge of illness and treatment, we may need to identify certain problems or needs for the patient as they may not realise that they exist or be aware of the importance of addressing those problems or needs. In some instances, a care pathway may already be in existence following standardised care as advocated by professional bodies and the government (for example, care as advocated by National Service Frameworks).

However, as the NMC (2004b, p.16) has highlighted, 'in keeping with the orientation towards holistic care, the emphasis must be one that avoids a narrow disease-orientated perspective and instead encompasses a health promotion and health education perspective'. Furthermore, 'all members of the profession must demonstrate an inviolable respect for persons and communities, without prejudice, and irrespective of orientation and personal, group, political, cultural, ethnic or religious characteristics' (NMC, 2004b, p.18). It may seem to some that avoiding a disease-orientated perspective may actually result in some aspects of a patient's care being neglected. However, one could argue that this is definitely not the case as all the problems and needs that arise with any given illness or disease can generally be addressed in at least one of the activities of living. For example, a diabetic patient will need a sugar-free diet and this can be included under 'eating and drinking'. They will also need to have regular blood sugar tests and be monitored for potential hypoglycaemic or hyperglycaemic attacks and these needs can be included under 'maintaining a safe environment'. Approaching your care planning in this manner will go a long way to ensuring your success in future assignments and examinations that revolve around the care of a patient.

Evidence-based practice and care planning

Another important aspect that must be considered is the use of evidence-based practice and ensuring that the care planned is up to date. Research is continually being performed in order to improve patient outcomes and to save time and money. Quality of care is at the forefront of the government's agenda for health care and, as registered nurses, it is a professional requirement that we continually develop our knowledge and skills and this should be reflected in our care planning. Indeed, the NMC (2004b, p.13) says that 'within the complex and rapidly changing health care environment, it is essential that the best available evidence informs practice'. Furthermore, the NMC's Code of Professional Conduct (2004a, 6.5) advocates that 'you have a responsibility to deliver care based on current evidence, best practice and, where applicable, validated research when it is available'. The Code also highlights that 'to practise competently, you must possess the knowledge, skills and abilities required for lawful, safe and effective practice without direct supervision. You must acknowledge the limits of your professional competence and only undertake practice and accept responsibilities for those activities in which you are competent' (NMC, 2004a, 6.2). In addition, any limitations should be addressed by appropriate training in order to acquire that requisite knowledge and skill (NMC, 2004a, 6.3).

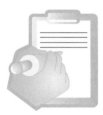

Activity 18.

When you have completed the Kardex from the last exercise, use the Roper, Logan and Tierney Model of Living (1980) to assess and plan the care of this patient. Ensure that you address each of the 12 activities of living and identify what care should be implemented in order to improve these activities. You may find it useful throughout this exercise to refer back to the information already given in this chapter and to apply the principles highlighted in many of the other relevant chapters in this book.

Implementation

Once the assessment and care planning has been completed, the interventions highlighted in the care plan for each need and/or problem need to be implemented. The timing of this process will vary according to the intervention, its appropriateness at that given time, whether it is a priority and the availability of the necessary resources for each particular intervention. For example, it may be necessary to perform an ultrasound scan but this will have to be ordered and there may be some specific preparation that needs to be done beforehand. The priority of the intervention is extremely important and the skill that is needed in order to prioritise effectively comes with experience. A simple example of priority of intervention is treating a patient's pain before attending to their hygiene needs. Certain interventions may be performed in isolation (as in the ultrasound scan) and others may need to be done repeatedly (as in the recording of observations).

Following the care plan ensures continuity of care, provided that the care given is documented accordingly or verbally passed on to all the members of the multidisciplinary team. By doing this, all the necessary people are aware of what care has been given and which aspects of care are still outstanding (see the NMC (2004c) *Guidelines for records and record keeping* for more information).

Again, the care implemented must be evidence based and the NMC reiterate this by saying 'safe and effective practice requires a sound underpinning of the theoretical knowledge, which informs practice, and is in turn informed by that practice' (NMC, 2004b, p.13).

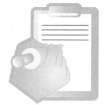

Activity 19.

1.   When next in clinical practice, ask your mentor to go through a care plan for one of your patients and explain how and why this particular plan of care has changed and developed over time.

2.   Consider our scenario patient George. As his abdominal pain turned out to be a perforated ulcer and he needed an emergency operation to repair the perforation, how would his initial care plan on admission change before and after his operation?

Evaluation

As patients improve or deteriorate their problems and needs change and this has to be highlighted in their plan of care. Reviewing the care planned is therefore imperative and this is performed by evaluating the individual's care on a regular, if not continual, basis. This phase is the last in the cyclical approach to the nursing process before the cycle starts again with assessment.

Summary

From the information given in this chapter it is clear to see that the assessment procedure within nursing is an extremely important and ongoing process. It starts at admission and is followed by continual assessment, planning, implementation and evaluation.

Having the necessary skills in order to consider every aspect of a patient/client's needs is something that needs to be developed with experience. This experience is twofold and involves gaining essential communication and cultural skills and also the underpinning knowledge of differing diseases, illnesses and treatments in order to tailor the assessment to each and every individual.

This experience is not gained overnight and much patience and practice is needed. Furthermore, the issues and recommendations addressed in this chapter are not an exhaustive list and further reading on the topic is strongly recommended.

Further reading

Holland, K., Jenkins, J., Solomon, J. and Whittam, S. (2004) *Applying the Roper, Logan, Tierney model in practice*. Edinburgh: Churchill Livingstone

References

Bellman, L.M. (1996) 'Changing nursing practice through reflection on the Roper, Logan and Tierney model: the enhancement approach to action research'. *Journal of Advanced Nursing*, 24(1): 129–38

Fawcett, J. (1989) *Analysis and evaluation of conceptual models of nursing*, 2nd edn. Philadelphia: F.A. Davis

Fitzpatrick, J. and Whall, A. (1989) *Conceptual models of nursing: analysis and application*, 2nd edn. Norwalk, CT: Appleton & Lange.

Heartfield, M.R.N. (1996) 'Nursing documentation and nursing practice: a discourse analysis'. *Journal of Advanced Nursing*, 24(1): 98–103

Moores, Y. (1996) *Just for the record (NHS Training Directorate)*. London: NHS Training Directorate

Nursing and Midwifery Council (2004a) *Code of Professional Conduct*. London: NMC

Nursing and Midwifery Council (2004b) *Standards of proficiency for pre-registration nursing education*. London: NMC

Nursing and Midwifery Council (2004c) *Guidelines for records and record keeping*. London: NMC

Nursing and Midwifery Council (2006) *Essential skills clusters*. London: NMC

Roper, N., Logan, W. and Tierney A.J. (2000) *The Roper, Logan, Tierney model of nursing based on the activities of living*. Edinburgh: Churchill Livingstone

Sturdy, D. and Carpenter, I. (1995) 'Right plan for elderly care?' *Nursing Management*, 2(7): 16–18

Yura, D. and Walsh, M.B. (1978) *The nursing process: assessing, planning, implementing and evaluating*. New York: Appleton Century Crofts

Chapter 3

TRANSFERRING AND DISCHARGING PATIENTS

Renette Ellson

Throughout this chapter reference will be made to the Nursing and Midwifery Council (NMC) Essential Skills Clusters (ESCs). Transferring and discharging patients are extremely important aspects of nursing care and, as such, the NMC has identified several subsections within two of the Essential Skills Clusters titled 'Care, Compassion and Communication' and 'Organisational Aspects of Care' that relate to these necessary skills. However, note that virtually all the Essential Skills Clusters relate in one way or another to these processes.

Patients/clients can trust a newly registered nurse to:

Section 11   Act to safeguard those requiring support and protection.
Section 13   Promote continuity when their care is to be transferred to another service or person.
Section 14   Be confident in their own role within the multidisciplinary/multi-agency team and to inspire confidence in others.
Section 15   Safely delegate care to others and to respond appropriately when a task is delegated to them.
Section 16   Safely lead, co-ordinate and manage care.
Section 18   Identify and safely manage risk in relation to the patient/client, the environment, self and others.

Patient transfers

In order to ensure that the best possible and most appropriate care is given, many patients are transferred from one department to another. Transfers may be transient in that the patient spends only a short time in a different department for either an investigation or minor or major procedure. Other transfers may be more permanent. For example, a patient may be admitted with what provisionally appears to be a medical condition that then turns out to be surgical one. Alternatively, a patient may be admitted with either a medical or surgical condition that is treated, but then the patient's need changes to one of rehabilitation or palliative care. In this situation they need to be transferred to the appropriate area for this type of care. In these instances, many hospitals have a specific transfer form that needs to be completed, and the requirements therein adhered to prior to the actual transfer. Not all patients need to be transferred, but for those who do, for whatever reason, effective communication skills are essential to ensure patient safety and to make sure continuity of care is maintained.

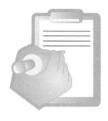

Activity 1.

When you are next in clinical practice, ask your mentor for a copy of the transfer form (if such a form exists) so that you can familiarise yourself with any necessary requirements or procedures. If the form is difficult to understand or follow then ask your mentor if he or she would kindly explain those issues to you in more depth.

Short-term transfers

If the transfer is extremely short term such as, for example, to a department for a simple investigation, then the most important aspect of care involves communicating the process to the patient, ensuring that they fully understand what is going to happen and that all the legal aspects of consent have been adhered to. Another important aspect of care is ensuring that the transfer is safe. This includes making sure the correct patient is actually transferred, that appropriate transportation aids are used and that the patient's notes and a nurse accompanies them to the relevant department.

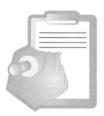

Activity 2.

Consider our scenario patient, George. What specific short-term transfers may be relevant to him? Think about the investigations that he is likely to need.

Transfers to theatre

Another short-term transfer may be a transfer to theatre for an operation or another form of invasive procedure. In this instance the preparation for transfer begins well before the actual transfer takes place. Again, communication skills are essential. Giving the patient a full explanation of the operation or procedure is vital and legally required as part of the requirements of consent. As a general rule this communication is usually performed by the consenting doctor. However, the nurse does have the responsibility of being able to reiterate the facts to the patient and/or relatives if needed (though, in some cases, there are ethical and legal principles involved in giving information to the patient's relatives and you must have the patient's consent to do this). Indeed, even though the capacity to understand is a legal requirement of consent, and many patients/clients give the impression that they do understand, this may not necessarily be the case. As Lunde (1993) has demonstrated, patients may still hold radically different views from the doctor about what is happening or what has been discussed during a medical consultation (as cited in Jarrett and Payne, 1995).

Reflection

Think about your own life in this regard. Have you ever found yourself saying that you understand something when, in reality, you haven't really understood a word? If this was the case, did you make it known that you didn't understand? If not, why didn't you say that you couldn't understand? What was it about the information you were given that made it difficult for you to understand it? Discuss your findings with fellow students and try to identify the significance of such occasions or events within the nursing profession.

The safety issues that are involved include preparing the patient physically for whichever operation they are having. This might entail starving the patient for a length of time before surgery if requested by the surgeon, bathing or shaving the patient, getting them into a theatre gown, giving them a particular medicine or preparation, preparing the bed and bed area and completing the consent form, to name but a few. (See also Chapter 20.) Immediately prior to transfer the nurse needs to ensure that the consent form has been fully completed as this may be the only source of some information once the patient is in theatre and anaesthetised. Generally, checking the consent form involves ensuring the following.

See also Chapter 20.

❑ The patient understands what is going to happen during and after the operation.

❑ They have signed the consent form.

❑ Any specific preparations have been done.

❑ The patient's observations, urinalysis and generally their most recent haemoglobin have been recorded.

❑ They have been starved appropriately.

❑ Any crowns, false teeth or hearing aids have been recorded.

❑ Any allergies have been recorded.

❑ The patient is properly attired (which includes removing jewellery and nail varnish).

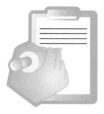

Activity 3.

When next in clinical practice, ask your mentor to show you a patient consent form so that you can familiarise yourself with any necessary requirements or procedures. If the form is difficult to understand or follow then ask your mentor if he or she would kindly explain those issues to you in more depth.

The patient's identity is then ensured by checking their name and hospital number on their wristband against the name and hospital number on the consent form. The importance of this safety aspect can never be underestimated and, because of this, the patient's identity will be checked time and time again by different people in the operating department. Another safety aspect is the use of appropriate transportation, which may depend upon the patient's condition at the time of transfer. In the light of recent health and safety developments regarding the moving and handling of patients, many hospitals actually allow their patients to walk to theatre (provided of course that their dignity is maintained). If this is not possible then a theatre trolley with an accompanying nurse and theatre porter/orderly may be necessary.

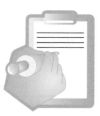

Activity 4.

1.   When next in clinical practice in a surgical setting, ask your mentor to allow you to observe the pre-operative process, from checking the consent form to escorting the patient/client to theatre.

2.   Consider George, our scenario patient. What specific safety aspects would need to be considered when he is transferred to theatre for his operation?

Reflection

Have you ever had an operation yourself? If so, try to remember the procedure that was followed. Did you wonder why certain things were performed or checked? If so, what were these things? Can you now understand why they were necessary?

Transferring a patient from accident and emergency to their admitting ward

Many hospital admissions are admitted via the accident and emergency department (A&E) and patients are then transferred to an admitting ward. When a patient is transferred from A&E it is important that all the necessary assessments are taken to the admitting ward with them. It is also important that the patient is escorted by the A&E nurse, who can then give a detailed report about the patient to the ward nurse who will be responsible for admitting that patient. However, for the purpose of this chapter we shall concentrate on the transfer of a patient/client from ward to ward and from ward to another hospital.

Transferring patients from ward to ward or to another hospital

Transferring a patient to another ward or hospital happens quite often and is performed in order that the patient receives the most appropriate care. This will sometimes be a planned decision or it may be an emergency decision. In either case it is important to communicate information about the transfer to the patient/client, to their relatives and to the receiving ward or hospital. If the transfer is planned then this makes this communication task a little easier as time is not an issue. This is not the case, unfortunately, in an emergency and, in these instances, it is essential to employ team work, together with exceptional leadership skills, to ensure as seamless a transfer as possible. Information needs to be given to the patient and their relatives as to where exactly they are being transferred and why they are being transferred. Time must be given to allow those involved to ask questions and to ensure consent.

Transfer forms

Communicating with the members of the receiving department can be improved by completing a transfer form, and many hospitals have adapted a format/checklist to ensure that all the necessary information is communicated. Quite often these forms provide a summary of the care that the individual patient has received and what their present needs are. The forms also ensure that all the necessary preparatory tasks have been done by listing these in order and allowing the transferring nurse to tick them off as they have been addressed.

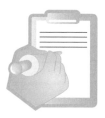

Activity 5.

When next in clinical practice, ask your mentor to show you a patient transfer form so that you can familiarise yourself with any necessary requirements or procedures. If the form is difficult to understand or follow then ask your mentor if he or she would kindly explain those issues to you in more depth.

Nursing and medical records

Transferring the patient's nursing and medical records is extremely important as they include the whole of the patient's information to date. From a nurse's perspective it is vital that he or she ensures that the care plan and Kardex have been updated immediately prior to the transfer and that all the necessary arrangements for the transfer have been documented. Another important role of the transferring nurse, immediately prior to transfer, is that he or she ensures that the bed-state and the admissions and discharges books are completed. In many instances this may be delegated to the ward clerk, but it is an important task as it ensures that the right number of patients are on the ward and that the number of available beds is also correct at any given time. It also allows you to locate patients should the need arise.

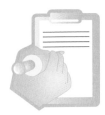

Activity 6.

When next in clinical practice ask your mentor to show you the bed-state and the admissions and discharge books and to explain to you how these documents are completed. If possible, ask him or her if you can work alongside the ward clerk for part of a shift to gain an insight into the administrative duties that need to be carried out on the ward.

Personal effects and valuables

All personal effects and valuables need to be packed up and taken with the patient to the new ward or hospital. This may involve signing certain valuables back out to the patient if they are being kept safe on the ward. Where medicines are concerned, inter-department transfers of medicines dispensed for the individual patient should not occur, although, depending on the time of the transfer and the importance of the medication, this can sometimes cause a dilemma. However, in these instances, the transferring nurse can advise the staff on the new ward of the patient's medication needs as soon as the patient is transferred thus allowing the new ward the opportunity to receive their own stock of any particular medication. Alternatively, if the transfer is out of pharmacy hours, then the new ward may be able to get an emergency supply of that medication from the emergency drugs cupboard or, as a last resort, the emergency out-of-hours pharmacist could be contacted.

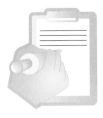

Activity 7.

When next in clinical practice, ask your mentor to show you the procedure for getting an emergency supply of drugs from the emergency drugs cupboard.

Transportation and comfort

Transporting your patient to another ward or hospital needs to be done safely and comfortably. If the transfer is within the same hospital, a porter and a suitable mode of transport will need to be arranged. The mode of transport will depend upon the patient's condition at the time of transfer. If the patient is very poorly then a hospital trolley (with sides) and a porter may be needed. However, if appropriate, the patient may be transferred using a wheelchair with the help of a porter, or it may even be possible for the patient to walk with the transferring nurse to the ward to which they are being transferred. The mode of transfer should be decided by the transferring nurse and it should never compromise the safety of the patient.

Where a transfer to another hospital is concerned, the mode of transport also needs to be considered. In some instances the patient may need a paramedic and nurse escort or an ambulance escort (with or without a nurse) or, if appropriate and the patient's condition allows, hospital transport may be used. Again this all depends upon the patient's condition at the time of transfer. When an ambulance is needed, consideration also needs to be given to whether the patient will need a trolley or a wheelchair for their transfer.

To ensure comfort, it is vital that the correct mode of transport is chosen and that blankets or personal clothing are used to make sure the patient is kept warm throughout their journey. The escorting nurse can also ask the patient if they are comfortable at regular intervals and address any issues as they arise. Analgesia may also be required prior to the transfer to ensure that the patient remains pain free.

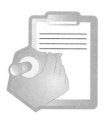

Activity 8.

Consider our scenario patient, George. Following his operation he needs to be transferred to a surgical ward. What specific considerations will there be in order for this to be done successfully?

When he had recovered from his operation it was decided that he was in need of some rehabilitation and this was arranged at a different hospital. What issues would need to be considered with regard to his transport? What arrangements would need to be made to ensure a safe transfer? What is your reasoning for this? What differences are there between the two transfers?

Introductions to new staff

Upon arrival at the new ward it is important that the transferring nurse introduces the patient to the staff. He or she must also provide an in-depth history of the patient's care and needs to the receiving staff to ensure continuity of care. The responsibility of care is then transferred to the new ward and the new named nurse must settle the patient into their new environment, review the patient's care and needs and update any documents accordingly (including the bed-state and the admissions and discharges books). Certain other issues may also need to be considered and addressed such as, for example, the fact that the patient may have missed a meal or their medications because of the transfer.

Patient discharges

> The planning of a patient/client's discharge is an ongoing process that should start prior to admission for planned admissions, and as soon as possible for all other admissions. (Department of Health, 2003, p.2)

Discharges can be complicated and quite often require the full involvement of all the members of the multidisciplinary team. Of course, this is not always the case and some discharges can be extremely straightforward, especially those following less complicated illnesses and with patients who have very few needs, are younger or have plenty of family back-up. All hospitals should have a discharge policy that needs to be adhered to in order to ensure that the discharge is successfully completed and that the possibility of needing to readmit the patient is prevented. Indeed, as Kee and Borchers (1998) highlight, many hospital admissions are actually readmissions caused by early discharge or inadequate care during and after hospitalisation.

The Single Assessment Process

The House of Commons Health Committee (2001–2) stated that one of the main problems that cause delay in discharges is a failure of communication between health and social care. Some of the major problems with the process include that 'discharges are too early or are delayed, they are poorly managed from the patient/carer perspective or that the patient/client is discharged to an environment that is unsafe' (Department of Health, 2003, p.2). An important development to improve this problem was advocated in Standard 2 of the National Service Framework for Older People (Department of Health, 2001). This Standard highlights the need for a Single Assessment Process (SAP) in order to standardise the assessment process and care management system for older people (Department of Health, 2001). The aim of this Standard is to ensure that individual needs are met appropriately, regardless of the boundaries between health and social services. Guidance on how this can be achieved can be found from page 23 onwards in the National Service Framework for Older People (Department of Health, 2001), although it is advised that you read the whole of the document. The key issues involve inter-agency responsibilities, person-centred assessment and care planning, the training of health care professionals in order to perform these assessments and plan care, information sharing and IT support for SAP and, finally, care co-ordination (Department of Health, 2004b). The Department of Health also advocated that, from 1 April 2004, the systems and processes needed to underpin this assessment process should be in place in local health and social care systems (Department of Health, 2004a). Furthermore, as a small proportion of cases, perhaps in the region of 10–20 per cent, will have needs so complex and/or require services so intense or prolonged, the government advocates the need for a named professional to co-ordinate the involvement of all the professionals and services involved in assessments and care planning. They highlight that the 'professionals who act as care co-ordinators should play a prominent role in assessments and reviews, determine eligibility for services, put together packages of care, and act as a source of information and advice' (Department of Health, 2004b, p.6). Also, in some instances, a discharge may be delayed because of the patient's mental health and therefore the National Service Framework for Older People has also identified this as a standard (Standard 7) with specific guidelines highlighted to address this issue.

Activity 9.

For more information on the SAP have a look at the following website: **www.cpa.org.uk/sap/sap_home.html**. You can also order a film called *Listen to what I am saying* that shows health and social care professionals working directly with individuals and their carers, and shows the difference that a person-centred approach makes to individuals with many/complex needs. It outlines key principles of person-centred care that are evolving including holistic assessment, personalised care plans, sharing information, continuity and co-ordination and self-care/self-management (Centre for Policy on Ageing, 2007).

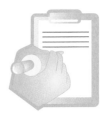

Documents and guidance relating to patient discharge

Other important documents have been produced to improve the process of discharges and ensure that discharges are timely, safe and successful. They cover many aspects and include planning discharges, promoting communication and co-operation between different organisations, addressing the funding of discharges, ensuring patient choice where discharge is concerned and addressing the needs of carers. Unfortunately, the information contained in these documents is too vast to cover in any depth and therefore you are advised to read the documents listed under Further Reading at the end of this chapter.

See this chapter pages 77–82.

Specific discharge considerations

As already mentioned, the discharge planning of a patient is started upon admission. Discharge planning tools should be in place and many will begin with a 'Risk Assessment Screen' that is completed for all patients. These risk assessments appear to vary slightly between different hospitals although many do appear to have similarities and are based upon the Blaylock Assessment.

The Blaylock Risk Assessment Screening Score

The Blaylock Risk Assessment Screening Score (BRASS) index contains ten items and each item is assessed individually and allocated a score by the nurse, depending upon which option most relates to the patient. The ten items that are assessed are:

❑ age;

❑ living situation/social support;

❑ cognition;

❑ functional status;

❑ behaviour pattern;

❑ mobility;

❑ sensory deficits;

❑ the number of previous admissions/ER (emergency room) visits;

❑ the number of active medical problems;

❑ the number of drugs that the patient is presently prescribed.

The higher the score, the more in-depth the patient/client's discharge needs are likely to be and, if the patient scores above ten on this assessment, then a referral should be made to the discharge planning co-ordinator or discharge planning team.

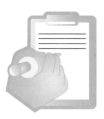

Activity 10.

1. When next in clinical practice ask your mentor if their ward uses this type of assessment. Ask if you can have a copy of the assessment and, if necessary, ask your mentor to explain it to you.

2. Consider our scenario patient George. Using the blank assessment sheet that you have been given, assess George and complete the form to find out what his overall score is. The information needed to complete the assessment is provided in the scenario.

Referral to members of the multidisciplinary team

Following assessment, the co-ordination of needs can be arranged by referring the patient to the relevant multidisciplinary team (MDT) members. Deciding who to refer the patient to will depend upon what the patient's needs are, and how complex they are. In some instances it may be necessary for a case conference to be organised in order that all the necessary MDT members, including the patient and their relatives, liaise to discuss the patient's needs and what services can be put in place to address them. Members of the MDT team may include the following.

Physiotherapists

> Physiotherapy is a healthcare profession concerned with human function and movement and maximising potential. It uses physical approaches to promote, maintain and restore physical, psychological and social well-being, taking account of variations in health status. It is science-based, committed to extending, applying, evaluating and reviewing the evidence that underpins and informs its practice and delivery. The exercise of clinical judgement and informed interpretation is at its core (Chartered Society of Physiotherapy, 2002, p.19).

Physiotherapists work in a wide variety of health settings and their role covers far more than fixing musculoskeletal sports injuries, although that is perhaps the most common perception of the profession (Chartered Society of Physiotherapy, 2007). Indeed, they may be involved in the treatment of conditions such as asthma, back pain, fractures, heart conditions, incontinence, nerve disorders, pain relief, cerebral vascular attacks and even tinnitus. For more in-depth information on the role of the physiotherapist see the Chartered Society of Physiotherapy (CSP) website, particularly **www.csp.org.uk/director/physiotherapyexplained/whatis physiotherapy.cfm** which allows you to go through an A to Z of conditions that they may be involved in, with access to information of what exactly they do for each different condition. See also the Chartered Society of Physiotherapy (2002) *Curriculum framework for qualifying programmes in physiotherapy*, at: **www.csp.org.uk/uploads/documents/ CFforQPP.pdf**.

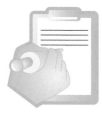

Activity 11.

1.   Research the specific roles of the physiotherapist and discuss your findings with other students. When next in clinical practice ask your mentor if you can spend some time with the physiotherapist to see exactly what their role entails.

2.   Following further reading on the roles of a physiotherapist, assess what needs our scenario patient George might have that the physiotherapist may be able to help him with. Consider his needs throughout his entire patient journey, from admission to discharge.

Occupational therapist

'Occupational therapy enables people to achieve health, well-being and life satisfaction through participation in occupation' (British Association/ College of Occupational Therapists, 2007). As with physiotherapists, occupational therapists can work in a wide variety of health settings and they may be involved in addressing individual patient needs such as providing adaptations within the home or helping patients to learn new ways of doing things. They may also be involved with the treatment of a vast array of conditions such as disabilities, injuries following accidents, Alzheimer's disease and even substance abuse. For more in-depth information on the role of the occupational therapist see the website of the British Association/College of Occupational Therapists (BAOT/COT) at: **www.cot.org.uk**, and also have a look at their information leaflet at: **www.cot.org.uk/members/promoting/CareersLeaflet.pdf.**

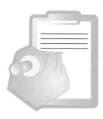

Activity 12.

1.   Research the specific roles of the occupational therapist and discuss your findings with other students. When next in clinical practice ask your mentor if you can spend some time with the occupational therapist to see exactly what their role entails.

2.   Following further reading on the roles of an occupational therapist, assess what needs our scenario patient George might have that the occupational therapist may be able to help him with. Consider his needs throughout his entire patient journey, from admission to discharge.

District nurse

District nurses are qualified nurses who provide care, support and education to their patients and their relatives in the patient's home environment. In some instances the patient may need basic nursing care so the district nurse may delegate this care to an unqualified member of the district nursing team. The more advanced types of nursing care will be solely the responsibility of the qualified district nurse.

A checklist of quality criteria was established by Vafeas (2000) to help ensure that referrals to the district nursing service are made appropriately and properly (as cited in Royal College of Nursing, 2002). The specific duties of a district nurse are quite vast and include a wide range of nursing duties such as performing dressings, monitoring and assessing wounds, administering specific medications or tube or intravenous feeds and care of the dying, to name but a few.

A district nursing referral needs to be completed that provides the following information:

❑ the patient's ward;

❑ consultant;

❑ date of discharge;

❑ name, address and telephone number;

❑ date of birth;

❑ general practitioner's (GP) name, address and telephone number;

❑ any out-patient appointment details;

❑ next of kin details;

❑ details of where the patient is going to be discharged to.

Brief summaries are also needed to highlight the patient's condition, the treatment or care required and details of their pressure areas. A brief assessment of the patient's capabilities on discharge should also be provided together with a list of any other services that are needed. As a rule, four copies of the referral will be made; one is filed with the patient's notes and the others are distributed to district nurse liaison, the patient's general practitioner and the patient themselves.

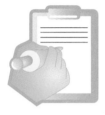

Activity 13.

1.   Research the specific roles of the district nurse and discuss your findings with other students. When next in clinical practice ask your mentor if they will show and explain a district nurse referral form to you.

2.   Following further reading on the roles of a district nurse, assess what needs our scenario patient George might have that the district nurse may be able to help him with.

Social services

The Social Work Recruitment Campaign (2007) says that social workers form a variety of relationships, such as that of an adviser, an advocate, a counsellor or a listener, with clients, their families and friends. They help people to live more successfully by helping them find solutions to their problems. However, in order to access these services it is important that the discharge co-ordinator completes a section 2 referral as advocated by the Community Care (Delayed Discharges etc.) Act (2003) to give notice of the patient's likely need for community care services.

Where the discharge of patients is concerned the social worker may need to work alongside people with mental health problems or learning difficulties, people with HIV/AIDs, children with long-term illnesses and with older people to sort out problems with their health, housing or benefits. This may include arranging alternative accommodation for the patient (including warden controlled accommodation, a home for the elderly or a nursing home) or arranging meals on wheels, a home help, day care, help with personal hygiene or helping the patient and/or their carers to claim for financial help. For more in-depth information on the role of the social worker see the Social Work Recruitment Campaign's website at: **www.socialworkandcare.co.uk/ socialwork**, and the General Social Care Council's website at: **www.gscc.org.uk/Home.**

A social services referral, based on a section 2 referral, needs to be completed. This includes the following information:

❑ the patient's ward;

❑ consultant;

❑ date of admission;

❑ name, address and telephone number;

❑ date of birth;

❑ NHS district number;

❑ general practitioner's name, address and telephone number;

❑ next of kin details.

The nurse must document whether a patient contact assessment has been completed, whether the patient has consented and, if not, why. Also, the nurse must ascertain whether the patient has been considered for fully funded NHS continuing care and whether they have been referred to therapy services (with details if this is the case). The reason for admission, the likely social care needs and the reason for referral also need to be disclosed. The expected date of discharge also needs to be highlighted and then the referral is sent or faxed to the relevant social services department.

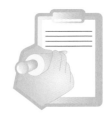

Activity 14.

1.   Research the specific roles of the social worker and discuss your findings with other students. When next in clinical practice ask your mentor if they will show and explain a social services referral to you.

2.   Following further reading on the roles of a social worker, assess what needs our scenario patient George might have that the social worker may be able to help him with.

Specialist nurses

Many hospitals have specialist nurses and patients can be referred to these nurses depending upon their condition and needs. As their name suggests, they are nurses that have a particular expertise in their field of nursing and they can provide extensive advice about their subject and offer specialist care both in hospital and following discharge. Specific specialities include diabetes, cardiac problems and stoma care to name but a few.

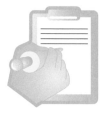

Activity 15.

1. Research the different types of specialist nurse and discuss your findings with other students. When next in clinical practice ask your mentor if you can spend some time with any of the specialist nurses that they may refer their patients to.

2. Following further reading on the different types of specialist nurse, assess the needs of our scenario patient George and decide which of these specialist nurses, if any, he might need to be referred to and why.

Communicating with patients and relatives about discharge

Continued communication with the patient and their relatives throughout the discharge process is vital. They must be involved at all times, with particular reference being made to their own perceived needs. Care must be discussed fully and, ideally, a hospital discharge leaflet that lists all the contact numbers to call in the event of any problems should be provided prior to discharge. Providing health education and health promotion and checking patient understanding is also important as this may be the difference between a successful discharge and an unsuccessful discharge. Again, if possible, leaflets should be provided to reiterate this advice.

Details of the exact discharge date should be communicated well in advance to allow outdoor clothes to be brought in from home, previous services to be recommenced, transport to be arranged if using their own transport (if hospital transport is required then this is usually booked on the day of discharge), and the heating to be switched on at the patient's home if needed. It is also important to ensure that a supply of food is available to the patient on their return and that they have access to their property.

Activity 16.

What communication problems may arise with our scenario patient George and how might they be addressed?

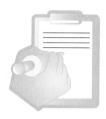

Discharge forms and bed-state

As with transfers, the bed-state and admissions and discharges books need to be completed on discharge. Some form of discharge planning document should also be completed and, following the Department of Health's guidelines, this form should be completed on a continual basis from admission. One of the first items to complete on this document is the nurse's estimate of a date of discharge and that the patient has been advised of this. Quite often these forms have an assessment on them to determine whether the patient is likely to have complex needs on discharge, with the opportunity to reassess this throughout their hospital stay. Specific referrals will also need to be documented including information on who the patient has been referred to, their contact details, the date they were referred, who referred them and dates/notes of any meetings between those professionals and the patient. Details of the patient's home circumstances and any care already being received should also be documented.

Other considerations regarding discharge

Medication

The patient's discharge prescription can be ordered, dispensed and locked away for safe keeping until the day of discharge. Instructions on how to take medication and discussion around side effects and contra-indications can be performed in advance of discharge and reiterated on the day of discharge to ensure that the patient and/or relatives/carers fully understand.

Confirmation of service requirements

Checks should be made to ensure that all the specific services provided by other members of the multidisciplinary team (for example, equipment, alterations to the home, care packages, benefits, etc.) have already been arranged or will definitely be arranged in preparation for the discharge date.

The discharge checklist

A specific checklist will also need to be completed, usually on the day of discharge, to ensure that every eventuality has been catered for. This checklist may include confirmation of the following.

❏ The patient's discharge prescription has been given to them, and any dressings or specific equipment have been handed over.

❏ A discharge leaflet, carer's pack or any written advice has been given to the patient or carers.

❏ Any verbal advice previously given to the patient has been reiterated.

❏ Hospital transport has been booked, highlighting an estimated time of pick up and the type of transport arranged. Should the patient need to take any specific equipment home with them then the type of transport needs to be considered and those transporting the patient also need to be made aware of this need.

❏ The district nurse has been informed by telephone that discharge is imminent.

❏ A letter for the patient's GP has been given to the patient or, if this is not possible, that arrangements will be made to fax or send this on to the patient's GP.

❏ Any property that is being kept safe for the patient has been returned to them.

❏ Any outpatient appointments have been made and given to the patient or, if not, that it/they will be made and sent on.

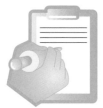

Activity 17.

1.   When next in clinical practice ask your mentor if they will show and explain their discharge checklists or forms to you.

2.   What discharge needs is our scenario patient George likely to have and how may they be addressed?

Summary

Transfers and discharges happen on a regular basis and, from a layperson's point of view, they may appear to be quite a straightforward occurrence. However, I hope, having worked through this chapter, you now realise that there are a lot of issues and considerations involved in these procedures in order to make them as smooth as possible.

Again, continued practice is the vital key to ensuring that the essential skills are mastered and that any transfers or discharges are completed safely and successfully with all the necessary patient/client's needs being addressed. This is also a very topical subject at the moment with many government initiatives being produced. It is therefore very important to be continually aware of the developments through reading and research.

Further reading

Adams T. (1996) 'Informal family caregiving to older people with dementia: research priorities for community psychiatric nursing'. *Journal of Advanced Nursing*, 24(4): 703–10

British Association/College of Occupational Therapists (2007) *The role of the occupational therapist*. See: **www.cot.org.uk/** (last accessed July 2007)

Carers UK (2006) *Looking after someone, a guide to carers' rights and benefits*. London: Carers UK

A guide to:

❑ financial help including carers' benefits, disability benefits, help with housing, fuel and health costs;

❑ practical help including social services and coming out of hospital;

❑ working and caring including flexible working, time off in emergencies and parental leave.

The Community Care (Delayed Discharges etc.) Act 2003. London: HMSO.

The Act includes guidance with regard to:

❑ determination of need for community care services on discharge:

  – notice of patient's likely need for community care services

  – notices under section 2: supplementary

  – duties of responsible authority following notice under section 2

  – duties of responsible NHS body following notice under section 2;

❑ delayed discharge payments:

  – liability to make delayed discharge payments

  – delayed discharge payments: supplementary;

❑ disputes:

  – ordinary residence

  – dispute resolution.

Department of Health (1998) *Modernising social services*. London: DoH

Includes coverage of issues on the following:

❏ services for adults such as independence, consistency and meeting people's needs;

❏ services for children including protection, quality of care and improving life chances;

❏ improving protection through new inspection systems and stronger safeguards;

❏ improving standards in the workforce by creating a General Social Care Council (GSCC) and improving training;

❏ improving partnerships to ensure better joint working for more effective services;

❏ improving delivery and efficiency and making sure it happens

Department of Health (2000) *The NHS plan: a plan for investment, a plan for reform*. London: DoH

Includes separate chapters on the following:

❏ the Department of Health's vision: a health service designed around the patient;

❏ the NHS at it was;

❏ options for funding health care;

❏ investing in NHS facilities;

❏ investing in NHS staff;

❏ changed systems for the NHS;

❏ changes between health and social services;

❏ changes for NHS doctors;

❏ changes for nurses, midwives, therapists and other NHS staff;

❏ changes for patients;

❏ changes in the relationship between the NHS and the private sector;

❏ cutting waiting for treatment;

❏ improving health and reducing inequality;

❏ the clinical priorities;

❏ dignity, security and independence in old age;

❏ the reform programme.

Department of Health (2000) *Patient and public involvement in the new NHS*. London: Department of Health.

Proposed government reforms including:

❏ Commission for Patient and Public Involvement in Healthcare;

❏ Patient Advocacy and Liaison Service;

❏ Independent Complaints and Advocacy Services;

❏ Patient and Public Involvement Forums.

Department of Health (2001) *Continuing care: NHS and local councils' responsibilities*, HSC 2001/015: LAC (2001)18. London: DoH (reviewed in 2003).

Addresses (among others) issues relating to the following:

❏ local policies for continuing care;

❏ NHS responsibilities for continuing care;

❏ continuing NHS health care;

❏ NHS services for people in nursing homes who are not receiving continuing NHS health care;

❏ NHS services in residential homes.

Department of Health (2002) *Making a difference: reducing burdens in hospital.* London: DoH

In this document there was a total of 40 issues identified to reduce the burdens in hospital. These issues broadly fit into 12 categories and the 12 categories were presented as three key themes: the patient journey, information flows and quality. Of the 12 categories those that relate specifically to discharge are:

❏ patient discharge – with regard to discharge planning and contact with social care, specific issues include:

   – Issue 8: Discharge to another locality

   – Issue 9: Discharge to another locality

   – Issue 10: Home authority status

   – Issue 11: Hospital discharge workbook

   – Issue 12: Model discharge documentation

   – Issue 13: Direction on choice

   – Issue 14: National assessment tools

   – Issue 15: National assessment tools

   – Issue 16: Single assessment process

   – Issue 17: Continuing care criteria

   – Issue 18: Communication of the discharge process to patients

   – Issue 19: Section 31 Partnerships and Care Trusts;

❏ patient discharge – with regard to medicines management, specific issues include:

   – Issue 20: National contract for bedside lockers

   – Issue 21: Self-administration and use of patient's own drugs

   – Issue 22: Dispensing for discharge

❏ patient records and hospital paperwork;

❏ requests for information and communications with hospitals;

❏ state benefits – with regard to requests for medical information, specific issues include:

   – Issue 33: Disability living allowance and attendance allowance forms

   – Issue 34: Incapacity benefit forms

❏ risk management;

❏ inspection, accreditation and audit.

Department of Health (2004) *Achieving timely 'simple' discharge from hospital: a toolkit for the multi-disciplinary team.* London: DoH

Contents include:

❏ tackling patient discharge: improving simple discharges;

❑ the myths and obstacles holding back timely discharge;

❑ what the multidisciplinary team can do to improve discharge;

❑ a step guide to making it work;

❑ case studies;

❑ practical tools to improve discharge.

Department of Health (2005) *The long-term (neurological) conditions national service framework*. London: DoH

Identifies key themes relevant to both neurological conditions and other long-term conditions relating to:

❑ independent living;

❑ care planned around the needs and choices of the individual;

❑ easier, timely access to services;

❑ joint working across all agencies and disciplines involved.

Department of Health (2006) *A new ambition for old age, next steps in implementing the national service framework for older people*. London: DoH

Includes ten programmes under the three themes of Dignity in Care, Joined-Up Care and Healthy Ageing. The specific programmes are:

❑ Dignity in care;

❑ Dignity at the end of life;

❑ Stroke services;

❑ Falls and bone health;

❑ Mental health in old age;

❑ Complex needs;

❑ Urgent care;

❑ Care records;

❑ Healthy ageing;

❑ Independence, well-being and choice.

Department of Health (2007) *A recipe for care – not a single ingredient*. London: DoH

Contents include:

❑ early intervention and assessment of old age conditions;

❑ long-term conditions management in the community integrated with social care and specialist services;

❑ early supported discharge whenever possible delivering care closer to home;

❑ general acute hospital care whenever the elderly need it combined with quick access to new specialist centres;

❑ partnership built around the needs and wishes of older people and their families.

Department of Health (2007) *Implementing care closer to home: convenient quality care for patients*. London: DoH

General Social Care Council (2007) Various internet pages. See: **www.gscc.org.uk/Home/** (last accessed July 2007)

The Health and Social Care Joint Unit Change Agent Team (2003) *Discharge from hospital: pathways, process and practice.* London: DoH

This document is extremely informative and includes:

❑ an introduction and overview covering (among others):
- delayed transfer of care
- improving discharge performance
- the government's policy

❑ background information of the policy context;

❑ developing a 'whole system approach' covering (among others):
- what are the characteristics of whole system working?
- who is included?
- whole system working for effective hospital discharge
- the contents, characteristics and components of a good inter-agency discharge policy
- action steps
- useful appendices:
    supporting the system
    transport
    discharge planning self-assessment tool

❑ involving patients and carers includes:
- an overview of the issues
- key features to achieve successful involvement
- assessing need
- useful appendices:
    carer's assessment checklist
    carer's assessment and care plan
    patient's and carer's leaflet

❑ co-ordinating the patient journey includes:
- an overview of the key issues
- the patient journey
- pre-admission assessment
- admission to the ward
- equipment provision
- discharge lounges
- transport
- multidisciplinary and inter-agency teamwork
- useful appendices:
    medicines management
    discharge checklist

> equipment provision
>
> discharge lounges
>
> discharge needs of people who are homeless
>
> admission of people with additional needs
>
> guidelines for the acute sector when caring for someone with a learning disability
>
> common problems and simple solutions

❑ intermediate care, transitional care and sheltered housing which covers:

- – intermediate care
- – transitional care
- – sheltered housing

❑ continuing health and social care which covers:

- – what continuing care is
- – who is responsible for providing and funding continuing care
- – where continuing care is provided
- – what effect the provision of continuing care has on delayed transfers of care
- – assessing the need for continuing health and social care
- – the direction on choice for accommodation
- – dealing with disputes.

Social Work Recruitment Campaign (2007) *The role of the social worker.* See: **www.socialworkandcare.co.uk/socialwork/** (last accessed July 2007)

Other important documents also include the following (though this is not an exhaustive list):

❑ The Carers and Disabled Children Act 2000. London: HMSO.

❑ The Carers (Recognition and Services) Act 2000. London: HMSO.

❑ The Health Act 1999. London: HMSO.

❑ The Health and Social Care Joint Unit Change Agent Team (2002) *Discharge from hospital – good practice checklist.* London: Department of Health.

❑ The Health and Social Care Joint Unit Change Agent Team (2003) *Discharge from hospital: getting it right for people with dementia, a supplementary checklist to help with planning the discharge from acute general hospital settings of people with dementia.* London: Department of Health.

References

British Association/College of Occupational Therapists (2007) *The Role of the Occupational Therapist.* See: **www.cot.org.uk** (last accessed July 2007)

Centre for Policy on Ageing (2007) *Single assessment process moving towards a common assessment process.* See: **www.cpa.org.uk/sap/sap_home.html** (last accessed 8 May 2007)

Chartered Society of Physiotherapy (2002) *Curriculum framework for qualifying programmes in physiotherapy.* London: CSP. See: **www.csp.org.uk/uploads/documents/CFforQPP.pdf** (last accessed July 2007)

Chartered Society of Physiotherapy (2007) See: **www.csp.org.uk/director/physiotherapy explained/whatisphysiotherapy.cfm** (last accessed July 2007)

Department of Health (2001) *National service framework for older people.* London: HMSO

Department of Health (2003) *Winning ways: working together to reduce health care associated infection in England.* London: DoH

Department of Health (2004a) *Single assessment process for older people: April 2004 milestone.* London: HMSO

Department of Health (2004b) *Single assessment process for older people, supplementary checklist for implementation.* London: HMSO

Jarrett, N. and Payne, S. (1995) 'A selective review of the literature on nurse–patient communication: has the patient's contribution been neglected?' *Journal of Advanced Nursing,* 22(1): 72–8

Kee, C.C. and Borchers, L. (1998) 'Reducing readmission rates through discharge interventions'. *Clinical Nurse Specialist, The Journal of Advanced Nursing,* 12(5): 206–9

Royal College of Nursing (2002) *District nursing – changing and challenging. A framework for the 21st century: guidance for nursing staff.* London: RCN

Chapter 4

PAIN MANAGEMENT

Renette Ellson

Refer also to Chapter 15, page 284.

Throughout this chapter reference will be made to the Nursing and Midwifery Council (NMC) Essential Skills Clusters (ESCs). Pain management and its subsequent nursing interventions are extremely important aspects of nursing care and, as such, the NMC has identified several subsections that are relevant to this skill within three of the Essential Skills Clusters titled 'Care, Compassion and Communication', 'Organisational Aspects of Care' and 'Medicines Management'. (Refer also to the Skills Clusters identified in Chapter 15 on the administration of medicines.)

Patients/clients can trust a newly registered nurse to:

Section 5   Provide care that is delivered in a warm, sensitive and compassionate way.

Section 8   Ensure that their consent will be sought prior to care or treatment being given and that their rights will be respected.

Section 9   Make a holistic and systematic assessment of their needs and develop a comprehensive plan of nursing care that is in their best interests and which promotes their health and well-being and minimises the risk of harm.

Section 10   Deliver and evaluate care against the comprehensive assessment and care plan.

Section 16   Safely lead, co-ordinate and manage care.

Section 18   Identify and safely manage risk in relation to the patient/client, the environment, self and others.

Section 20   Select and manage medical devices safely.

Section 35   Work as part of a team to offer a range of treatment options of which medicines may form a part.

The aetiology of pain

There is much to read about the aetiology of pain and the advances made in order to develop the ideal pain theory, so further reading on the subject is advised. However, in short, the theory is that a stimulus, such as tissue damage to your finger, activates the pain receptor nerve endings in the skin. These receptors are known as **nociceptors**, and pain caused by the stimulation of nerve endings is known as nociceptive pain (Rahman, 2004). The nociceptors convert the stimulus into nerve impulses by the transduction of chemicals, nerve fibres then transmit these impulses to the brain via the spinal cord (see Figure 1) and the brain interprets these impulses as pain. It has been recognised that a

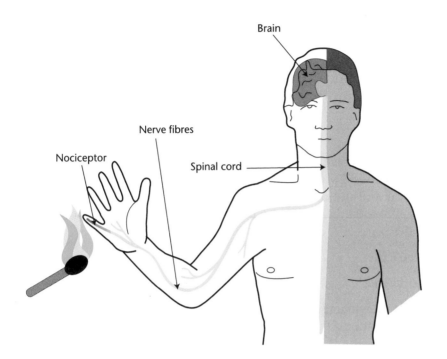

Figure 1
Pain transmission

break in the path the pain impulse takes may still result in an element of pain perception as, for example, with phantom limb pain. It is also acknowledged that stress and its physiological effects can play a major part in the perception of pain, particularly where the issue of chronic pain is concerned. Developments such as these in our understanding of the aetiology of pain have helped considerably with the overall management of pain, thus allowing the practitioner to treat their patient with the most suitable drug or non-drug therapies for that individual (Melzack and Wall, 2003).

Types of pain

When treating patients you will need to consider the type of pain that they are suffering. Pain can be described according to its duration and its source and has traditionally been separated into the two distinct categories: acute pain and chronic pain. However, in some instances, an individual may suffer from both – an acute on chronic pain. Acute and chronic pain may be caused by a variety of stimuli and these are classified as cutaneous (skin) pain, visceral (abdominal) pain, somatic (muscles, bones, etc.) pain and neuropathic (damage to nerves) pain. Cutaneous, visceral and somatic pain relate to the area of the body that has been injured. Neuropathic pain is described by the British National Formulary (2007) as that which arises as a result of damage to neural tissue, with the pain occurring in areas where there are sensory deficits.

Acute pain

Acute pain has been defined by Ready and Edwards (1992) as a 'pain of recent onset and probable limited duration, usually having an identified temporal and causal relationship to injury or disease' (as cited by the Clinical Standards Advisory Group, 2000, p.2). Examples of acute pain include:

❏ headache;

❏ toothache;

❏ pain following a physical injury (for example burns, sprains, fractures and lacerations);

❏ dysmenorrhoea;

❏ abdominal pain.

Acute pain as protection from harm

Ironically, when some incidences of acute pain occur, it may help to protect the individual from further or subsequent harm. For example, if a person is suffering from lower left-sided abdominal pain they are likely to have the pain investigated. Should the investigations reveal an inflamed appendix then the appendix will be surgically removed as an emergency and, hopefully, before the appendix perforates. If the pain had not resulted in the investigation and in the appendix being removed then the patient would be at serious risk of developing further, life-threatening complications such as peritonitis.

Behavioural psychology also plays a role in our response to pain. We learn how to avoid potential causes of pain like, for example, when the pain is caused by touching a sharp object. The perception of the pain felt is transferred to our memory and from this we learn not to touch that sharp object again.

Chronic pain

Chronic pain has been defined by the Clinical Standards Advisory Group (2000, p.2) as a 'pain that either persists beyond the point at which healing would be expected to be complete or that occurs in disease processes in which healing does not take place'. Chronic pain occurs with many different types of illnesses, injury or disease. Examples of chronic pain include:

- back pain;
- osteoarthritis;
- rheumatoid arthritis;
- cancer;
- diabetic neuropathy;
- post herpetic neuralgia;
- multiple sclerosis;
- post-surgical pain.

The Pain in Europe Survey (Fricker, 2003) (by NFO WorldGroup and sponsored by Mundipharma International) highlighted that long-term pain is a widespread problem in Europe and that many sufferers are not satisfied with the treatment that they are receiving for their pain. This pan-European study embraced over 46,000 people across 16 countries and revealed that one in five adults suffers from chronic pain and one in three households have at least one member who experiences pain. One-third of the individuals with chronic pain are suffering severe pain on a regular basis and most have suffered with pain for at least two years with one-fifth having been in pain for 20 years or more.

Furthermore, unemployment in this group is more than double the background rate, one in five chronic pain sufferers have lost a job as a result of their pain, those in jobs report losing an average of 7.8 working days due to pain in the last six months and at least one in five respondents had been diagnosed with depression as a direct result of their pain (Fricker, 2003, p.21).

From these statistics we can see that for the chronic pain sufferer life can become unbearable if their pain is not managed successfully. Indeed, if left untreated, chronic pain can affect the quality of life for sufferers and their carers, feelings of helplessness, isolation and/or depression may arise and, in some instances, family breakdown may occur (Clinical Standards Advisory Group, 2000). Luckily, the developments made with regard to pain management have helped to control chronic pain for many sufferers; these developments will be discussed later in the chapter.

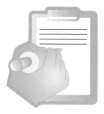

Activity 1.

1. Research cutaneous, visceral and somatic pain in a little more depth. Try to identify the specific areas of the body that may be affected, how severe the pain may be for each area and what types of injury may be presented when the sufferer is actually suffering from each individual type of pain.

2. Think about our scenario patient George. What type of pain, according to its duration, do you think he is suffering from? What is your reasoning for this? What type of pain, according to its source, do you think he is suffering from? What is your reasoning for this?

Symptoms of pain

A patient may express his or her feelings of pain verbally, but they may also show other non-verbal gestures or expressions that may indicate that they are suffering from some form of pain. Examples of non-verbal expressions of pain include:

❑ grimacing or other facial expressions;

❑ the patient's overall posture;

❑ guarding or holding the affected site;

❑ inactivity or a reluctance to move the affected site.

There are a vast number of physiological symptoms of pain (see Figure 2 for some examples), so further reading on this topic is advised. However, some physiological symptoms that can be measured by the nurse and/or doctor have been identified and one of these symptoms is an increase in the patient's respiratory rate. This is measured by counting the patient's respirations or by checking their blood gases for a rise in carbon dioxide and a reduction in oxygen levels. An increase in cardiac function is also a symptom of pain and this can be ascertained following a blood pressure check (which would be elevated) and a pulse check (which would also be elevated).

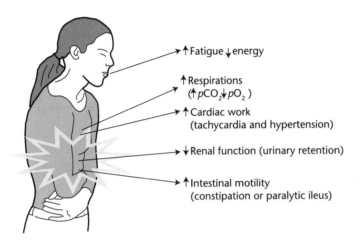

Figure 2
Symptoms of pain

↗↑Fatigue ↓energy

↑Respirations
($\uparrow pCO_2 \downarrow pO_2$)

↗↑Cardiac work
(tachycardia and hypertension)

↘↓Renal function (urinary retention)

↗↑Intestinal motility
(constipation or paralytic ileus)

However, it must be noted that elevated vital signs may occur for only a short time. The body will seek equilibrium, which could happen within an hour from the onset of the pain, and the vital signs will quite often return to the patient's normal rate even if the pain is still persistent (McCaffery and Robinson, 2002). Furthermore, other physiological conditions that affect the vital signs may actually manifest themselves through pain or occur at the same time as pain. Therefore relying on the monitoring of vital signs alone to identify symptoms of pain may be rather inconclusive.

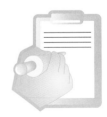

Activity 2.

1.   Think about a time when you or a friend or relative was in moderate to severe pain. How was this pain expressed? Think about two different people who have suffered from moderate to severe pain. Did they express their pain in the same way? If not, what were the differences?

2.   Think about our scenario patient George. How might he express his pain? What is your reasoning for this?

Pain management

A very important aspect in the management of pain is the fact that pain is very subjective and may be perceived differently by different individuals; we all have different pain thresholds. Therefore, as McCaffery and Robinson (2002) note, pain can neither be proved nor disproved. Indeed, as the Scottish Intercollegiate Guidelines Network (2000) highlight, there is no simple, direct measure of pain. It is therefore generally recommended that pain should be assessed by the patient and, as Portenoy and Lesage (1999) point out, 'because pain is inherently subjective, a patient's self-report is the gold standard for assessment' (as cited in the Royal College of General Practitioners and British Pain Society, 2004, p.37).

Several academics, including Allen *et al.* (2002) and McLean *et al.* (2004), have emphasised that pain is quite often the symptom that causes individuals to seek care in the hospital setting (as cited by Layman *et al.*, 2006). It would therefore seem fitting that we as nurses are able to deal with this problem appropriately. However, as Ferrell (1995) notes, even though pain can be quite easily treated, it is ironic that the treatment of pain is often cited as one of the failures of modern medicine (as cited by Mayer *et al.*, 2001). There are various reasons for this. One reason has already been mentioned and relates to the issues of recognising the non-verbal cues for pain and using the measurement of vital signs as a prerequisite for providing analgesia. Briggs (1995) states that there is a real need to discourage nurses from relying on signs and symptoms and, instead, advocate that the only true way of ascertaining whether a patient is in pain or not is to ask them directly.

The management of pain in children and the older person

The ability to recognise and assess pain is particularly important when it comes to children and the elderly. Indeed, Blomqvist (2003) says that staff should provide treatment and care on a needs basis irrespective of their own preferences. However, Pasero and McCaffery (1997) note that many elderly people are stoic and may be reluctant to report pain. Therefore, making an assumption that the patient is comfortable just because they haven't verbalised their pain is a breach of the nurse's duty of care. Archer Copp (2006) says that failing to treat a patient in pain, with the result of pushing them beyond their endurance, could actually be an act of negligence. In addition to this, it could also be a breach of that person's human right not to be subjected to inhumane and degrading treatment and torture (Human Rights Act 1998, Article 3).

Where children are concerned, Jacob and Puntillo (1999) feel that the nursing assessment of their pain is quite often ineffective and, following a survey in one study, they identified that almost half of those surveyed were unaware that a patient's self-report of pain was the single most reliable indicator of the existence of pain (as cited in Simons and Roberson, 2002). Simons and Roberson (2002) go on to say that poor communication with parents and knowledge deficits in this area of care are the main causes of this ineffectiveness and it is imperative that these obstacles are addressed. The Royal College of Paediatrics and Child Health (RCPCH) (2001) have published some guidelines on identifying the best method for recognising and assessing pain in children and on identifying reliable and valid measures of pain by means of pain scales appropriate for use with children depending upon their age group and level of development.

Prescribing medication for children

The National Prescribing Centre (2000) highlights that children are not 'mini adults' and therefore the dose of medications for children should never be calculated from the adult dose and that an up-to-date paediatric dosage reference text, such as *Medicines for Children* by the Royal College of Paediatrics and Child Health or *The Children's British National Formulary* by the Paediatric Formulary Committee, should always be used. The European Commission has also produced 'the paediatric regulation' (which is derived from Regulation (EC) No. 1901/2006, amending Regulation (EEC) No. 1768/92, Directive 2001/20/EC, Directive 2001/83/EC and Regulation (EC) No. 726/2004) which came into force on 26 January 2007. This regulation aims:

❏ to facilitate the development and accessibility of medicinal products for use in the paediatric population;

❏ to ensure that medicinal products used to treat the paediatric population are subject to research of high quality and are appropriately authorised for use;

❏ to improve the information available on the use of medicinal products in the various paediatric populations.

These objectives should be achieved without subjecting the paediatric population to unnecessary clinical trials and without delaying the authorisation of medicinal products for other age populations (European Commission, 2007, p.3).

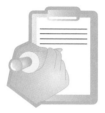

Activity 3.

1. Take a look at the Department of Health website at **www.dh.gov.uk** and find and read up on the following documents: *The NHS end of life care programme* (2004) and *The National Service Framework for Long-term Medical Conditions* (2005).

2. Think about our scenario patient George. If he cannot verbally express that he is in pain, and any changes in his vital signs have settled down, how could you ensure that he remains pain free?

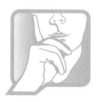

Reflection

Have you ever suffered with pain and had no analgesia with you to be able to treat it? How did you feel at that time? How would you feel if you went to visit a close relative in hospital and they told you that they have been in a lot of pain and the nurse had not offered them any analgesia?

Pain assessment

As I have said above, pain management needs to be based upon the individual pain sufferer's perception, and not on our perception of what the pain should be for that individual's particular injury or illness. For example, if we have suffered a particular injury in the past but were able to cope with the pain that the injury caused without some form of analgesia, we should not assume that someone else with the same injury would also be able to cope with the pain with no analgesia. Indeed, as

Lisson (1989) notes, assessing a patient's level of pain in this way and then basing your decision of whether to relieve the pain or not solely on your own morals and values hardly resembles a professional judgement (as cited by Archer Copp, 2006). Furthermore, as McCaffery and Robinson (2002) highlight, this approach results in an inconsistent assessment of the patient's pain which results in inconsistent pain relief and an increasing risk of under-treatment.

Several assessment tools have been developed to assist the health care professional with the task of taking a patient/client's history of their pain. No one individual tool has been advocated and any are acceptable as long as the process used is detailed and methodical.

The PQRST assessment method

One method that is quite easy to remember is the PQRST method for assessing pain, as advocated by Rahman (2004). This method includes establishing that a patient has pain and, for each episode of pain, the following five characteristics need to be discussed with them (some example questions for each are given):

P = Provokes. What causes the pain? What makes it better/worse?

Q = Quality. What does it feel like? Can you describe the pain – is it sharp/dull/stabbing/cutting/burning/achy/crushing/tightness, etc.?

R = Radiates. Does the pain go anywhere else? Does it move around?

S = Severity. How bad is the pain? There are various methods to evaluate this – e.g. pain scoring.

T = Time. When did the pain start? How long does it last? Is it constant or does it come and go?

(Rahman, 2004)

British Pain Society and RCGP method

Another similar method, as advocated by the British Pain Society and the Royal College of General Practitioners (2004), is assessing pain by considering the following issues:

❏ site: primary sites and patterns of radiation;

❏ quality: e.g. stabbing, burning;

❏ temporal features: how long the pain has been present, what pattern it follows, diurnal variation;

❏ factors that exacerbate or relieve the pain;

❏ impact of pain on sleep;

❏ emotional impact: e.g. anxiety, depression, etc.;

❏ severity: mild, moderate or severe or as indicated on a numerical rating scale or visual analogue scale;

❏ impact on quality of life: activities that are difficult to carry out or the patient has stopped doing or avoids, or manages but at a high cost to their pain.

(British Pain Society and the Royal College of General Practitioners, 2004, p.38)

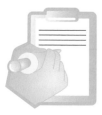

Activity 4.

1.   Think about the last time you were in moderate or severe pain. Answer the questions from one of these questionnaires based on your experience of the pain you suffered.

2.   Think about our scenario patient George. How effective are these questionnaires likely to be for him? What are your reasons for your answer?

Pain assessment tools

Several academics have designed assessment tools in order to help health care professionals and pain sufferers to assess pain. Examples of such tools include asking the patient or client to rate their pain on a visual scale by using lines ranging from 'no pain' to 'worst pain imaginable', or by rating their pain verbally as 'none', 'mild', 'moderate' or 'severe', or by rating their pain on a numerical scale of 1 to 10 with 10 being the worst pain possible. Questions may also be asked as part of the assessment tool to ascertain the effect of pain on the individual's quality of life or on their ability to carry out their activities of living. Questions are also used to help to identify the type of pain as this may help the health care professional to treat the pain accordingly and effectively. Jacox *et al.* (1994) point out that these assessment scales are very useful for eliciting responses from patients about their comfort or discomfort, thus enhancing clarity in communications and providing the basis for the ideal management programme for that individual. The assessment tool used very much depends upon the individual Trust's protocols and their pain management services. However, in view of recent developments in pain management, it is likely that some form of assessment tool will be used in most Trusts.

The British Pain Society has produced a series of pain scales to assist in the assessment of pain. These scales are also available in a variety of languages, which may be very useful if a translator is not at hand (British Pain Society, 2004, p.50). The pain scale translations are available on the British Pain Society's website at: **www.britishpainsociety.org**.

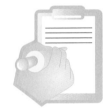

Activity 5.

1.   When you are next in clinical practice, ask your mentor about their pain assessment scale and compare and contrast it with other scales that can be found on the British Pain Society's website (**www.britishpainsociety.org**). If possible, ask your mentor if you can spend some time with the Trust's pain management team.

2.   Consider our scenario patient George. Of the assessment scales that you have looked at, which one do you think would be the most appropriate for him and why?

Specialised assessment scales

In view of the potential for some elderly people and children to be cognitively impaired, several academics have developed assessment tools specifically for these types of people. Examples include:

❑ The Abbey Pain Scale (see Figure 3) (Abbey *et al.*, 2004);

❑ ADD – the Assessment of Discomfort in Dementia Protocol (Kovach *et al.*, 1999);

❑ DS-DAT – the Discomfort Scale – Dementia of the Alzheimer's Type (Hurley *et al.*, 1992);

❑ PAINAD – Pain Assessment in Advanced Dementia Scale (Warden *et al* ., 2003);

❑ the Wong-Baker FACES Pain Rating Scale (more specifically for children) (Wong and Baker, 2001).

Figure 3
The Abbey
Pain Scale

Abbey Pain Scale

For measurement of pain in people with dementia who cannot verbalise.

How to use scale: While observing the resident, score questions 1 to 6

Name of resident: ....

Name and designation of person completing the scale: ....

Date: ....Time: ....

Latest pain relief given was...at ....hrs.

Q1.	**Vocalisation** e.g: whimpering, groaning, crying *Absent 0 Mild 1 Moderate 2 Severe 3*	**Q1**	☐
Q2.	**Facial expression** e.g: looking tense, frowning, grimacing, looking frightened *Absent 0 Mild 1 Moderate 2 Severe 3*	**Q2**	☐
Q3.	**Change in body language** e.g: fidgeting, rocking, guarding part of body, withdrawn *Absent 0 Mild 1 Moderate 2 Severe 3*	**Q3**	☐
Q4.	**Behavioural change** e.g: increased confusion, refusing to eat, alteration in usual patterns *Absent 0 Mild 1 Moderate 2 Severe 3*	**Q4**	☐
Q5.	**Physiological change** e.g: temperature, pulse or blood pressure outside normal limits, perspiring, flushing or pallor *Absent 0 Mild 1 Moderate 2 Severe 3*	**Q5**	☐
Q6.	**Physical changes** e.g: skin tears, pressure areas, arthritis, contractures, previous injuries *Absent 0 Mild 1 Moderate 2 Severe 3*	**Q6**	☐

Add scores for 1 – 6 and record here ⟹ **Total Pain Score** ☐

Now tick the box that matches the Total Pain Score ⟹

0 – 2 No pain	3 – 7 Mild	8 – 13 Moderate	14+ Severe

Finally, tick the box which matches the type of pain ⟹

Chronic	Acute	Acute on Chronic

Dementia Care Australia Pty Ltd
Website: www.dementiacareaustralia.com

Abbey, J. De Bellis, A. Piller, N. Esterman, A. Giles, L. Parker, D.and Lowcay, B.
Funded by the JH & JD Gunn Medical Research Foundation 1998 – 2002
(This document may be reproduced with this acknowledgment retained)

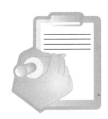

Activity 6.

1. Research the issue of specialised pain scales. Try to locate two or three different scales and compare and contrast them. You may find the following articles useful – Zwakhalen *et al.* (2006) and/or Zwakhalen *et al.* (2007).

2. Consider our scenario patient George. Look at the Abbey Pain Scale and assess whether this would be appropriate for him. Of the specialised assessment scales that you have looked at in response to Question 1, which one of these do you think would be the most appropriate for George and why?

The treatment of pain

Drug therapy

Various analgesic drugs can be used to alleviate pain but the choice of analgesia very much depends upon the nature and severity of the pain and, in some instances, on the actual cause of the pain. The following section will highlight the most commonly used drugs, the types of pain that they may be used for and the most prevalent side effects. However, further reading on these drugs is advised to ascertain the usual doses for each particular drug, other, less common side effects and knowledge of issues like contra-indications and drug interactions. An up-to-date version of the British National Formulary will provide all this information for you. Furthermore, continually updating your knowledge will ensure that you are aware of any important research changes around the issue of pain management and treatment.

Although initially developed by the World Health Organisation (WHO) for the treatment of cancer pain, the pain relief ladder (see Figure 4) has been adapted by health care professionals for routine treatment of acute and chronic pain. To calm fears and anxiety, WHO advocate that additional drugs (**adjuvants**) should be used.

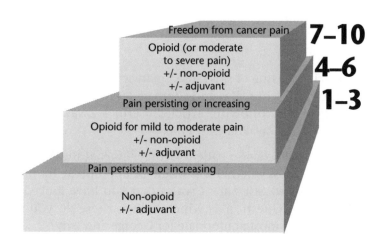

Figure 4 WHO's Pain Relief Ladder Reproduced with the permission of the World Health Organization. Original source: **www.who.int/ cancer/palliative/ painladder/en**

Figure 4 shows that the WHO advocates that the first line of treatment if the pain is mild (1–3 on a numerical scale) should be a non-opioid drug such as paracetamol or aspirin, with or without an adjuvant. If the pain persists or increases or is moderate in the first instance (4–6 on a numerical scale) then the drug of choice should be a mild opioid such as codeine, with or without the non-opioid and/or adjuvant. The next step on the ladder, should pain persist or increase to a level of moderate to severe or is severe in the first instance (7–10 on a numerical scale), is the use of strong opioids such as morphine, again with or without a non-opioid and/or adjuvant. The WHO also advocates that to ensure total pain control treatment should be given regularly at prescribed intervals and not on demand.

Non-opioid analgesics

Aspirin

Aspirin is given for mild to moderate pain by mouth or by rectum in the form of a suppository. The side effects of aspirin include gastro-intestinal irritation, though this may be prevented by prescribing enteric coated preparations. Bleeding times may also be increased as aspirin has an anti-platelet effect, so care should be taken with patients who are already receiving anti-coagulation treatment. Hypersensitivity, mainly in the form of bronchospasm or rashes, may also occur so care should be taken with asthmatic patients.

Paracetamol

Paracetamol is given on its own for mild to moderate pain or with stronger analgesia for moderate to severe pain. It is given by mouth, intravenously or by rectum in the form of a suppository. Side effects of paracetamol are rare but may include rashes or blood disorders. However, care should be taken not to exceed the stated dose as this could lead to liver damage. This can sometimes happen by accident if other preparations are given or taken at the same time without the knowledge that they also include paracetamol.

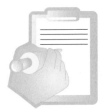

Activity 7.

1. Research these drugs to ascertain the less common side effects, their contra-indications and drug interactions.

2. Think about our scenario patient George. How effective are these drugs likely to be for him at each separate stage of his patient journey? What other considerations may need to be taken into account where these drugs are concerned, especially given the fact that he has been admitted as an emergency with abdominal pain?

Opioid analgesics

Morphine

Morphine is administered for severe acute and post-operative pain by subcutaneous or intramuscular injection, or via patient-controlled analgesia (PCA). It is also given by slow intravenous injection for myocardial infarction and acute pulmonary oedema. For severe chronic pain sufferers the ideal administration route is oral (this includes sublingually or by oral modified release every 12–24 hours, according to the brand), but morphine may also be administered by subcutaneous injection (though this is not suitable for oedematous patients), by intramuscular injection or via the rectum in the form of suppositories.

The most prevalent side effects of opiates include nausea and vomiting (particularly in the initial stages of treatment) so it is important to monitor your patient for this and, if need be, the doctor can prescribe an anti-emetic to prevent it occurring. Constipation is another possible side effect and, again, you need to monitor your patient for this and provide laxatives as required. Drowsiness may also occur so, if this is the case, it is important that you ensure safety for your patient by supervising them closely. Larger doses of opiates may produce respiratory depression and hypotension so it is extremely important that the patient's vital signs are observed during their treatment and that there is easy access to the antidote (naloxone/Narcan), especially when the treatment is first initiated.

Diamorphine

Diamorphine is given for very severe acute and chronic pain by subcutaneous or intramuscular injection. It is also given for myocardial infarction and acute pulmonary oedema by slow intravenous injection (though the dose is usually lower than that for morphine). The side effects are the same as those for morphine.

Pethidine hydrochloride

Pethidine is given for moderate to severe acute or post-operative pain by mouth, by subcutaneous injection, by intramuscular injection or by slow intravenous injection. In some instances it may also be given as a premedication before an operation though this use is now quite rare. It is more commonly used for pain control during labour. The side effects are the same as those for morphine, though convulsions have been reported in cases of overdose.

Buprenorphine

Buprenorphine is given for moderate to severe acute or chronic pain by sublingual administration, by intramuscular injection or in the form of a self-adhesive patch (the dose adjustment for the patch has strict guidelines and can vary between preparations). It may also be given as a premedication by sublingual administration or by intramuscular injection, or given intra-operatively by slow intravenous injection.

The side effects are the same as those for morphine. However, should respiratory depression occur, the effects of the antidote (naloxone/Narcan) are only partial. Mild withdrawal symptoms may also occur and care must be taken with patients who have had patches prescribed as the patches can sometimes cause skin reactions. Treatment should be stopped if an allergic reaction with severe inflammation occurs.

Dihydrocodeine tartrate

Dihydrocodeine is given for moderate to severe pain by mouth (including modified release), or by deep subcutaneous or intramuscular injection. The side effects are the same as those for morphine.

Tramadol hydrochloride

Tramadol is given for moderate to severe acute or chronic pain and for post-operative pain by mouth (including as an effervescent lemon-flavoured, sugar-free powder), by intramuscular injection or by intravenous injection (over two to three minutes) or by intravenous infusion.

The side effects are the same as those for morphine but there is also the risk of abdominal discomfort, diarrhoea, hypo/hypertension, paraesthesia, anaphylaxis and confusion. Patients taking this medication need to be observed closely for all these potential risks and either treated accordingly and/or reviewed for a more suitable analgesic. This is particularly important where anaphylaxis is concerned as this type of reaction is potentially fatal.

Codeine phosphate

Codeine is given for mild to moderate pain by mouth (including as a syrup) or by intramuscular injection. The side effects are the same as those for morphine.

The risk of addiction to opioids

A major concern among health care professionals is that using morphine, diamorphine or morphine derivatives may cause the patient to become addicted. However, according to McCaffery and Robinson (2002) various studies over the last 20 years have shown that the likelihood of addiction occurring is rare (probably less than 1 per cent), even for those taking the drug for long periods of time.

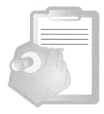

Activity 8.

1.   Research these drugs to ascertain the less common side effects, their contra-indications and drug interactions.

2.   Think about our scenario patient George. How effective are these drugs likely to be for him at each separate stage of his patient journey? What other considerations may need to be taken into account where these drugs are concerned? In this regard, especially consider the fact that he has been admitted as an emergency with abdominal pain. If you were to administer one of these drugs, which one is it likely to be?

Compound analgesics

Compound analgesics contain a weaker analgesic, such as aspirin or paracetamol, and also an opioid derivative such as codeine phosphate. The research on these drugs has not yet substantiated their overall effectiveness. Furthermore, because the two drugs are part of a compound there is no scope for the health care professional to titrate the individual drug dosages according to patient need. Therefore it may be more beneficial to give the drugs separately. There are numerous compound preparations available and these include Cocodamol 8/500, Cocodamol 15/500, Cocodamol 30/500, Codydramol and Remedeine. The side effects of each very much depends upon the individual drugs that are in them.

Non-steroidal anti-inflammatory drugs (NSAIDs)

NSAIDs are given for mild to moderate pain including dysmenorrhoea, post-operative pain and migraine. If taken regularly they have both an analgesic and an anti-inflammatory effect, which makes them particularly useful for musculoskeletal and/or joint diseases, though the anti-inflammatory effect may take up to three weeks.

The most prevalent side effects are gastro-intestinal discomfort, nausea, diarrhoea and, occasionally, bleeding and ulceration. Therefore care must be taken and patients should be advised to take the medication with food or a glass of milk. Should ulceration occur then the drug should be discontinued if possible. For those at risk of ulceration another form of medication to prevent ulceration should be prescribed alongside the NSAID to help to reduce the risk (see the NICE (2001) guidelines).

There are various NSAIDs available but the most commonly used drug is ibuprofen as it has fewer side effects than other drugs in this category. However, its anti-inflammatory properties are weaker than those of other drugs. Other preparations include naproxen, fenbufen, fenoprofen, ketoprofen, tiaprofenic, diclofenac, aceclofenac, diflunisal, etodolac, indometacin (indomethacin), mefenamic acid, meloxicam, nabumetone, piroxicam, sulindac and tenoxicam.

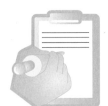

Activity 9.

1. Research these drugs to ascertain the less common side-effects, their contra-indications and drug interactions. Have a look at the *Musculoskeletal services framework* (Department of Health, 2006) on the following website for further information on musculoskeletal problems: **www.18weeks.nhs.uk/Public/ default.aspx?main=true&load=ArticleViewer&ArticleId=612.**

2. Think about our scenario patient George. How effective are these drugs likely to be for him on admission? What other considerations may need to be taken into account where these drugs are concerned? Consider, especially, the fact that he has been admitted as an emergency with abdominal pain.

Tricyclics and anticonvulsants for pain management

Tricyclics (gabapentin and pregabalin) and anticonvulsants (amitriptyline hydrochloride) are usually given orally as adjuvents to another form of licensed analgesic for neuropathic pain. They have many side effects and you are advised to research these in order to gain a better understanding of the drugs.

If these types of drugs are prescribed it is very important that informed consent is given by the patient. This entails a full explanation of the rationale for the use of any of these drugs and in-depth advice as to the side effects. Furthermore, some of these drugs (for example amitriptyline) do not have product licences for treating neuropathic pain and are used outside their product licence. The British Pain Society booklet on *The use of drugs beyond licence in palliative care and pain management* (2002) offers valuable advice on this subject (British Pain Society and the Royal College of General Practitioners, 2004).

Specific post-operative pain relief

All patients should have a full pain assessment after an operation. In many instances, especially with major operations, the anaesthetist will discuss pain relief in depth with the patient before the operation. This is especially important with patients who are likely to have either 'patient-controlled analgesia' or an 'epidural'. It is important to ensure that the patient understands the treatment regime, firstly to promote compliance and, secondly, to prevent any distress that they may have when they see an extra piece of equipment attached to them on their return from theatre.

Patients undergoing major operations will benefit from the use of these types of analgesic delivery systems for several reasons.

❑ They allow a continual/almost continual supply of analgesia and thus prevent the chance of breakthrough pain occurring, which is very reassuring to the patient.

❑ They allow the patient and/or the health care professional to titrate the amount of analgesia required, while still ensuring an adequate level of pain control.

❑ They help to avoid the patient having to have injection after injection.

❑ Because the patient's pain is controlled, the patient is likely to comply with their post-operative recovery regime, which will help to prevent many post-operative complications.

Patient-controlled analgesia

See also Chapter 20, page 448.

Patient-controlled analgesia (PCA) is an opioid administered parenterally via an infusion pump (see Figure 5) which allows the patient to administer their own analgesia depending upon their own requirements. (See also Chapter 20, page 448.) In order for PCA to be successful the patient has to be able to understand that they need to press a button in order to deliver the analgesia. The pump can be set to deliver a background infusion, but this on its own may not be enough to control the patient's pain totally, so the patient still needs to be able to comply. In some instances, this method is unsuitable such as, for example, with patients who are cognitively impaired or are unable to operate the handset.

Because an opioid is being administered, it is extremely important that the staff on the ward area have a good understanding of the contra-indications and side effects of opioids, and that they are able to monitor and observe their patients appropriately. Specific observations should include the patient's sedation level, their blood pressure, their pulse, their respiration rate and their oxygen saturations (especially important as opioids affect the respiratory centre in the brain and may cause a depression of the respirations resulting in the need for an antidote like naloxone/Narcan). A regular assessment of the patient's pain should also be carried out. Opiates may cause nausea and it may therefore be necessary to administer an anti-emetic. They may also cause confusion or even hallucinations, especially in the elderly, so this should also be monitored. Caution should also be taken with patients who have renal impairment, liver failure or a head injury.

See this chapter, page 99.

The infusion is administered via a peripheral intravenous line so it is important that the site of entry is checked regularly for any signs of **extravasation** or infection, and that the line is checked to ensure that it is patent. Knowledge of the PCA pumps is also important to avoid the risk of overdosing. The pumps should be lockable and should include alarms that warn of any excessive doses.

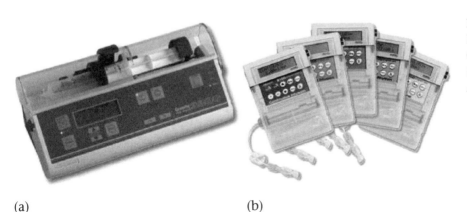

(a)   (b)

Figure 5
PCA pumps: (a) Graseby 3300 pump; (b) Graseby 9300 Ambulatory PCAs

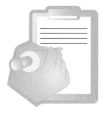

Activity 10.

1. Research PCA in a little more depth. What are the main benefits and disadvantages of this type of post-operative analgesia? What knowledge does the nurse need in order to care for a patient with this form of analgesic treatment?

2. Think about our scenario patient George. Following his operation, how effective is PCA likely to be for him? What are the considerations that the nursing staff would need to take into account where this type of treatment is concerned?

Epidural analgesia

See also Chapter 20, page 447.

An epidural allows the administration of analgesia to specific nerve receptors in the spine (see also Chapter 20, page 447). The exact insertion site will depend upon where in the body the analgesic affect is required. The use of epidurals within any given area depends upon the abilities and knowledge of the trained staff working in that area to manage the device safely and effectively. The recent guidelines *Good practice in the management of continuous epidural analgesia in the hospital setting* (2004) have been produced jointly by the Royal College of Anaesthetists, the Royal College of Nursing, the Association of Anaesthetists of Great Britain and Ireland, the British Pain Society and the European Society of Regional Anaesthesia and Pain Therapy, and you are strongly advised to read this document for further information.

Non-pharmacological options for pain management

Physical therapies

In order to manage a patient's pain effectively referrals may be made to other health care professionals such as physiotherapists, occupational therapists and chiropractors. They will perform their own assessments and use their knowledge to help the individual with their pain. For example, a physiotherapist may suggest exercises to increase mobility and educate the patient to take control of the pain. An occupational therapist may offer the individual specific aids that may help with certain activities of living.

Cognitive behavioural pain management programmes

The British Pain Society (2007) highlights that several academics, including Koes *et al.* (2006) and Hoffman *et al.* (2007), as well as the European Commission in their *Guidelines* (2004) have provided good evidence that cognitive behavioural pain management programmes can improve the patient's pain experience, their mood, their ability to cope, their negative outlook on their pain and also their activity levels. In light of this evidence the British Pain Society developed and published *Recommended guidelines for pain management programmes for adults* in April 2007 (which builds on the concepts in their previous document *Desirable criteria for pain management programmes* published in 1997). These guidelines state that, in some instances, chronic pain cannot be resolved by conventional pain relief methods and so a pain management programme may be a suitable method to restore the sufferer's life to as near normal as possible. A multidisciplinary approach is advocated which includes the following:

❑ a medical specialist – to assess and manage medical needs, provide education and training;

❑ a chartered clinical psychologist – to assess and implement psychological principles and provide cognitive behavioural therapy, education and training;

❑ a state registered physiotherapist – for physical reactivation;

❑ an occupational therapist – for group work, goal setting, planning and pacing a return to activities, retraining and return to work;

❑ a state registered nurse – for medication review, rationalisation and reduction when agreed, health education and liaison with patient's family and other agencies;

❑ a pharmacist – for education and planning of medication adjustment;

❑ assistant psychologists – for data collection and analysis, implementing graded exposure programmes;

❑ administrative staff – for all administrative duties;

❑ a graduate patient – for patient education and serving as a role model.

(British Pain Society, 2007, pp.18–19)

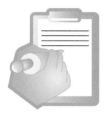

Activity 11.

Think about our scenario patient George. How effective is this type of programme likely to be for him? Look at all the different aspects of the programme and assess their suitability for George.

Complementary therapies

As the title suggests, complementary therapies should complement and work alongside traditional medicine. There are many different types of complementary therapies that can be tried to assist with the treatment of pain. Unfortunately, for some of these therapies, research into their efficacy is inconclusive. However, this is not the case for all complementary therapies as Table 1 shows (overleaf).

Transcutaneous electrical nerve stimulation

Transcutaneous electrical nerve stimulation (TENS) machines work by stimulating areas of the skin (via a pair of electrodes) with an electric current. They are most frequently used by patients who have chronic pain.

Patient support groups

Patients with long-term chronic pain may find a support group beneficial as it will enable them to discuss and share their concerns and coping strategies with others. The support group may also help with the emotional aspects of chronic pain and may help to improve the patient's overall mood and psychological state of mind.

Patient information

Various leaflets are available for patients who suffer from acute or chronic pain. These include the following.

❏ Action on Pain (available at: **www.action-on-pain.co.uk**):

- *Understanding chronic pain;*
- *Managing your pain;*
- *Have pain will travel;*
- *Planning to start exercising – but need some advice;*

Name	Principle	Conditions used for	Efficacy	Safety	Risk-benefit balance
Acupuncture	Needle insertion into acupuncture points for health purposes	Used as a panacea in China, in the West predominantly for pain control	Encouraging data	Serious adverse effects are rare, mild ones occur in 7% of cases	Positive for some conditions
Alexander technique	Training process of ideal body posture and movement; developed by F. M. Alexander	Musculoskeletal problems, e.g. back pain	Few clinical trials exist, no final verdict possible	No serious adverse effects	Uncertain
Aromatherapy	Application of essential oils usually through gentle massage techniques; developed by R. M. Gattefoss	Relaxation, chronic pain	Systematic review was inconclusive	Allergic reactions to oils	Uncertain
Autogenic training	Form of self-hypnosis for relaxation and stress reduction; developed by J. Schultz	Stress management, chronic pain	Encouraging evidence	No serious adverse effects	Positive for stress, uncertain for pain
Chelation therapy	Intravenous infusion of ethyline diamine tetra-acetic acid (EDTA) used for 'deblocking' arteries from arteriosclerotic lesions	Circulatory disorders, e.g. intermittent claudication (ischaemic pain)	Repeatedly shown in rigorous clinical trials to be ineffective	Serious adverse effects reported	Negative
Chiropractic	Popular manual therapy based on the assumption that most health problems are due to malalignments of the spine and treatable through spinal manipulation; developed by D. D. Palmer	Back pain, neck pain	Conclusions of systematic reviews of chiropractic for back pain are not uniform. The methodologically best are not positive	Serious adverse effects have been reported, their exact incidence is not known	Negative
Herbal medicine	Medical use of preparations containing exclusively plant material	Various, including pain	Some herbs have been shown to be effective, e.g. Devil's Claw	Depends on specific herb (e.g. toxicity, herb–drug interaction)	Positive for some herbs

Name	Principle	Conditions used for	Efficacy	Safety	Risk-benefit balance
Homeopathy	Medical use of diluted remedies according to the 'like cures like' principle	Various benign, chronic conditions associated with pain, e.g. headache	No sound evidence	No serious adverse effects	Negative
Hypnotherapy	Induction of trance-like state to influence the unconscious mind	Chronic pain	Encouraging evidence	Adverse effects probably infrequent	Positive
Massage	Various techniques of manual stimulation of cutaneous, subcutaneous or muscular structures	Musculoskeletal pain, e.g. back pain	Encouraging evidence	Few serious adverse effects	Positive
Osteopathy	Various techniques of spinal mobilisation; developed by T. Still	Back pain, neck pain	Systematic reviews of osteopathy for back pain are inconclusive	Adverse effects less than with chiropractic	Inconclusive
Reflexology	Internal organs correspond to areas on the soles of the feet and can be influenced through massaging these	Relaxation, chronic pain	Inconclusive	No serious adverse effects	Inconclusive
Spiritual healing	Umbrella term for techniques of channelling 'healing energy' through a healer into a patient	Chronic pain	Clinical studies highly contradictory; the best recent studies are negative	No serious adverse effects	Negative
Yoga	Meditative, postural and breathing techniques from ancient India	Various conditions associated with pain, e.g. back pain	Inconclusive	No serious adverse effects	Inconclusive

Table 1 Examples of complementary medicine used for pain control
Reproduced with permission. This data is based on systematic reviews published in Ernst *et al.* (2001).

- *Pacing;*
- *Relaxation;*
- *Step into my World – Understanding Pain in Children.*

❏ The Neuropathy Trust:
- *Peripheral Neuropathy and Neuropathic Pain Under the Spotlight;*
- *Diabetic Neuropathy under the Spotlight.*

Both are 28-page booklets covering many aspects and can be bought for a minimal cost by accessing the website **www.neurocentre.com/cd.htm**.

❏ Pain Concern – several leaflets are available at **www.painconcern.org. uk/pages/page9.php.**

❏ Pain Relief Foundation – several leaflets are available at: **www.pain relieffoundation.org.uk/paininfo/paininfo.html.**

❏ The British Pain Society (leaflets available at **www.britishpainsociety. org/pubpatient.htm**):
- *Pain management programmes for adults: information for patients (2007);*
- *Pain and problem drug use: information for patients (2007);*
- *Using drugs beyond licence – information for patients (2005);*
- *Spinal cord stimulation for pain: information for patients (2005);*
- *Opioid medicines for persistent pain: information for patients (2004);*
- *Understanding and managing pain (2004).*

Activity 12.

1. Read some of these leaflets and analyse their appropriateness for a selection of patients of differing ages with differing illnesses. Are there any leaflets that you particularly like and would advocate for your patients?

2. Consider our scenario patient George. If he was discharged from hospital but was still suffering from mild to moderate pain, would any of the leaflets that you've just analysed be appropriate for him? If not, other than providing analgesia on discharge, how might you try to ensure that the necessary information and advice is provided to George?

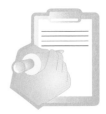

Summary

This chapter has briefly covered several aspects that relate to pain and its management. However, the information provided is, of necessity, rather concise and there are many other sources that will provide a deeper understanding of pain management. Therefore you are strongly advised to carry out further reading and research in order to consolidate and expand your knowledge.

Further reading

Association of the British Pharmaceutical Industry (2007) *Some questions and answers about pain*. See: **www.abpi.org.uk/publications/publication_details/targetpain/tp3_questions.asp** (last accessed April 2007)

Bucknall, T., Manias, E. and Botti, M. (2007) 'Nurse's reassessment of postoperative pain after analgesic administration', *Clinical Journal of Pain*, 23(1): 1–7

Department of Health (2004) *The NHS end of life care programme*. London: DoH

Department of Health (2005) *The national service framework for long-term medical conditions*. London: DoH

Hadjistavropoulos, T., Herr, K., Turk, D.C., Fine, P.G., Dworkin, R.H., Helme, R. *et al.* (2007) 'An interdisciplinary expert consensus statement on assessment of pain in older persons'. *Clinical Journal of Pain*, 23 (Suppl.): 1–43

Moore, A., Edwards, J., Barden, J. and McQuay, H. (2003) *Bandolier's little book of pain*. Oxford: Oxford University Press

Napp Pharmaceuticals (2002) *Pain and pain services in the NHS – an overview of current thinking and provision in the UK*. Cambridge: Napp Pharmaceuticals

Nursing Focus in Pain Management Working Party of the Pain Society, British Chapter of the International Association for the Study of Pain (2002) *Recommendations for nursing practice in pain management*. London: Pain Society

Patient's Association (2007) *Pain in older people – a hidden problem*. Middlesex: Patient's Association

Royal College of Anaesthetists and Pain Society (2003) *Pain Management Services*. London: Royal College of Anaesthetists and Pain Society

Royal College of General Practitioners (2001) *Clinical guidelines for the management of acute low back pain*. London: RCGP

Royal College of General Practitioners and British Pain Society (2004) *A practical guide to the provision of chronic pain services for adults in primary care*. London: RCGP and British Pain Society (this document includes information on the five pledges to help people living with persistent pain)

Royal College of Paediatrics and Child Health (1999) *Medicines for Children*. London: RCPCH Publications

Scottish Intercollegiate Guidelines Network (SIGN), Scottish Cancer Therapy Network (2000) *Control of pain in patients with cancer*. Edinburgh: SIGN

References

Abbey, N., Piller, A., De Bellis, A., Esterman, D., Parker, D., Giles, L. and Lowcay, B. (2004) 'The Abbey pain scale: a 1-minute numerical indicator for people with end-stage dementia'. *International Journal of Palliative Nursing*, 10(16): 6–14

Archer Copp, L. (2006) 'An ethical responsibility for pain management'. *Journal of Advanced Nursing*, 55(1): 1–3

Blomqvist, K. (2003) 'Older people in persistent pain: nursing and paramedical staff perceptions and pain management'. *Journal of Advanced Nursing*, 41(6): 575–84

Briggs, M. (1995) 'Principles of acute pain assessment'. *Nursing Standard*, 9(19): 23–7

British National Formulary (BNF) (2007) *British National Formulary*. London: BMJ Publishing

British Pain Society (1997) *Desirable criteria for pain management programmes*. London: BPS

British Pain Society (2004) *Recommendations for the appropriate use of opioids for persistent non-cancer pain*. London: BPS

British Pain Society (2007) *Recommended guidelines for pain management programmes for adults*. London: BPS

Clinical Standards Advisory Group (2000) *Services for patients with pain*. London: HMSO

Department of Health (2006) *Musculoskeletal services framework*. London: DoH See: **www.18weeks.nhs.uk/Public/default.aspx?main=true&load=ArticleViewer& ArticleId=612**

Ernst, E., Pittler, M.H., Stevinson, C. and White, A.R. (2001) *The desktop guide to complementary and alternative medicine*. Edinburgh: Mosby

European Commission (2007) *Commission guidelines on the format and content of applications for agreement or modification of a paediatric investigation plan and requests for waivers or deferrals and concerning the operation of the compliance check and on criteria for assessing significant studies*. See: **http://ec.europa.eu/enterprise/pharmaceuticals/paediatrics/** (last accessed 14 June 2007)

Fricker, J. (2003) *Pain in Europe – a report*. Cambridge: Mundipharma International. See: **www.paineurope.com/files/PainInEuropeSurvey_2.pdf** (last accessed 15 June 2007)

Hurley, A.C., Volicer, B.J., Hanrahan, P.A., Houde, S. and Volicer, L. (1992) 'Assessment of discomfort in advanced Alzheimer patients'. *Research in Nursing and Health*, 15(5): 369–77

Jacox, A., Carr, D.B., Payne, R., Berde, C.B., Brietbart, W., Cain, J. M. *et al.* (1994) *Management of cancer pain*, Clinical Practice Guideline No 9, AHCPR Publication No. 94-0592. Rockville, MD: Agency for Health Care Policy and Research, US Department of Health and Human Services, Public Health Service

Kovach, P.L., Weissman, D.E., Griffie, J., Matson, S. and Muchka, S. (1999) 'Assessment and treatment of discomfort for people with late-stage dementia'. *Journal of Pain Symptom Management*, 18(6): 412–19

Layman Young, J., Horton, F.M., Davidhizar, R. (2006) 'Nursing attitudes and beliefs in pain assessment and management'. *Journal of Advanced Nursing*, 53(4): 412–21

McCaffery, M. and Robinson, E.S. (2002) 'Your patient is in pain: here's how you respond'. *Nursing*, 23: 327–33

Mayer, D.D., Torma, L., Byock, I. and Norris, K. (2001) 'Speaking the language of pain'. *American Journal of Nursing*, 1001(2): 44–50

Medicines and Healthcare Product Regulatory Agency (2007) *Medicines and medical devices regulations: what you need to know*. London: HMSO

Melzack, R. and Wall, P.D. (2003) *Handbook of pain management: a clinical companion to Wall and Melzack's textbook of pain*. London and Edinburgh: Churchill Livingstone

National Prescribing Centre (2000) 'Prescribing for children'. *MeReC Bulletin*, 11(2): 5–8

NICE (2001) 'TA27 Osteoarthritis and rheumatoid arthritis – cox II inhibitors: guidance'. See: **http://guidance.nice.org.uk/TA27/guidance/pdf/English**

Pasero, C.L. and McCaffery, M. (1997) 'Overcoming obstacles to pain assessment in elders'. *American Journal of Nursing*, 97(2): 15

Rahman, M. (2004) *Cancer pain management: e-learning*. See: **www.cancerpain.org.uk** (last accessed 6 June 2007)

Royal College of Anaesthetists, Royal College of Nursing, Association of Anaesthetists of Great Britain and Ireland, British Pain Society and European Society of Regional Anaesthesia and Pain Therapy (2004) *Good practice in the management of continuous epidural analgesia in the hospital setting*. London and Redditch: joint publication between all authors

Royal College of Paediatrics and Child Health (2001) *Guidelines for good practice – recognition and assessment of acute pain in children*. London: RCPCH Publications

Simons, J. and Roberson, E. (2002) 'Poor communication and knowledge deficits: obstacles to effective management of children's post-operative pain'. *Journal of Advanced Nursing*, 40(1): 78–86

Wall, P.D. and Melzack, R. (2005) *Textbook of Pain*, 5th edn. Edinburgh: Churchill Livingstone

Warden, V., Hurley, A.C. and Volicer, L. (2003) 'Development and psychometric evaluation of the Pain Assessment in Advanced Dementia (PAINAD) Scale'. *Journal of the American Medical Directors Association*, 4(1): 9–15

Wong, D.L. and Baker, C.M. (2001) 'Smiling faces as anchor for pain intensity scales'. *Pain*, 89(2–3): 295–300

World Health Organisation (2007) *Cancer and palliative care pain ladder*. See: **www.who.int/cancer/palliative/painladder/en/** (last accessed July 2007)

Zwakhalen, S., Hamers, J. and Berger. M. (2007) 'Improving the clinical usefulness of a behavioural pain scale for older people with dementia'. *Journal of Advanced Nursing*, 58(3): 493–502

Zwakhalen, S., Hamers, J., Abu-Saad, H. and Berger, M. (2006) *Pain in elderly people with severe dementia: systematic review of behavioural pain assessment tools'*. See: **www.doaj.org/doaj?func=abstract&id=160440&recNo=3&toc=1**

Chapter 5

VENEPUNCTURE AND CANNULATION

Renette Ellson

Throughout this chapter reference will be made to the Nursing and Midwifery Council (NMC) Essential Skills Clusters (ESCs). In addition to the general skills of effective communication and compassionate care, there are several ESC subsections that are relevant to the skills of venepuncture and cannulation. (Refer also to the Skills Clusters identified in Chapter 15 on the administration of medicines.)

Refer also to Chapter 15, page 284.

Patients/clients can trust a newly registered nurse to:

Section 8   Ensure that their consent will be sought prior to care or treatment being given and that their rights will be respected.

Section 20   Select and manage medical devices safely.

Section 22   Maintain effective Standard Infection Control Precautions for every patient/client.

Section 25   Safely apply the principles of asepsis when performing invasive procedures and be competent in aseptic technique.

Section 32   Safely administer fluids when fluids cannot be taken independently.

Introduction

Venepuncture is the introduction of a needle into a vein to obtain a blood sample for haematological, biochemical or bacteriological analysis (Lavery and Ingram, 2005, p.55). Cannulation is where a tube is inserted into a body duct or cavity to provide access to an individual's circulation in order to administer some form of intravenous fluid or medication on a short-term basis (Scales, 2005).

Intravenous venepuncture and cannulation are procedures that are being carried out by more and more nurses. These procedures may cause trauma and discomfort to the patient, and this is even more likely if the person performing them is not very competent. In view of this, Chang *et al.* (2002) highlight that it is extremely important that nurses are well prepared by practising the procedures using simulation before performing them with patients. Both Dougherty (2000) and the Nursing and Midwifery Council (2004a) agree and say that if competence is to be maintained practice needs to be ongoing. Registered nurses who perform these procedures must have undergone intensive training in both theory and practice before they are able to use the skill on their patients. This is especially important when it comes to cannulation as, according to Dougherty (2000, p.61), up to 80 per cent of in-patients receive some form of intravenous therapy. She therefore feels that it is imperative that nurses have an extensive and comprehensive knowledge of all aspects of IV therapy.

Although you are unlikely to perform venepuncture and cannulation as a student, you will be involved in the care of patients who have these procedures performed and the information in this chapter will prepare you for this and for when you eventually do perform this role. For more information on the topics covered in this chapter, it is recommended that you read *Standards for infusion therapy* by the Royal College of Nursing (2003).

The structure of veins

Veins are important blood vessels that generally carry deoxygenated blood back to the heart (the exception is the pulmonary vein). They range from approximately 1 millimetre to 1.5 centimetres in diameter and consist of three layers: the tunica intima, the tunica media and the tunica adventitia (see Figure 1).

Figure 1
The structure of veins

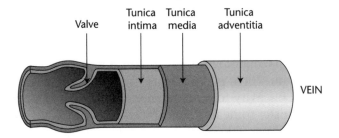

Tunica intima

The tunica intima is a smooth endothelial lining in which the cells create a smooth surface by sitting flat and close together. This minimises friction and clot formation of the blood, which helps to prevent the development of a thrombosis. Valves are also located within the tunica intima and they prevent any backflow of the blood thus ensuring a constant flow of blood to the heart (Scales, 2005).

Tunica media

The tunica media is the middle layer of the vein wall and this is constructed of a small amount of muscle tissue and elastic nerve fibres. The muscle tissue and elastic nerve fibres stimulate the vein to contract and relax during the processes of vasoconstriction and vasodilatation (Dougherty, 1996).

Tunica adventitia

The tunica adventitia is the outer layer of the vein and this is constructed of connective tissue which surrounds and protects the vessel (Dougherty, 1996).

The circulatory system

The circulatory system consists of arteries, arterioles, capillaries, venules and veins. Oxygen and nutrients in the blood are distributed to the tissues via the arteries, arterioles and capillaries. Metabolic waste products, such as carbon dioxide, are then carried away from the tissues by the venules and veins (see Figure 2).

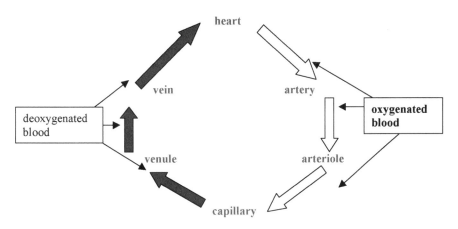

Figure 2
The circulatory system

Figure 3 highlights the general position of the veins within the body and these are coloured blue. The arteries are shown in grey and it is important to note that they quite often run alongside the veins so it is imperative that the nurse performing venepuncture or cannulation is aware of the arterial blood

Figure 3
The main veins and
arteries in the body

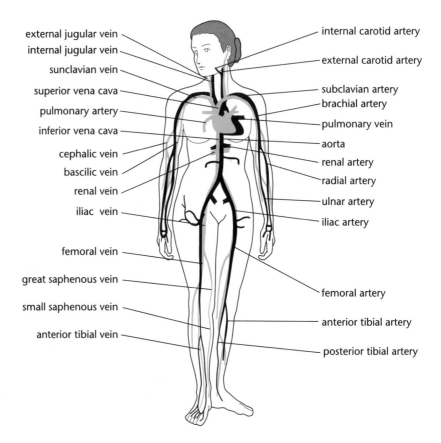

external jugular vein
internal jugular vein
sunclavian vein
superior vena cava
pulmonary artery
inferior vena cava
cephalic vein
bascilic vein
renal vein
iliac vein
femoral vein
great saphenous vein
small saphenous vein
anterior tibial vein

internal carotid artery
external carotid artery
subclavian artery
brachial artery
pulmonary vein
aorta
renal artery
radial artery
ulnar artery
iliac artery
femoral artery
anterior tibial artery
posterior tibial artery

supply and can differentiate between the two systems. This is especially important as some individuals may have an aberrant artery, which is an artery that is located superficially in an unusual place, as opposed to being positioned more deeply, as is usually the case with the arteries.

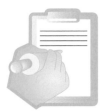

Activity 1.

Research all the major veins as shown in Figure 3 and look for their specific functions, identify their exact location in the body and what they connect to. Make a note of any problems that may arise with each individual vein.

Important considerations when performing venepuncture and cannulation

Ideal vein selection

As Davies (1998), Dougherty (1996) and Black and Hughes (1997) highlight, the superficial veins of the upper extremities of the body are generally used for venepuncture and cannulation because they are located just beneath the skin in the superficial fascia. As a last resort, it may be possible to use a patient's lower limbs. However, as Scales (1996) highlights, there is an increased risk of **thromboembolism** with the use of these veins for cannulation. Figure 4 shows which veins in the arm may be used. However, other issues may need to be taken into consideration and these issues will only be identified upon careful inspection of the patient/client's veins. Choosing a suitable and healthy vein may make the difference between being successful and not. These issues will be discussed later in the chapter.

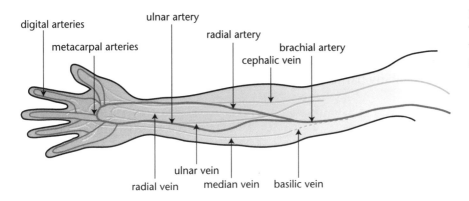

digital arteries
metacarpal arteries
ulnar artery
radial artery
brachial artery
cephalic vein
ulnar vein
radial vein
median vein
basilic vein

Figure 4
The position of the veins and the arteries in the arm

Belonephobia

Belonephobia is a fear of needles. Hamilton (1995) highlights that belonephobia may be an inherited **vasovagal reflex** of shock that is triggered by needle puncture. It may also be a condition that is learned from memory of previous experiences involving the individual themselves or close family members or friends. The physical symptoms of this phobia are vast and may include minor symptoms like sweating or more serious symptoms such as fainting, convulsions or even death. In view of this, it is very important to be aware that some patients may be affected by this condition and it is vital that you know how to deal with it if it happens. Furthermore, if the patient is anxious, this can lead to vasoconstriction and obtaining a sample of blood will therefore become much more difficult.

There are several ways in which to deal with belonephobia and, hopefully, to prevent any of the potential symptoms from occurring. Carlquist (1981), Dougherty (1994) and Sager and Bomar (1980) highlight that technical confidence, minimising pain, diversion, distraction and relaxation techniques and good communication skills all help to reduce the stress associated with this procedure (as cited in Davies, 1998), though some of these methods can be time-consuming. Minimising pain may be achieved by applying a local anaesthetic cream such as Emla. Technical confidence is reiterated by Weinstein (1997) who suggests that with patients suspected of having a needle phobia it is best if the procedure is undertaken by someone who constantly performs the task as this will make the process less traumatic for the patient (as cited by Davies, 1998).

Another important issue to remember is that identified by Inwood (1996), who rightly says that the patient may have had venepuncture and/or cannulation performed on them in the past. It is therefore imperative to involve the patient in the procedure as they may be able to tell you which site has been the easiest previously and whether there have been any particular problems.

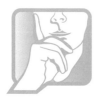

Reflection

Have you ever had blood taken or a cannula inserted into yourself? How did you feel at the time? If you have had this done more than once, was there any difference in how you felt each time and, if so, why?

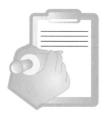

Activity 2.

Think about our scenario patient George. What difficulties might occur when trying to perform venepuncture and cannulation on him? How might you address these issues?

Present injuries, disease or treatment

Always consider the patient as an individual by taking any injuries, disease or treatment into consideration. In some instances, the venous access sites of certain limbs may be inaccessible because of injury, treatment or disease (for example, fractures that have been put into plaster of paris or amputated limbs) or contraindicated for some patients (for example, the affected side of the patient who has had a cerebral vascular accident or a patient's limb that has lymphoedema).

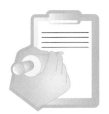

Activity 3.

Research the examples mentioned above and find out why it is important to bear these issues in mind when performing venepuncture or cannulation.

The present medical condition of the patient

The present medical condition of the patient also needs to be considered as this may impede the processes of venepuncture and cannulation. For example, if a patient is suffering from any type of serious shock it is likely that their peripheral venous system will start to 'shut down'. In these instances, the patient is likely to need urgent cannulation in order to treat the cause of whichever shock the patient is suffering from and, ultimately, to prevent any potential fatality. In this case it is especially important that the person attempting the procedure is extremely competent in doing so, as a failure to be successful on the first attempt may result in a severe lack of other suitable veins.

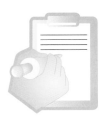

Activity 4.

1. Examples of shock include hypovolaemic shock, cardiogenic shock, septic shock, anaphylactic shock or neuropathic shock. Research all these types of shock for their causes, signs, symptoms and necessary treatment.

2. Think about our scenario patient George. What medical conditions may be present that could impede his vascular access?

Present medications

Being aware of the medications that the patient is presently taking is also useful. Some medications can affect the condition of the veins themselves or they may increase some of the risks that are involved in venepuncture and cannulation. Two particular types of drug therapies that are relevant are steroids and anticoagulants.

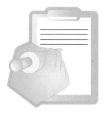

Activity 5.

Research steroids and anticoagulants and find out why they may cause problems with venepuncture and cannulation. When next in clinical practice see if you can identify any patients who are on these types of medication and ask them what problems, if any, they have had when it comes to performing these procedures.

The patient's age and weight

The age and weight of the patient may affect your choice of vein. Young children have short fine veins and the elderly tend to have prominent yet fragile veins. Patients who are malnourished and underweight also tend to have fragile veins and those who are particularly overweight may have veins that are difficult to find because of the extra subcutaneous tissue that they have.

Environmental factors

Environmental factors include ensuring that the patient is warm as this will promote venous dilation. If the patient is cold this will promote vasoconstriction, which will impede the process. Positioning your patient so that the chosen limb is easily accessible and supported is also important. A good source of lighting is imperative as this will assist with the selection of the vein and the actual procedure.

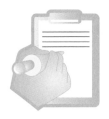

Activity 6.

When next in clinical practice, put a tourniquet around your own arm and look at your own veins; assess and palpate them for suitability.

Venepuncture and cannulation

Equipment required for venepuncture and cannulation

The Medicines and Healthcare Products Regulatory Agency (MHRA) is a government body that was set up in 2003 to bring together the functions of the Medicines Control Agency (MCA) and the Medical Devices Agency (MDA). The Agency's regulatory decisions are impartial and based solely on the extensive evidence of quality, safety and efficacy required for each product. Different products are treated differently but the MHRA considers the particular characteristics, drawbacks and advantages of each one (Medicines and Healthcare Product Regulatory Agency, 2007). These standards ensure that equipment is manufactured to meet a high level of safety. However, in selecting equipment, it is the nurse's responsibility to ensure that the products used are appropriately packaged and undamaged and that they are in date.

Usual equipment for venepuncture (Figure 5)

❑ Personal protective equipment: gloves, disposable apron, eye protection

❑ Clinically clean tray or **receiver**

❑ Tourniquet

❑ **Steret** containing isopropyl alcohol 70 per cent or a swab with chlorhexidine gluconate

❑ 21 g multi-sample monovette needle

❑ Monovette blood sample tubes as directed by blood request form

❑ Gauze swabs

❑ Plasters

❑ Sharps bin

❑ Blood request forms

Figure 5
Usual equipment for
venepuncture

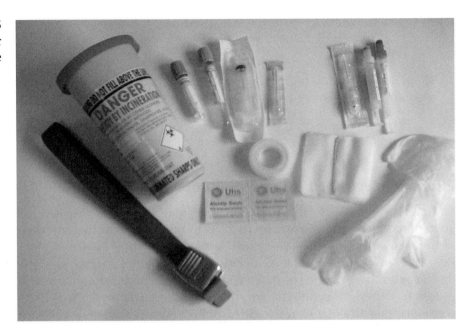

Usual equipment for cannulation (Figure 6)

❑ Personal protective equipment: gloves, disposable apron, eye protection

❑ Clinically clean tray or receiver

❑ Tourniquet

❑ Steret containing isopropyl alcohol 70 per cent or a swab with chlorhexidine gluconate

❑ Intravenous cannula – size according to clinical circumstances

❑ Gauze swabs

❑ Sterile occlusive dressing

❑ 5 ml syringe containing 0.9 per cent sodium chloride flush

❑ Injection cap

❑ Sharps bin

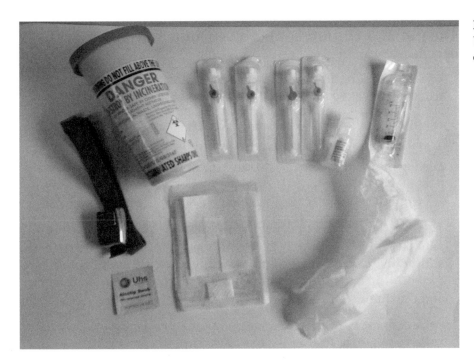

Figure 6
Usual equipment for cannulation

Introduction to the procedure

Although there do not appear to be any universal guidelines on these procedures, many individual Trusts have written their own. It is therefore important that you make sure that you follow the guidelines that your own Trust has implemented, although research shows that many of the Trust guidelines are a variation on a theme and are very similar indeed. Furthermore, many academics have written articles or guidelines for these procedures, and some of these guidelines are very detailed and include rationales for each step in the procedure. It is therefore advised that you read the in-depth descriptions of these procedures to gain a detailed understanding of these important processes.

In view of it being unlikely that you will have the opportunity to perform these procedures as a student, the following guidelines are very concise, but they will give you a brief explanation and demonstration of what is involved. The first parts of both procedures are exactly the same and therefore these will only be covered once.

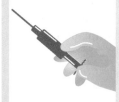

The initial procedure for both venepuncture and cannulation

1. The first important aspect is to gain consent from your patient and this is achieved by following the legal requirements:

   ❑ ensuring capacity;

   ❑ explaining the full procedure calmly and confidently;

   ❑ allowing your patient to ask any questions about the procedure, and about the potential consequences or risks associated with it, before they decide if they wish to consent to the procedure.

   This is the ideal opportunity to discuss any problems with venepuncture which may have arisen previously for the patient and/or to ascertain which veins are likely to be the most appropriate for both the patient (to ensure comfort and promote management) and the nurse (to ensure success).

2. Once consent has been gained, it is important to prepare yourself fully before going back to your patient to perform the procedure. Assemble the necessary equipment (see Figures 5 and 6), ensuring that all the packaging is undamaged and that the equipment is in date. Place all the equipment on a tray or receiver and take the equipment to the patient. Then wash your hands and put your apron on.

3. Ensure that the chosen limb is supported and that there is adequate lighting, ventilation and privacy and that your patient is in a comfortable position.

4. Assess the veins for suitability. In order to do this effectively it is important to improve venous access and this is most often done by applying a tourniquet. However, there are other methods of improving venous access.

   ❑ **Tourniquets** – applying a tourniquet (see Figure 7) helps to impede venous return and therefore promotes venous distension. The tourniquet should not be applied too tightly as this may restrict the arterial blood flow (Dougherty, 1996).

   ❑ **The use of gravity** – lowering the arm below heart level (see Figure 8) will also increase the blood supply to the veins and therefore promote venous distension (Dougherty, 1996).

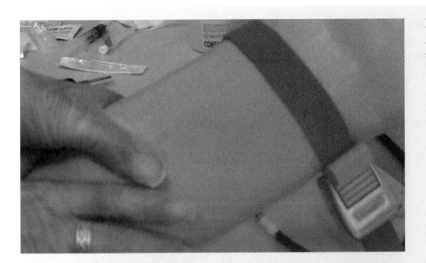

Figure 7
Applying a
tourniquet

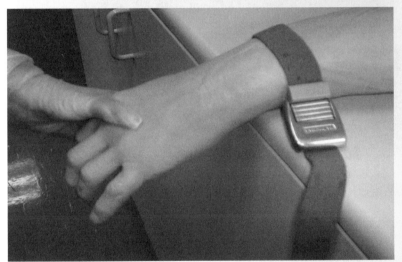

Figure 8
Using gravity to
improve venous
access

❏ **Fist clenching by the patient** – ask the patient to open and close
their fist (see Figure 9) as this helps the muscles to force blood into
veins and promotes venous distension (Dougherty, 1996).

❏ **Stimulating the vein** – light tapping and stroking of the vein (see
Figure 10) may be useful but can be painful and, in some cases,
may cause subsequent bruising (Dougherty, 1996).

❏ **Less frequently used methods** – as Dougherty (1996) highlights,
venospasm may be caused by a change in temperature, mechanical

Figure 9
Fist clenching to
promote venous
distension

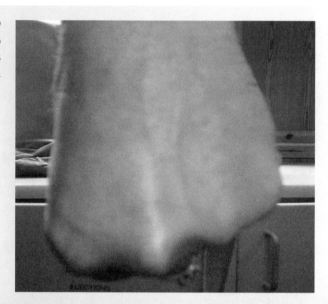

Figure 10
Stimulating the vein

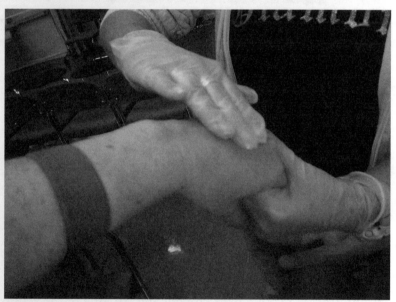

irritation or chemical irritation and this may impede blood flow
and cause pain. The application of heat may prevent these
problems, relieving both spasm and pain. This can be achieved by
immersing the patient's arm in a bowl of warm water for ten

minutes. Other solutions include using a local anaesthetic cream as this will prevent pain when the needle is inserted and will therefore help to reduce any patient anxiety. Some creams also have a mild vasodilatory effect (Scales, 2005). As a last resort, glyceryl trinitrate patches may be applied to facilitate venous dilation.

5. Once venous dilation has been improved it is important to visually inspect and palpate the veins in order to choose the most appropriate vein (see Figure 11). Remember to listen to your patient as they may be able to give you some invaluable advice on which of their veins has been successful in the past. Observe the limbs and ascertain the best site. Certain sites are best avoided:

❑ extensive scars from burns and surgery;

❑ limbs with any oedema;

❑ areas where there is a haematoma, dermatitis or cellulites;

❑ limbs affected following a cerebral vascular attack;

❑ limbs that already have an intravenous therapy/blood transfusion sited or a cannula/fistula/heparin lock.

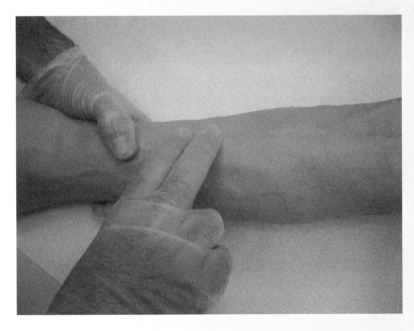

Figure 11
Palpating the vein

Trace the path of veins, try to ascertain their condition and differentiate between the veins and the arteries. It is also important to be aware of the potential risk of inserting the needle at the site of a vein valve as this will compress the lumen of the vein, resulting in a prevention of blood flow through the needle. Should this occur the process must be reattempted elsewhere or above the valve area.

Characteristics of a healthy and suitable vein

❑ Visible
❑ Bouncy
❑ Straight
❑ Well supported.

Characteristics of an unsuitable vein

❑ Fragile
❑ Hard
❑ Thrombosed
❑ Mobile.

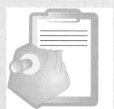

Activity 7.

Research the issues around vein selection. Identify why certain areas should be avoided, what problems are associated with choosing unsuitable veins and what the benefits are of choosing suitable veins. Read the article by Scales (2005) and ascertain why the antecubital fossa is not the ideal position in which to site a cannula for intravenous therapy.

6. Once the ideal vein has been selected, release the tourniquet and either rewash your hands (if your hands are soiled), or apply an alcohol hand rub. When your hands are dry, put on your gloves and protective eyewear. The selected site must then be cleaned. Franklin (1999) studied several pieces of research relating to the need to cleanse the skin site prior to venepuncture and cannulation and what

exactly the site should be cleansed with. She concluded that, although there was some controversy about whether cleansing was necessary or not, the ideal cleanser should be a 70 per cent isopropyl alcohol swab (see Figure 12). More recently, the Royal College of Nursing (2003) has identified that the ideal cleansing agent should be chlorhexidine gluconate. However, both are in agreement that a cursory wipe is not effective and that at least 30 seconds of cleansing is required. Once cleansing has been performed, it is important that the site is not touched by the nurse or the patient as this would make the cleansing process futile and recleansing would need to be performed. The site should also be allowed to dry naturally before any device is inserted, otherwise the cleaning solution may sting the patient and, if you are taking bloods, it may interfere with the results.

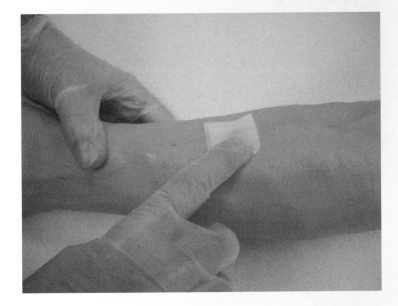

Figure 12
Cleansing the patient's skin

7. Your equipment should then be inspected carefully when out of its packaging, the tourniquet reapplied and the selected vein anchored by your thumb just below the selected insertion site.

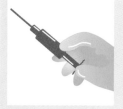

Venepuncture

1. For venepuncture the needle is then inserted smoothly at an angle of approximately 30 degrees. The angle is then reduced slightly as you feel the puncture of the vein wall. If possible, the needle should be advanced into the vein slightly to improve anchorage and prevent the needle tip from coming out of the vein before all the necessary samples have been collected (see Figure 13).

Figure 13
Inserting the needle

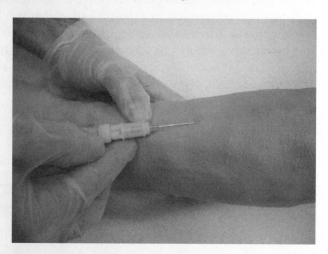

2. Withdraw the required amount of blood using the vacuum collection system (see Figure 14).

Figure 14
Withdraw the required amount of blood

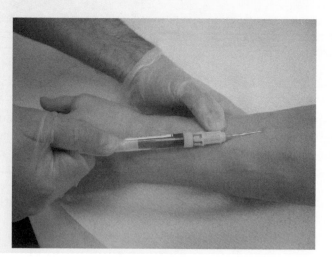

Try to keep the needle in position throughout the procedure, ensuring that no pressure is applied as this may push the needle further into the vein, puncturing the back of it. Disconnect the first sample bottle and attach the next, depending upon which bloods need to be collected. Always be mindful that there is an 'order of draw' that involves using sample bottles without any additives first because the additives in some sample bottles might affect the laboratory analysis. The order of draw is especially important when taking blood for culture (the aerobic culture should be drawn before the anerobic) as the aerobic culture is for bacteria that grow in the air whereas the anerobic is for bacteria that do not grow in the air.

3. When all samples have been collected you then release the tourniquet. Note that the procedure is slightly different if you are collecting certain bloods such as, for example, calcium due to haemostasis. You must ensure that the last vacuum collecting sample bottle has been disconnected before you remove the needle as, otherwise, the bottle will continue to vacuum the blood and there is more likelihood of bruising. Apply a swab and remove the needle, applying pressure to prevent bleeding once the needle has been removed fully (see Figure 15). Continued digital pressure may then be applied by the patient. Applying pressure by bending the elbow is not advocated as this may increase the blood flow and result in bruising. The needle should be discarded appropriately as soon as it is disconnected.

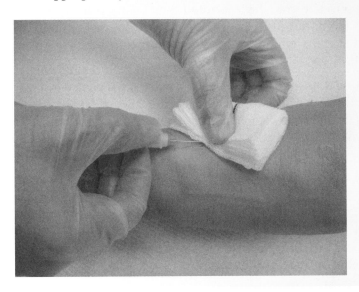

Figure 15
Removing the needle

4. Sample bottles should then be mixed if needed, labelled with the necessary patient details while you are at the side of the patient and then placed in the relevant sample bag with the request form. The patient's puncture site should be checked again for bleeding and, if all is well, a plaster can then be applied to the puncture site, provided of course that the patient is not allergic to plaster. If they are allergic then an alternative dressing may be applied. Throughout the procedure it is important to act calmly and confidently and ensure that your patient is comfortable at all times.

Cannulation

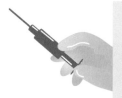

1. Follow the initial procedure for venepuncture and cannulation as described previously. Once the ideal vein has been chosen you need to select the appropriate cannula. Smaller cannulas are advocated as they can reduce potential problems such as pain and chemical and mechanical **phlebitis**, while still providing a sufficiently high flow rate to deliver most therapies (Scales, 2005). Manufacturers colour code their devices with reference to size, but the colours used are not necessarily the same for all manufacturers so it is important to check the information provided on the individual packaging to be sure of using the correct size.

2. Once selected, your device should then be inspected carefully for any faults when out of its packaging, the tourniquet reapplied and the selected vein anchored by your thumb just below the selected insertion site.

3. Inserting the cannula can be done in three ways: (a) you could approach from the top, or (b) approach from the side, or (c) you could tunnel through the tissue before entering a vein that is only partially palpable and visible. However, for the purpose of this chapter we will concentrate on the most common approach of cannulating from the top.

When approaching from the top of the vein you need to insert the cannula, bevel side up, at a 5–15 degree angle (see Figure 16). Keep the vein immobilised with the thumb of your other hand and either insert the cannula carefully and quickly directly into the selected vein, or perforate the skin and then reposition the cannula tip over the vein wall before inserting.

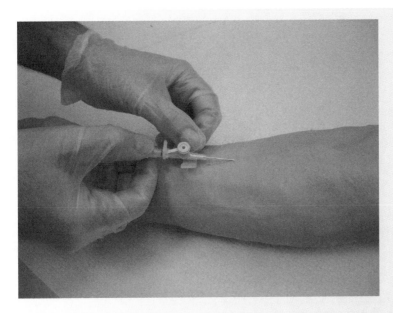

Figure 16
Inserting the cannula

4. As soon as there are any signs of blood in the cannula, the angle of the device must be reduced so that the back of the device is almost touching the skin. Forgetting to do this could result in the cannula going all the way through the back of the vein. If there are no signs of blood then the vein has not been punctured or it is already thrombosed and clotted (Scales, 2005). The cannula is then advanced, the stylet is withdrawn slightly and the chamber at the back of the cannula should then fill with blood. If this fails to happen then the cannula is no longer in the vein (Scales, 2005).

5. The cannula is then fully advanced off the stylet and pushed into the vein. The tourniquet is released and digital pressure is applied to the vein above the cannula tip to prevent blood loss. The stylet is removed and disposed of immediately in the sharps bin (see Figure 17).

6. The device is then capped or attached to an administration set (that has been run through with the prescribed intravenous fluids) and then flushed slowly with 0.9 per cent sodium chloride (see Figure 18). During this process it is important that the nurse checks the site for any signs of swelling or leaking and asks the patient if there is any pain or discomfort while he/she is flushing. If all is well, the wings of the cannula are opened out and the cannula is then secured by a

Figure 17
Removing the stylet

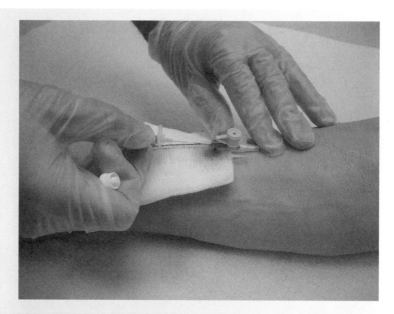

Figure 18
Flushing the
cannula

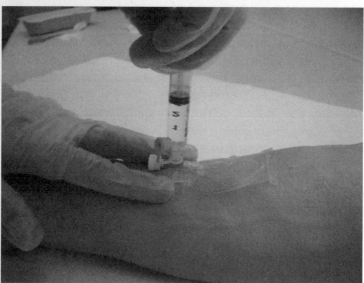

clear occlusive dressing to allow the insertion site to be observed
regularly for any problems (see Figure 19).

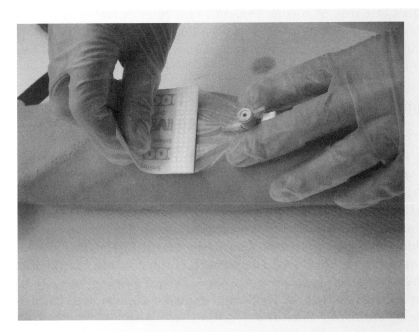

Figure 19
Securing the
cannula

7. All waste material and protective equipment is then disposed of
   appropriately according to health and safety policies.

Documentation

When performing venepuncture or cannulation it is vital that
all information is documented immediately following completion.
Documentation should include:

❏ that the patient's consent was obtained;

❏ the site of venepuncture or cannulation;

❏ the size and type of cannula used;

❏ the type of dressing applied;

❏ factual details of any problems encountered;

❏ the samples taken.

Good record-keeping is a mark of a skilled and safe practitioner (NMC,
2004b). It is important to remember that any record documenting

patient care may be used as evidence by a court of law or as part of an investigation or complaints procedure. For more information on documentation please refer to the *Guidelines for records and record keeping* by the Nursing and Midwifery Council (2004b).

Complications of venepuncture and/or peripheral cannulation

Infection control

See also Chapter 21 on Infection Control

The Department of Health (2006) is firmly committed to reducing health care-associated infection (HCAI). It has produced a number of documents – *Getting ahead of the curve* (Department of Health, 2002b), *Winning ways: working together to reduce health care associated infection in England* (Department of Health, 2003) and *Towards cleaner hospitals and lower rates of infection: a summary of action* (Department of Health, 2004) – as guidance to reduce HCAI. The most recent documents, *Saving lives: a delivery programme to reduce health care associated infection including MRSA* (Department of Health, 2005) and *Essential steps to safe, clean care: reducing health care associated infection* (Department of Health, 2006a), provide guidance on moving toward compliance with these policies, best practice and evidence-based care. Participation in this programme will help demonstrate compliance with the Health Act 2006 *Code of practice for the prevention and control of healthcare associated infections* (Department of Health, 2006b, p.10) (the Code). The Code highlights that specific policies to prevent and control infection must be in place in all NHS Trusts. The specific policies that are particularly relevant to venepuncture and cannulation are:

❑ standard (universal) infection control precautions;

❑ aseptic technique;

❑ safe handling and disposal of sharps;

❑ prevention of occupational exposure to blood-borne viruses (BBVs), including prevention of sharps injuries;

❑ management of occupational exposure to BBVs and post-exposure prophylaxis.

(Department of Health, 2006b, p.7)

According to the Department of Health (2003) and the Royal College of Nursing (2005) over 60 per cent of blood infections are introduced by intravenous devices because micro-organisms on the patient's skin (natural or acquired) enter into the patient's system during the process of insertion. In view of this, local policies on the use of indwelling devices should be followed and adhered to. The use of aseptic technique, observation of universal precautions and product sterility are also advocated (Royal College of Nursing, 2003, p.9). Furthermore, intravenous cannula insertion will only be carried out by trained and competent staff using strict aseptic techniques (Department of Health, 2003)

Wearing gloves

The Department of Health (2001b) advocates the need for gloves during venepuncture and cannulation as the necessary risk assessment highlights that there is the potential for exposure to blood and there could be contact with non-intact skin during these invasive procedures. Gloves must also be discarded after any of the procedures to prevent the transmission of micro-organisms to other sites on that individual or to sites on other patients.

Hand washing

Another important aspect of infection control is hand washing and guidelines for this should be adhered to at all times (see Chapter 21). Indeed, the World Health Organisation (2007), in its *Patient safety solutions* preamble, Volume 1, Solution 9, highlights the need for improved hand hygiene to prevent HCAI and says that proper hand-washing techniques are a fundamental part of ensuring patient safety.

See Chapter 21, pages 455–8.

Tourniquets

Golder *et al.* (2000) have studied the issue of infection being transferred via tourniquets and highlight the need for stringent efforts by the practitioner to prevent this. Tourniquets that are soiled with blood are a potential source of infection and the use of disposable tourniquets has been suggested.

Cannulation and infection control

Should the first attempt at cannulation be unsuccessful then the nurse in question must dispose of the present vascular device and reattempt the procedure with an entirely new device. This is reiterated by the Infusion Nurses' Society and MHRA among others (Royal College of Nursing, 2003). Also, once a device is *in situ* and has been stabilised with the necessary dressing, it is important to visually inspect the site on a regular basis for any signs of infection. Furthermore, should a device migrate externally for whatever reason, it is extremely important that the device is not re-advanced into the patient (Royal of College of Nursing, 2003). This is because the external area of the device may have been exposed to micro-organisms. If the device is then re-advanced, those micro-organisms may be introduced into the patient.

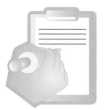

Activity 8.

When next in clinical practice, find your local Trust's policies on venepuncture and cannulation, as well as any policies on the use of indwelling devices, and read them. Observe the practice in your clinical placement. Are the Trust's policies followed and adhered to?

Specific patient infections caused by cannulation

The most common infection is phlebitis and so this is the focus of this section. However, patients may also be affected by bacteraemia and septicaemia, which are very serious conditions. In view of this, it is strongly advised that you research these conditions in order to improve your knowledge.

As Perdue (2001) notes, phlebitis occurs following inflammation of the tunica intima, while Lamb (1999) and Lister (2004) state that the three main types of phlebitis are mechanical, chemical and infective (as cited in Royal College of Nursing, 2003). Mechanical phlebitis is caused by the actual cannula itself being *in situ* and this is why it is important to use the smallest cannula possible. Chemical phlebitis is caused by the fluids or medications that are being infused, so care should be taken when preparing the solutions to ensure that they are at the correct strength and they should also be checked when they are being administered. Infective phlebitis is caused by infection entering the site and therefore strict aseptic techniques should be maintained at all times.

Unfortunately, as Ung *et al.* (2002) have identified, in some instances the reported phlebitis rates for patients receiving intravenous therapy have been as high as 80 per cent (as cited in Davies, 1998). In view of this, it is important to understand the problem and be able to identify the signs and symptoms. Signs of phlebitis include:

❑ redness/erythema to the cannula site;

❑ pain near the site or along the path of the cannula;

❑ swelling;

❑ induration;

❑ a palpable venous cord;

❑ pyrexia.

The Royal College of Nursing (2003) advocate that the treatment for phlebitis should follow the phlebitis scale as produced by Jackson (1998) (cited in RCN, 2003) and this can be found in Appendix 1 of the RCN (2003) document.

As Villani *et al.* (1995) highlight, septic thrombophlebitis is a potentially devastating complication of venous infusion therapy (as cited by Katz *et al.*, 2005). Prevention is therefore imperative and, because of this, the Department of Health (2003) has advocated that insertion sites are checked regularly for any signs of infection and that the cannula is removed immediately if infection is suspected. Furthermore, peripheral intravenous cannulae should be removed at once if they are no longer needed and they must be changed every 72 hours, irrespective of the presence of infection. Administration sets will also have a time limit, with those for a blood transfusion or intravenous feed being changed immediately following completion or at 24 hours (whichever is sooner). Where sets for clear fluids are concerned the change will occur at 72 hours. The dates of any insertions, removals or changes should be documented in the patient's clinical records as a matter of routine. Note that this guidance is from the Department of Health. Other sources have advocated different times for the removal of the cannula. For example, the Royal Infirmary, Lothian University Hospitals NHS Trust's policy advocates reviewing and re-siting each cannula every 48 hours (as cited in Lavery, 2003) and the Centers for Disease Control and Prevention (CDCP (2002) advocate a change of polyurethane cannulae every 96 hours (as cited in Scales, 2005).

Lavery (2003), among others, also advocates that patients need to be involved in the care of their intravenous site. They need to be encouraged to inform nursing staff of any signs of phlebitis, as mentioned previously, and patients should be given advice on not touching the site/cannula, minimising the movement of a limb if a cannula is sited in an area where flexion may occur and also taking extra care when dressing/undressing.

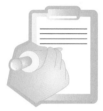

Activity 9.

1. Read the following articles: 'Peripheral intravenous cannulation and patient consent' (Lavery, 2003); 'Vascular access: indications and implications for patient care' (Gabriel *et al.*, 2005); and 'Peripheral intravenous therapy: key risks and implications for practice' (Ingram and Lavery, 2005). Complete the 'Time Out' exercises and answer any questions found in the articles.

2. Think about our scenario patient George. If he complained of slight pain and there was a little bit of redness around his cannula site what, according to the Phlebitis Scale (RCN, 2003, Appendix 1), should you do? Would you do anything different if he complained of pain, swelling and redness around the site?

Needlestick injuries

Nurses who perform venepuncture and/or cannulation are professionally accountable for the safe disposal of the sharps that are used during these procedures. This is also a legal requirement. Should any other individual suffer harm as a result of sharps not being disposed of appropriately a nurse could find themselves in a civil court of law on the grounds of negligence.

Lipley (2001) refers to evidence from the Royal College of Nursing's Exposure Prevention Information Network (EPINet) study involving 14 sites across the UK, which shows that 40 per cent of the staff members injured over a six-month period were nurses and that venepuncture and cannulation were procedures that rated among the highest for risk.

Pearce (2001) is a little more specific, highlighting that 100,000 UK nurses are affected by needlestick and other sharps injuries each year. The major risk associated with these injuries is that the sufferer may become infected from a contaminated needle. A Department of Health study in 2001 found the risk of transmission following a needlestick injury to be one in three for hepatitis B, one in thirty for hepatitis C and one in three hundred for HIV (Moffatt, 2003). In view of these statistics, one can only agree with May and Brewer (2001) when they say that all health care staff performing clinical procedures should constantly observe their Trust's written policies and procedures and observe the relevant government regulations. The EPINet study is ongoing, with more than 40 sites in the UK and Ireland taking part. The study gives up-to-date information on the management of sharps injuries and can be found on the following website: **www.needlestickforum.net.** However, a worrying thought is the fact that several academics have highlighted that it is likely that these statistics are an underestimate of actual injuries by as much as 50 per cent, due to a failure of institutes to report the incidents. What is even more worrying is the fact that all sharps injuries are considered to be potentially preventable (Department of Health, 2001).

The Epic Project (Department of Health, 2001) has made several recommendations in order to help prevent the occurrence of sharps injuries.

❑ Sharps must not be passed directly from hand to hand and handling should be kept to a minimum.

❑ Needles must not be bent or broken prior to use or disposal.

❑ Needles and syringes must not be disassembled by hand prior to disposal.

❑ Needles should not be recapped.

❑ Used sharps must be discarded into a sharps container (conforming to UN 3291 and BS 7320 standards) at the point of use. These must not be filled above the mark indicating that they are full. Containers in public areas must not be placed on the floor and should be located in a safe position.

❑ Consider the use of needlestick-prevention devices where there are clear indications that they will provide safe systems of working for health care practitioners.

❑ Conduct a rigorous evaluation of needlestick-prevention devices to determine their effectiveness, acceptability to practitioners, impact on patient care and cost-benefit prior to widespread introduction.

Where the issue of needlestick-prevention devices is concerned, the World Health Organisation firmly backs this idea up saying that new injection technologies and needle-less systems should be considered (WHO, 2007, Volume 1, Solution 8). For more information on needlestick-prevention devices please see Health Devices (2000).

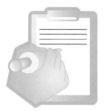

Activity 10.

Research the issues of hepatitis B, hepatitis C and HIV and identify the potential consequences for a nurse who has contracting these diseases. Take a look at the Department of Health document (2002) *Getting ahead of the curve: a strategy for combating infectious diseases (including other aspects of health protection)* for in-depth information of the statistics and prevalence of these and other diseases. As May and Brewer (2001) highlight, there are many ways in which the health care professional can minimise the risk of sharps injuries. Find and read their article 'Sharps injury: prevention and management', and work through the 'Time Out' boxes and multi-choice self-assessment found in the article.

Extravasation and infiltration

'Extravasation is defined as the inadvertent administration of vesicant medication or solution into the surrounding tissue instead of into the intended vascular pathway' (Royal College of Nursing, 1998; Oncology Nursing Society, 2000; Intravenous Nurses Society, 2000; Perdue, 2001; Stanley, 2002 – all as cited by the Royal College of Nursing, 2003). When this happens the infusion infiltrates the surrounding tissue. Several academics, including Davies (1998), Intravenous Nurses Society (INS) (2000) and the RCN (2003), state that the first symptoms of both infiltration and extravasation include swelling/oedema around the infusion site, blanching of the skin, coolness of the skin, leakage around the cannula and/or pain. Treatment should be initiated at once, the infusion should be discontinued and, if the therapy is still required, then the cannula should be re-sited on another extremity (INS, 2000, as cited by RCN, 2003) or proximal to the inflamed site to prevent the therapy being infused through damaged veins (Scales, 2005).

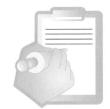

Activity 11.

1. Find the RCN's (2003) document *Standards for infusion therapy* and look at Appendix 2. What are the clinical criteria for grade 4 infiltration?

2. Think about our scenario patient George. If he complained of pain around his cannula site and there was oedema, his skin was cool to touch and his skin was blanched, what grade of infiltration would he have?

Adequate nursing knowledge of intravenous therapy

Every year over 15 million infusions are carried out in the NHS (National Patient Safety Agency, 2004a, p.1). In view of this, as Hand (2001) rightly notes, 'Nurses have a professional and legal responsibility to understand the rationale for the use of prescribed fluids. Safe administration requires an understanding of the role of electrolytes and water and of the mechanisms of movement between different body compartments' (p.47). Some of these issues are covered in Chapter 10 on Nutritional support, hydration and fluid balance (page 216). However, you are advised to research this issue in more depth and Hand's article (2001), 'The use of intravenous therapy', is a very good place to start.

See Chapter 10, page 216.

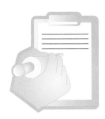

Activity 12.

1. Read the article by Hand (2001) and then answer the multiple-choice self-assessment at the end of the article.

2. Consider our scenario patient George. Bearing in mind that he may be **hypovolaemic** on admission due to his perforated duodenal ulcer and that he will require surgery in order to repair this perforation, what type of intravenous fluids is he likely to need?

Problems with infusion devices

The MHRA receives over 700 reports of problems with infusion devices every year and, on average, 19 per cent of these are due to mistakes by those using the devices (National Patient Safety Agency, 2004a, p.1). The mistakes include administering fluids/medicines too quickly or too slowly and administering fluids/medicines via an incorrect route, all of which could lead to some harm to, or even the death of, the patient.

Using the wrong route quite often happens when a patient has several infusion lines at once and they are connected to the wrong site. In order to prevent this the Department of Health (2003, p.13) advocates that 'the number of lines, lumens and stopcocks will be kept to the absolute minimum consistent with clinical need'. Indeed, the World Health Organisation (2007), in their *Patient safety solutions* preamble, Volume 1, Solution 7, has highlighted that misconnections of catheters and tubing should be avoided at all times, especially since one consequence of misconnections is that the patient may receive their medication through the wrong route and this could result in serious injury or death. Suggested actions include the following.

❑ Only clinical staff should connect or disconnect any devices.

❑ Labels are used to identify differing lines.

❑ Attachments are verified by staff at all times.

❑ Communication between shifts is improved.

❑ All new equipment is risk assessed.

❑ Hazard training is given to all staff.

❑ Equipment should be purchased that helps to improve the safety aspects for the patient.

Incorrect patient identification

Between November 2003 and July 2005 the UK National Patient Safety Agency reported 236 incidents and near misses related to missing wristbands or wristbands with incorrect information (World Health Organisation, 2007). The World Health Organisation (2007) has also said that a failure to identify the correct patient could result in numerous errors. Where venepuncture and cannulation are concerned, one of the main issues is that the results of a blood test could be attributed to the wrong patient and, therefore, subsequent treatment may be incorrect. This is especially serious when it comes to transfusing blood because if the wrong blood group is being administered to a patient then this may result in serious anaphylactic shock or even death. Another possible error resulting from incorrect patient identification is that the wrong infusion may be administered to a patient. In view of these facts it is extremely important that patients are clearly identified at all times, ideally through the use of two identifiers. Also, sample bottles should be labelled in the presence of the patient to avoid any potential confusion.

Summary

It can be seen from the information given in this chapter that venepuncture and cannulation procedures carry several risks to the patient. In view of this, informed consent is an absolute must and, in the event of any harm occurring to a patient following these procedures, it is imperative that this is documented and a patient safety incident report is completed to document the incident (National Patient Safety Agency, 2004b).

Given that there are so many complications that may arise from these procedures, especially peripheral intravenous cannulation, one has to agree with Davies (1998) that it is paramount that nurses performing these procedures are competent to do so. Furthermore, the importance of nurses having an in-depth knowledge and understanding of these procedures cannot be overemphasised, and this includes students who are not going to be performing the actual procedures. In view of this, it is strongly advised that further reading around the subject is carried out, especially as this chapter has really only touched the tip of the iceberg. There is a vast array of invaluable research available that has not been included in the chapter.

Further reading

Department of Health (1995) *Hospital infection control*, Health Service Guidance HSG (95) 10. London: DoH

Ingram, P. and Lavery, I. (2005) 'Peripheral intravenous therapy: key risks and implications for practice'. *Nursing Standard*, 19(46): 55–64

National Patient Safety Agency (2005) *Wristbands for hospital inpatients improve safety*, Safer Practice Notice 11. See: **www.npsa.nhs.uk/site/media/documents/1440_Safer_Patient_Identification_SPN.pdf**

References

Black, F. and Hughes, J. (1997) 'Venepuncture'. *Nursing Standard*, 11(41): 49–53

Chang, K.K., Chung, J.W. and Wong, T.K. (2002) 'Learning intravenous cannulation: a comparison of the conventional method and the CathSim Intravenous Training System'. *Journal of Clinical Nursing*, 11(1): 73–8

Davies, S.R. (1998) 'The role of nurses in intravenous cannulation'. *Nursing Standard*, 12(17): 43–6

Department of Health (2001) *The Epic Project: developing national evidence-based guidelines for preventing health care associated infections.* London: DoH

Department of Health (2002) *Getting ahead of the curve: a strategy for combating infectious diseases (including other aspects of health protection).* London: DoH

Department of Health (2003) *Winning ways: working together to reduce health-care associated infection in England.* London: DoH

Department of Health (2004) *Towards cleaner hospitals and lower rates of infection: a summary of action.* London: DoH

Department of Health (2005) *Saving lives: a delivery programme to reduce health care associated infection (HCAI) including MRSA.* London: DoH

Department of Health (2006a) *Essential steps to safe, clean care: reducing health-care associated infection.* London: DoH

Department of Health (2006b) *Code of practice for the prevention and control of health-care associated infections.* London: DoH

Dougherty, L. (1996) 'Intravenous cannulation'. *Nursing Standard*, 11(2): 47–54

Dougherty, L. (2000) 'Changing tack on therapy'. *Nursing Standard*, 14(30): 61

Franklin, L. (1999) 'Skin cleansing and infection control in peripheral venepuncture and cannulation'. *Nursing Standard*, 14(4): 49–50

Gabriel, J., Bravery, K., Dougherty, L., Kayley, J., Malster, M. and Scales, K. (2005) 'Vascular access: indications and implications for patient care'. *Nursing Standard*, 19(26): 45–52

Golder, M., Chan, C.L.H., O'Shea, S., Corbett, K., Chrystie, I.L. and French, G. (2000) 'Potential risk of cross-infection during peripheral-venous access by contamination of Tourniquets'. See: **www.gbo.com/documents/Potential_risk_of_crossinfection.pdf** (last accessed 6 July 2007)

Hamilton, J.G. (1995) 'Needle phobia: a neglected diagnosis'. *Journal of Family Practice*, 41(2): 169–76

Hand, H. (2001) 'The use of intravenous therapy'. *Nursing Standard*, 15(43): 47–55

Health Devices (2000) *Needlestick-prevention device selection guide – special report.* Plymouth Meeting, PA: ECRI

Hyde, L. (2002) 'Legal and professional aspects of intravenous therapy'. *Nursing Standard*, 16(26): 39–42

Inwood, S. (1996) 'Designing a nurse training programme for venepuncture'. *Nursing Standard*, 10(21): 40–2

Katz, S.C., Pachter, H.L., Cushman, J.G., Roccaforte, J.D., Aggarwal, S., Yee, H.T. and Nalbandian, M.M. (2005) 'Superficial septic thrombophlebitis'. *Journal of Trauma (Injury, Infection and Critical Care)*, 59(3): 750–3

Lamb, J. (1993) 'Guidelines on intravenous therapy'. *Nursing Standard*, 9(30): 32–5

Lavery, I. (2003) 'Peripheral intravenous cannulation and patient consent'. *Nursing Standard*, 17(28): 40–2

Lavery, I. and Ingram, P. (2005) 'Venepuncture: best practice'. *Nursing Standard*, 19(49): 55–65

Lipley, N. (2001) 'Incidence of sharps injury "unacceptable", says RCN'. *Nursing Standard*, 15(35): 7

May, D. and Brewer, S. (2001) 'Sharps injury: prevention and management'. *Nursing Standard*, 15(32): 24–54

Medicines and Healthcare Product Regulatory Agency (2007) *Medicines and medical devices regulations: what you need to know*. London: HMSO

Moffatt, L. (2003) *House of Commons Hansard Debate*. See: **www.publications. parliament.uk/pa/cm200203/cmhansrd/vo030226/debtext/30226-05.htm** (last accessed 6 July 2007)

Murray, W. and Glenister, H. (2001) 'How to use medical devices safely'. *Nursing Times*, 97(43): 36–8

National Patient Safety Agency (2004a) *Summary*, Safer Practice Notice. London: Department of Health

National Patient Safety Agency (2004b) *Seven steps to patient safety*. London: DoH

Nursing and Midwifery Council (2004a) *Code of professional conduct*. London: NMC

Nursing and Midwifery Council (2004b) *Guidelines for records and record keeping*. London: NMC. See: **www.nmc-uk.org/aDisplayDocument.aspx?DocumentID=223**

Nursing and Midwifery Council (2006) *A to Z on record keeping*. See: **www.nmc-uk.org/aDisplayDocument.aspx?DocumentID=1587**

Pearce, L. (2001) 'Silent epidemic'. *Nursing Standard*, 15(35): 16–17

Royal College of Nursing (2003) *Standards for infusion therapy*. London: RCN

Royal College of Nursing (2005) *Good practice in infection prevention and control: guidance for nursing staff*. London: RCN

Scales, K. (1996) 'Legal and professional aspects of intravenous therapy'. *Nursing Standard*, 11(3): 41–8

Scales, K. (1997) 'Practical and professional aspects of IV therapy'. *Professional Nurse*, 12(8, Suppl.): 53–5

Scales, K. (2005) 'Vascular access: a guide to peripheral venous cannulation'. *Nursing Standard*, 19(49): 48–53

Ung, L., Cook, S., Edwards, B., Hocking, L., Osmond, F. and Buttergieg, H. (2002) 'Peripheral intravenous cannulation in nursing: performance predictors'. *Journal of Infusion Nursing*, 25(3): 189–95

World Health Organisation (2007b) *Patient Safety Solutions*. Geneva: World Health Organisation

Part

2 PERSONAL CARE

This part includes the following chapters:

6   Personal hygiene
7   Catheterisation (male and female)
8   Bowel care, suppositories and enemata
9   Skin integrity assessment and pressure area care

Scenario: Abdullah Akhtar

Mr Abdullah Akhtar is a 50-year-old man who has been admitted to an acute medical ward from accident and emergency, having suffered a stroke. On admission to the ward, Mr Akhtar is unconscious and has a marked right-sided weakness. Though he is able to maintain his own airway, he is currently dependent on nursing staff to meet his complete care needs.

Mr Akhtar is married to Shamina Akhtar and they have three children. He works as an accountant for a local Primary Care Trust. He smokes twenty cigarettes per day but drinks no alcohol.

Activity 1.

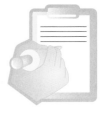

1.   When undertaking Mr Akhtar's admission to the ward, what information is required by the nurse in order to plan his complete care needs? Consider these four main areas within your assessment:

   – social needs;

   – psychological needs;

   – physical needs;

   – spiritual needs.

2.   Consider the following questions in relation to Mr Akhtar's needs.

– What information is required?

– From whom should this information be obtained?

– Why is this information important?

Information about Mr Akhtar

Previous medical history

- ❑ Insulin-dependent diabetes mellitus (IDDM) since 1972
- ❑ Hypertension (high blood pressure)
- ❑ Hypercholesterolaemia (high levels of cholesterol in the blood)

Observations on admission

- ❑ Blood pressure: 170/110
- ❑ Pulse: 101
- ❑ Respiration rate: 14 / min (laboured)
- ❑ Oxygen saturations (SaO_2): 88% on air
- ❑ Weight: 108 kg
- ❑ Height: 1.6 m
- ❑ Blood sugar: 15.5 mmol/l
- ❑ Glasgow coma scale: 10/11
- ❑ Right-sided flaccidity

Drug history

- ❑ Atenolol 100 mg daily
- ❑ Bendrofluazide 2.5 mg daily
- ❑ Simvastatin 20 mg at night

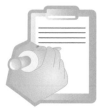

Activity 2.

Look at the above information in relation to Mr Akhtar and identify four risk factors he has for stroke.

Chapter 6

PERSONAL HYGIENE

Lizi Hickson

The Nursing and Midwifery Council has set standards to measure your performance. The Essential Skills Clusters covered in this chapter include Sections 1, 3, 4, 5, 22, 26 and, specifically, **Section 2**:

Patients/clients can trust a newly registered nurse to:

i. Actively involve the patient/client in their assessment and care planning.
ii. Determine patient/client preferences to maximise comfort and dignity.
iii. Actively encourage patient/client to be involved in and/or ensure they are supported in own care/self care.
iv. Support a patient/client to identify their goals.
v. Assess a patient's/client's level of capability for self care.
vi. Provide care (or make provision) for those who are unable to maintain own personal care (e.g. mouth care, elimination, bathing, care of skin, cleaning teeth, hair washing, cleaning eyes and cleaning and cutting nails).

Introduction

Personal cleansing and dressing is one of the activities of daily living. From early on in life, we all perform this activity according to our own preferences and, usually, in private. During illness, however, our patients are sometimes unable to wash and dress themselves, and may feel extremely embarrassed about it, especially if a nurse has to do it for them. This chapter will guide you through some of the methods we use to assist our patients with their hygiene needs while maintaining their individuality and dignity. While reading this chapter and caring for your patients in placement, try and imagine yourself in their position and consider how you would wish to be treated in similar circumstances.

Scenario review

After Mr Akhtar's admission to the ward his hygiene plan was structured and designed to meet his individual needs. It is important to remember that personal hygiene enhances a patient's physical and emotional well-being. Mr Akhtar has become dependent on the nursing staff and such a sudden reduction in independence and liberty can result in a loss of self-esteem. By enabling Mr Akhtar to feel fresh and clean and to look his best, you can boost his morale. However, prior to any contact with Mr Akhtar it is imperative that you take some important factors into consideration. These factors are moral and ethical issues and hygiene.

Moral and ethical issues

First of all, is Mr Akhtar fully aware of the procedure he is to take part in and can he consent? For example, if you are a female nurse, can you ask Mr Akhtar if it would be appropriate to undress him or if he would prefer you to ask a male nurse to attend to him? As Mr Akhtar has right-sided weakness it can be assumed that he has suffered a left-sided stroke. This is an abnormal condition of the brain characterised by occlusion by an embolus, thrombus or cerebrovascular haemorrhage, resulting in **ischaemia** of the brain tissue that would normally be perfused by the damaged vessels. The result of the damage can be the absence of or difficulty in speech because the speech domain is found in the inferior frontal gyrus and the loss of speech is a characteristic of a left-sided bleed. Therefore, Mr Akhtar may be fully aware of conversation but be unable to convey his wishes and feelings. As a result, in order to assist with his wishes, it may be appropriate to involve his family. They will be able to offer advice, and they may feel it befitting that a male nurse attends or assists Mr Akhtar. It is professional and crucial that such ethical issues are considered prior to beginning the procedure.

Once Mr Akhtar is fully aware of what is about to be done, you must involve him in the procedure by talking to him, even if he is unable to respond. A patient with limited speech can still make themselves understood by means of facial expression and body language, and you need to observe Mr Akhtar carefully when explaining your actions to make sure he understands and consents. Having and demonstrating patient empathy goes a long way to developing patient trust.

Hygiene

See Chapter 21, page 454.

The second factor to consider is your own hygiene. It is vital to remember that micro-organisms are carried on hair, skin and clothes, and that cross-contamination between patients can be limited if a nurse takes responsibility for his or her own hygiene behaviour (see also Chapter 21).

Modes of infection transmission

Modes of infection transmission include:

❏ airborne particles carrying bacteria;

❏ direct contact;

❑ indirect contact via:

- – clothing;
- – communal sharing;
- – inadequate cleaning;
- – transferring host, usually inadequate hand washing.

Reflection

❑ What infection control strategy is implemented in your local hospital?

❑ Should only appointed staff be responsible for infection control?

❑ What documentation would be appropriate to confirm that the standard of hygiene has been achieved?

❑ Who should oversee this?

Preparation for a bed bath

Having made the appropriate provision for Mr Akhtar to have his bed bath in terms of gaining his consent and arranging for appropriate staff, it is then essential to gather all the necessary equipment and allow reasonable time to deliver the service. Making proper preparation will stop any delay during the bed bath and will limit the time that Mr Akhtar is undressed. If this is the first time Mr Akhtar has had a bed bath he will be anxious and feel vulnerable. You need to be conscious of this, show kindness and sympathy and be gentle. Actions such as talking over the patient to a colleague will increase patient trepidation and this must be avoided. Remember to maintain Mr Akhtar's dignity at all times and never allow this to be compromised. If his first bed bath is an experience that Mr Akhtar can reflect back on without any concerns then he will view it as a positive experience that can be repeated without anxiety.

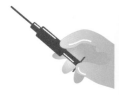

Bed bath

Gather together all equipment that is to be used. If there is a ward checklist of the necessary requirements then use this to make sure you have collected the right equipment. Also consider the environment in which the bed bath is to take place. Close curtains and windows to eliminate draughts and choose a good time of day – visiting time or ward rounds is not an appropriate time for giving a bed bath. Raising the bed will eliminate any need for over-reaching or stretching. Remember infection control procedures and make sure that you and your colleagues wash your hands and wear protective aprons to cover your uniforms before you start the bed bath. The equipment that you will need is as follows.

❑ Towels – use the patient's own if available. Patients feel more comfortable using their own personal belongings and the smell of a familiar conditioner can add to feelings of comfort.

❑ Separate wash cloths for face, torso and genital regions.

❑ Soap and toiletries. If these are from the ward check that the patient is not allergic to these products. Check with the patient's notes to determine beliefs and cultural practices. Some soap is unacceptable to vegans and vegetarians because they may contain animal products.

❑ Light sheets to cover the patient as you bathe them.

❑ The water should be delivered just prior to beginning. Use warm water at approximately 40°C. This water should be replaced as it cools or gets dirty. The same water should not be used for the facial area and genitals.

Reflection

❑ How did you feel before undertaking your first bed bath?

❑ How did you feel afterwards?

❑ Would you do anything differently, and why?

❑ Did you feel you were adequately prepared and supported?

❑ Did you make your patient aware this was your first bed bath? If so, why did you do so?

Washing the patient

1. During the bed bath encourage the patient to be as independent as possible. Mr Akhtar may be able to assist by using his non-affected side. Encourage him to wash his own face as this not only allows him to be part of the procedure, but also enhances his motor skills and his own sense of independence. Continue to be soothing and supportive throughout. Use the whole process to communicate with your patient, answer his questions and develop a therapeutic relationship.

2. When assisting or washing a patient, wash the face first. Do not use soap unless the patient has directed you to do so. Work away from the mid-line and avoid getting water into the eyes by asking the patient to tilt their face towards the pillow. Putting a towel under the face will catch any water. Wash in a gentle action up to the hairline and dry as you go using a soft face towel. Take care not to allow water to get into the ears.

3. If your patient is male, make sure that he is given the opportunity to shave, using either shaving soap and a razor or an electric shaver. If your patient is unable to shave himself, you must do it for him. A clean shaven man may feel extremely uncomfortable with stubble, and may give his relatives the impression that he is not being cared for even if that is not the case.

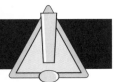

'Communal' electric razors were once common in hospital wards. Do not use a communal razor on your patients, as this is a way of spreading infection.

4. Once the face is clean begin on the torso. Start with the arm furthest away from you (to avoid dripping dirty water on areas that have already been cleaned) and soap it. Rinse the arm and then dry it thoroughly. Then do the same with the chest and abdomen, followed by the arm closest to you. Uncover only the area you are washing, and take care to wash thoroughly under the arms (axilla) and in any skin folds.

5. Once the upper torso is dry gently turn the patient onto their side and, with a colleague supporting the patient, wash the back and buttocks. This is a perfect opportunity to check for any developing pressure ulcers or reddening of the skin. If these are present then this should be

documented and action taken if necessary. If the patient has provided skin conditioner rub this in prior to repeating the action on the opposite side.

6. Change the water prior to washing the genitals. If possible, encourage the patient to assist with this most sensitive area. Then dry thoroughly and cover with the sheet as soon as possible.

7. After washing the genitals, change the water again and move down the body to the legs. While you are washing the feet, observe their colour and feel their temperature. Report and document any changes or delayed capillary refill.

8. Dress the patient in their own night attire if they have it. If they do not have their own night clothes, use a hospital nightdress or pyjamas, but take care to choose the right size. Wearing clothes that are too tight or too big diminishes the patient's own individuality and dignity.

Reflection

What have you learnt from this procedure? List key learning points and reflect on any previous experience of giving a bed bath. How might your practice change in future?

Hair care

It is important that a patient's hair is kept clean because dirty hair can feel extremely uncomfortable, especially if you are confined to bed. During the bed bath, the nurse is in a position to determine if the hair requires washing. Washing a patient's hair in bed can be very difficult, as their confinement, disability or loss of movement can create problems with water containment.

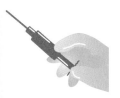

Washing a patient's hair

1. Absorbent towels and waterproof sheets must be placed around the patient's head. Another nurse must take control of the patient's head so that the patient does not feel insecure. This nurse can then communicate and keep eye contact with the patient.

2. Remove the head of the bed and store it safely. Placing a basin on the floor below the patient's head, keep the shoulders and head at the edge of the bed. Use jugs of warm water to wet the hair and then gently massage the shampoo into the hair. As with bed bathing, you need to consider which hair care products you are going to use before you start to wash the patient's hair to ensure they are suitable and the patient is not allergic to them.

3. After shampooing, rinse the hair thoroughly and dry. Try to comb or brush the hair into the style the patient normally prefers. Hair should be brushed from roots to tips, and care should be taken not to irritate the patient's scalp.

4. If at all possible, wash a patient's hair in a shower, at a wash-basin or during an immersion bath as this will be much easier.

5. Long-term patients may require their hair to be cut. Never be tempted to do this yourself. It is not within the remit of any nurse, and may be deemed as a form of assault. Instead, with your patient's permission, find out if there is a hair-dressing service in the hospital.

Nail care

Fingernails and toenails are made from a tough protein called keratin. The free part of the nail that grows beyond the nail plate has no nerve endings. Nails grow at approximately 0.1 mm each day. Nails in middle age begin to discolour, thin or thicken depending on health and physiological imbalances.

Nail care is important to ensure that bacteria do not enter the nail bed and cause infection. It is helpful to soak nails for five minutes to loosen dirt and germs and soften them prior to cutting. If nails are allowed to grow they can dry out and patients may be tempted to bite their finger nails. Biting nails can result in the transportation of germs that are buried in the surface of the nail into the mouth. Biting can also result in abnormal wearing of tooth enamel.

The cutting of a patient's nails must be undertaken by a professional manicurist or podiatrist using sterile equipment. This prevents infection being transferred to patient groups. However, it is the responsibility of the nurse to identify when a patient's nails need cutting. This should then be documented and appropriate action taken.

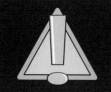

Cutting the toenails of diabetic patients like Mr Akhtar is extremely hazardous and should not be done by a nurse. This is because the circulation to the feet may be impaired in patients with diabetes. Therefore, if the skin is inadvertently nicked and an infection sets in, it may develop into gangrene and ultimately lead to amputation.

Oral care

The care of the mouth is very important. The mouth allows us to take in food and is also the way we verbally communicate and show emotion through smiling or grimacing. When we have a bad taste in our mouths we clean our teeth but this simple comfort measure is one that bed-bound patients do not have access to. It is therefore the responsibility of the nurse to meet this need. Oxygen therapy and many drugs cause the mouth to dry, and this can lead to infections such as oral thrush and ulceration. Oral care is part of the personal care that the nurse must routinely offer the patient.

The best way to remove decay-causing plaque is by brushing and cleaning between the teeth every day. Plaque produces substances that irritate the gums, making them red and tender or causing them to bleed easily. In time, gums may pull away from the teeth and pockets will form and fill with bacteria. If the gums are left untreated the bone around the teeth can be destroyed, and the teeth will become loose and may have to be removed. Periodontal disease is the main cause of tooth loss in adults.

Assisting with oral hygiene

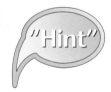

1. Use a soft-bristled brush. The size of the brush should fit easily into the patient's mouth. Remember that Mr Akhtar has weakness and this may mean his face has less muscle tone on his affected side.

2. Support the patient's head and place a bowl under their chin. Place an absorbent towel under the bowl.

3. Put toothpaste onto the brush and place the brush at a 45° angle against the gum.

4. Move the brush back and forth in short strokes.

5. Brush the outer, inner and chewing surfaces of the teeth.

6. Gently brush the tongue to remove bacteria and freshen breath.

7. Look out for blood stains on the toothbrush, and for any signs that the patient is experiencing discomfort.

8. Assist the patient to rinse their mouth, and hold a towel against their chin while they are doing so.

Hint

Find a willing volunteer such as a member of your family or a colleague and, using a clean toothbrush, practise cleaning their teeth. It is not as easy as it seems!

Dentures

9. Removing the upper plate. Hold the inner and outer surface on both sides of the plate. Insert forefingers over the upper edge of the palate and press until the seal breaks between the dentures and the gums. Pull the plate forward to remove.

10. Removing the lower plate. Hold the inner and outer surface with the thumb and forefinger. Turn slightly and pull the denture up and out.

11. Cleaning dentures. Put a towel in a basin half-filled with warm water. Using a tooth brush and denture paste, clean carefully and rinse well.

12. Inserting dentures. Wet dentures with cool water. Apply even, gentle pressure on both sides of the upper palate and gently place into position. Insert lower dentures last.

13. Report ill-fitting dentures, as these may cause ulceration within the oral cavity.

14. Food trapped between the plate and gums can be extremely uncomfortable and may lead to ulceration.

Immersion bath

As Mr Akhtar's condition improves he will become well enough to be assisted in an immersion or 'proper' bath. The feeling of lying in warm water is a form of relaxation therapy and, even with assistance, patients should be encouraged to have a bath as soon as they are able.

Assisting with an immersion bath

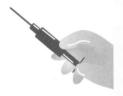

1. As with the bed bath, Mr Akhtar will need to be informed about the procedure and the intervention that may be required, and his consent must be sought.

2. Prepare the bath. The water temperature should not exceed 38°C. Mr Akhtar should be escorted to the bathroom and offered assistance to undress.

See Chapter 11, pages 244–52.

3. Mr Akhtar should test the water himself to confirm the temperature. This helps to give the patient a sense of control. The nurse will help to position him into the bath. A hoist or seating aid may be needed and staff and the patient should have a full understanding of the use of this equipment prior to undressing (see Chapter 11).

4. Mr Akhtar should be encouraged to wash himself with soap and any help should be given as required. His dignity can be retained by using small wash cloths to cover the genital region.

5. Help with back washing and hair care can be offered, particularly with patients with limb deficits.

6. Once Mr Akhtar is bathed, towels should be placed around him while he steps from the bath onto a non-slip mat (or while he is hoisted out).

7. Full assistance should be given with drying while he is seated in a chair and toiletries, such as deodorant or talcum powder, should be offered. Remember that if a patient feels clean and smells nice, this will help to boost their self-esteem and aid their recovery.

8. A full immersion bath allows the body to be exposed to the water, thus allowing all parts to be cleansed more thoroughly and should, therefore, be offered in preference to a bed bath if at all possible.

9. Some patients may prefer a shower to a bath, either for personal or cultural reasons. Such preferences should always be taken into account and noted on the patient's care plan.

Bed making

When Mr Akhtar is out of bed it is important to clean and remake his bed ready for his return.

Bed making

1. Put on a protective apron over your uniform.

2. Bring a linen-skip to the bedside, in preparation for bed stripping.

3. Remove all linen. Soiled linen should be placed in a red linen bag and labelled accordingly.

4. Wash the bed with detergent and rinse. Dry off and allow to fully dry. This need not be done on a daily basis, but should be a priority if the bed frame or mattress becomes soiled. The whole bed should be cleaned thoroughly between patients. This will not necessarily be the nurse's job (check your local policy), but it will be the nurse's responsibility to make sure it is done.

5. Change your apron and wash your hands. Disposable aprons should be changed after each bed is made to avoid cross-contamination.

6. Organise clean sheets, a duvet, pillow cases and a draw sheet.

7. Put the clean bottom sheet on the bed and put the centre fold of the bottom sheet in the middle of the mattress.

8. If the bottom sheet is fitted, fix the corners of the sheet on the side of the mattress nearest to you. Walk round to the other side of the bed and fix the other two corners.

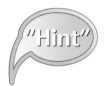

9. If the bottom sheet is not fitted, lift the top two corners and hold them away from the mattress (see Figures 1 and 2). Do not flap the sheet as this encourages the movement of air particles. Place the sheet under the mattress and tuck in the corners.

Figure 1
Arranging the bottom sheet

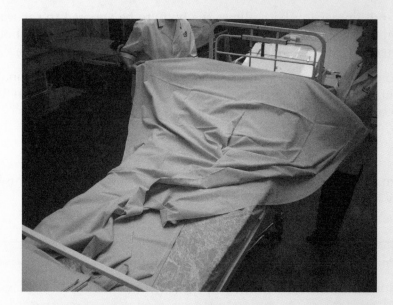

Figure 2
Mitred corners (on bottom sheet)

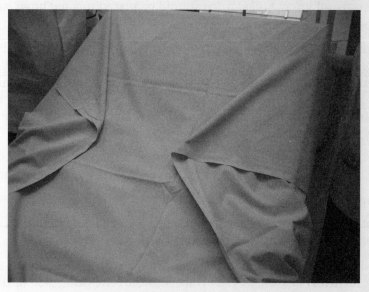

10. Place the bottom of the sheet under the mattress. It is important to avoid excess folds of sheet as this will be uncomfortable for the patient and will encourage bed sores. Create tension and tuck in the corners. (See Figures 3 and 4.)

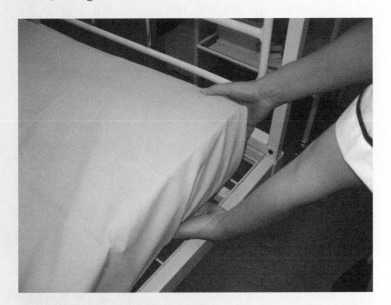

Figure 3
Tucking in the
'hospital corners'

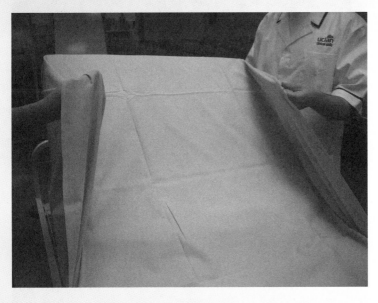

Figure 4
Repeat the
procedure at the
foot of the bed

11. Put the top sheet with the centre fold along the middle of the bed. Line up the top part of the sheet with the top part of the mattress. Then put the bedspread or duvet over the top sheet with the centre fold along the middle of the bed. Mitre the corners of the top sheet and the bed spread at the foot of the mattress. Pull the top linens up at the end of the bed to make a pleat (see Figure 5). This allows room for the patient's feet to move. It may also help to avoid skin sores or foot drop.

Figure 5
Pleating the top
sheet at the foot of
the bed

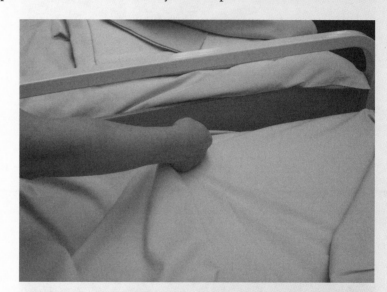

Figure 6
Arranging the
blanket and
counterpane (1)

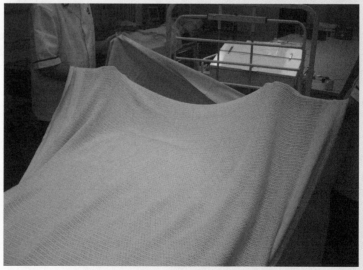

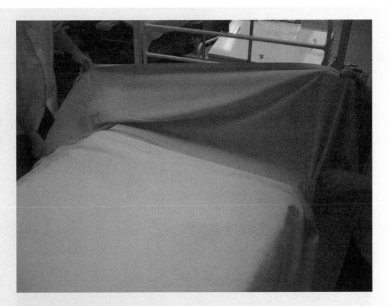

Figure 7
Arranging the
blanket and
counterpane (2)

12. Put on fresh pillow cases and place the pillows against the back rest
(see Figure 8).

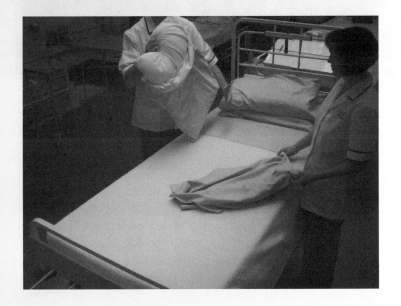

Figure 8
Putting on fresh
pillow cases

13. After changing the bed, remove the bed locks, place the bed in its original position and lower the bed to allow patient to enter safely. The newly made bed is shown in Figure 9.

Figure 9
A newly made bed

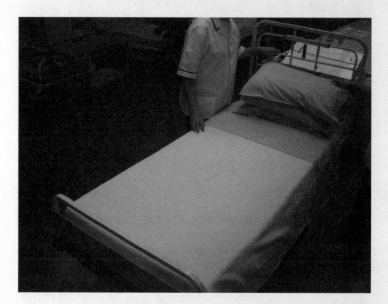

14. It is important to check on the condition of the linen on your patient's beds throughout the day. This is to keep them tidy and/or to replace soiled linen.

15. Prior to the improvement in Mr Akhtar's condition that enabled him to get out of bed, the bed had to be changed while he was still on it. The most appropriate time to do this is after his bed bath, so that any damp sheets can be removed and replaced with clean, dry ones.

16. The procedure is to roll the patient on to his side and feed the soiled linen out from under him using the natural curves of the body. You then roll the patient back onto clean sheets and tuck them in correctly using the three-point envelope technique. This technique helps to prevent the movement of the bedding when the patient moves about in bed. (For more details on moving and handling bed-bound patients, see Chapter 11).

See Chapter 11, page 235.

17. Make sure you check your local ward policies and procedures in relation to assistance with personal hygiene.

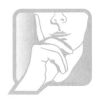

Reflection

After you have washed Mr Akhtar and changed his bed, address the following questions regarding the tasks.

❑ What would you do differently the second time you cared for this patient?

❑ What factors would influence your decision?

❑ Would any physical changes in you or your patient alter your plan of care?

❑ What is your conclusion on the methods used?

❑ Did you follow all safety regulations and provide good patient care?

❑ What would you propose for improvement of the recommended procedures?

Summary

Mr Akhtar has the right to help plan his nursing care. In order for him to do this, you must, if possible, communicate with him in order to assess his hygiene needs and reach agreement with him (or his family) on how the nursing staff will assist him. You must learn about the patient's illness, injury and treatment options as this will assist you in the care planning process. It is important for you to work with the patient and their family, keeping them involved and fully up to date with issues and concerns. Try to create a two-way communication and respond to your patient's changing needs in order to maintain a bond of trust.

Key points

❑ It is a vital part of the nurse's role to assist patients with their hygiene needs. These individual needs should be assessed on admission and reviewed at regular intervals.

❑ A high standard of personal hygiene is necessary to minimise the risk of infections, but also to enhance the comfort and self-esteem of your patients.

❑ Independence should be encouraged, and assistance given only when required.

❏ Washing is usually a very private process, so be aware of this when providing assistance. Be discrete and maintain your patient's dignity at all times.

❏ The daily washing routine is a good opportunity to talk to your patients and to build up an effective therapeutic relationship. Do not underestimate the value and importance of talking to your patients.

Chapter 7

CATHETERISATION (MALE AND FEMALE)

Robin Richardson

The Nursing and Midwifery Council has set standards to measure your performance. The Essential Skills Clusters covered in this chapter include Sections 1, 3, 4, 5, 22, 26 and, specifically, **Section 2**:

Patients/clients can trust a newly registered nurse to:

i. Actively involve the patient/client in their assessment and care planning.
ii. Determine patient/client preferences to maximise comfort and dignity.
iii. Actively encourage patient/client to be involved in, and/or ensure they are supported in own care/self care.
iv. Support a patient/client to identify their goals.
v. Assess a patient's/client's level of capability for self care.
vi. Provide care (or make provision) for those who are unable to maintain own personal care (e.g. mouth care, elimination, bathing, care of skin, cleaning teeth, hair washing, cleaning eyes and cleaning and cutting nails).

Introduction

Following his stroke, you notice that Mr Akhtar is not passing urine. Palpation of his lower abdomen reveals a distended bladder, which is then confirmed by an abdominal ultrasound scan. Commonly, most people who suffer strokes actually become incontinent of urine. This is due to the following factors.

❏ physiological factors:

   – an inability to communicate needs effectively, due to **dysphasia** and/or **dysarthria**;

   – short-term memory loss;

   – loss of mobility;

❏ neurological factors:

   – disruption to the parasympathetic branch of the autonomic nervous system through:

   i damage to the **micturition** centres (in the frontal lobe and brain stem);

ii an inability to inhibit bladder contraction, despite being aware of the need to void (a condition known as **detrusor hyperreflexia**);

❑ medicinal factors:

– muscle relaxants – sometimes prescribed in stroke patients to counteract muscular spasticity;

– antihypertensives – can cause night-time incontinence (nocturnal enuresis);

– diuretics – often prescribed to combat immobility-induced oedema.

Current research into the treatment of post-stroke incontinence has shown that many patients regain the ability to control their bladders within eight weeks and that this happens spontaneously (Nzarko, 2007). Therefore, the catheterisation of stroke patients should be avoided in all but the most exceptional of cases.

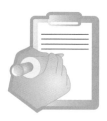

Activity 1.

Why do you think urinary catheterisation should be avoided if at all possible? Try and think of three reasons.

Mr Akhtar, however, is in urinary retention. This is due to a condition known as **detrusor sphincter dyssynergia**. In this condition, when the detrusor muscle of the bladder contracts (in order to empty the bladder), the urethral sphincter does not relax. This can either cause incomplete bladder emptying or acute retention of urine, as in the case of Mr Akhtar. The doctor requests that Mr Akhtar is catheterised with an indwelling Foley catheter. Helen, a second-year student nurse, is asked to set up a catheterisation trolley in preparation for the procedure.

What is urinary catheterisation?

Urinary catheterisation involves the insertion of a narrow tube into the urethra, which is then passed up into the urinary bladder. An indwelling catheter has a balloon at the end that is inflated in order to anchor the catheter in the bladder (see Figure 1). An intermittent catheter does not have a balloon, as it is only required for very short-term use. Reasons for catheterisation include:

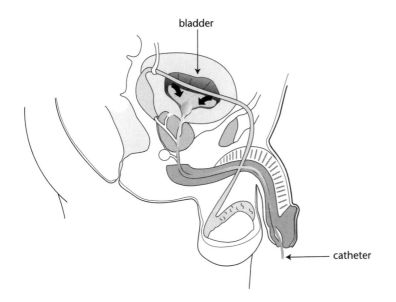

bladder

catheter

Figure 1
A catheter *in situ* in
the male bladder

❑ the retention of urine (acute or chronic);

❑ the administration of certain drugs;

❑ prior to and following certain types of surgical operation such as, for example, abdominal surgery, certain gynaecological procedures and any surgery that necessitates keeping a very close eye on urine output in the post-operative period;

❑ for bladder irrigation following urological procedures.

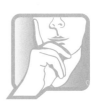

Reflection

Consider how you would feel if you had to have an indwelling urinary catheter inserted.

❑ Who would you want to perform the procedure?

❑ Where would you want the procedure to take place?

❑ What information would you require from your nurse prior to the procedure?

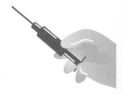

Male catheterisation

Equipment required

❑ A stainless steel trolley that has been cleaned according to local hospital/Trust policy.

❑ A catheter pack that contains:

– a **sterile field**;

– equipment required to clean the penis (disposable forceps, **gallipot**, cotton wool/sponge cubes/gauze swabs);

– a receptacle in which to contain the sterile catheter and for urine to drain into initially.

❑ Cleansing solution – this will vary according to Trust policy, but chlorhexidine solution or normal saline is adequate. Some Trusts advocate the use of plain soap and water for washing the genitals.

❑ A Foley catheter of an appropriate size and length should be selected. The external diameter of a urinary catheter is measured in Charriere units (Ch), with one Charriere being equivalent to 0.33 mm. Therefore, a 12 Ch catheter has an external diameter of slightly less than 4 mm. Generally speaking, the smallest diameter catheter that will do the job should be selected, as this will reduce trauma to the urethra. Catheter sizes 12 and 14 Ch should be adequate to drain clear urine. If the urine is cloudy or contains sediment, a larger size (16–18 Ch) may be required.

When catheterising an adult male, a longer length catheter must be selected as men have a longer urethra than women. An adult female catheter is 250 mm in length, while an adult male catheter is 450 mm in length. The type of catheter selected will also depend on how long it will be required for and whether or not the patient is allergic to latex. Figures 2 and 3 illustrate some of the more common types of urinary catheter you may experience in the clinical area.

❑ Local anaesthetic lubricating gel. This tends to be supplied in pre-filled syringes containing between 6 and 15 ml of gel. This will both lubricate the urethra and dull any sensation.

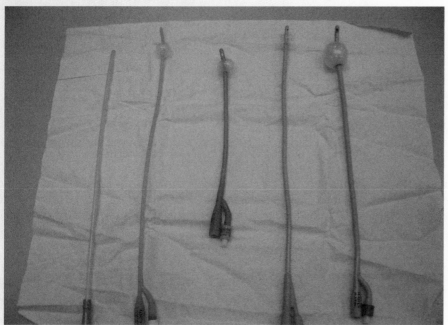

Figure 2
Types of catheter (with balloons inflated where appropriate).

From left to right:
- ❏ Intermittent catheter
- ❏ Silicone foley (16 Ch)
- ❏ Silicone coated foley (12 Ch)
- ❏ Silastic foley (18 Ch)
- ❏ Teflon coated latex foley (female) (16 Ch)

❏ Water for injection (10 ml). This is to fill the catheter's retaining balloon. The balloon should not be filled with air, as it will cause the balloon to float in the bladder. Normal saline should not be used as it may crystallise and tap water should not be used as it is not sterile. Note that some specialist catheters require the balloon to be inflated with more than 10 ml water – see catheter packaging for details.

❏ 10 ml syringe to draw up the water for injection.

❏ Drainage bag. This will be connected to the catheter following successful insertion.

Procedure for male catheterisation

1. The patient should have the procedure explained to him carefully, and you must make sure that he understands. This will enable you to gain informed consent prior to performing the catheterisation.

Figure 3
Types of catheter

Catheter type	Length of use	Comments
Latex catheter (Teflon coated)	Up to four weeks	Not to be used in patients with latex allergies. Teflon coating reduces trauma on insertion, and helps reduce encrustation.
Latex catheter (Hydrogel coated)	Up to 12 weeks	Not to be used in patients with latex allergies. Hydrogel coating allows the longer-term use of this type of indwelling catheter.
Silicone catheter (Hydrogel coated)	Up to 12 weeks	Suitable for those with latex allergies. Rigidity may cause discomfort.
Silicone	Up to 12 weeks	Suitable for those with latex allergies. Wide lumen provides better drainage.
Latex catheter (coated with silicone elastomer, aka Silastic)	Up to 12 weeks	Not to be used in patients with latex allergies. Can help reduce encrustation.
PVC (polyvinyl chloride)	Up to seven days	Rigidity may cause discomfort. Inflexible. May be used without a balloon for intermittent self-catheterisation.

When selecting the most appropriate catheter for your patient, it it important to consider:
❏ Is your patient allergic to latex?
❏ How long will this catheter be required for?
❏ What is the most appropriate size?

Remember:
❏ A large diameter will provide better drainage.
❏ A small diameter will cause less irritation to the urethral wall.

2. Ideally, the procedure should be carried out in a private treatment room if one is available and it is large enough to accommodate a bed. If this facility is not available, you should ensure that privacy is maintained and that the patient is not unduly exposed.

3. The patient should be made comfortable, in a supine position, with his legs extended.

4. Put on a disposable apron.

5. Wash your hands using bactericidal solution, using an effective hand-washing technique (see Chapter 21, page 455).

See Chapter 21, page 455.

6. Take your trolley to the patient's bedside and prepare your equipment, opening any supplementary packs and dispensing any required solutions using an aseptic technique. The catheter should be removed from its outer wrapper, but not from its inner wrapper. A trolley set up for catheterisation is shown in Figure 4.

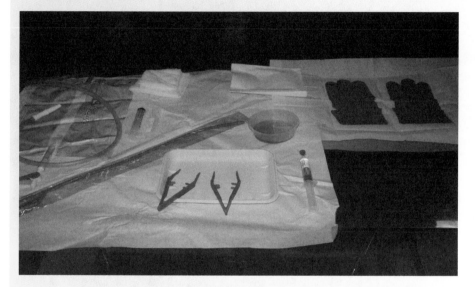

Figure 4
A catheterisation trolley

7. Before cleaning the penis, place an absorbent pad between the patent's legs to protect the bedclothes. Put on a pair of gloves, take hold of the penis with your non-dominant hand and retract the foreskin (if present). With your dominant hand, clean the glans penis carefully (see Figure 5).

8. Take the syringe of lubricating anaesthetic gel and insert the nozzle into the urethral opening. Gently inject the gel into the urethra until the syringe is empty (see Figure 6). Discard the syringe and use your non-dominant hand to prevent the gel escaping from the penis. The gel should be given about five minutes to take effect.

9. At this point, discard the gloves you are using and re-wash your hands. Put on a pair of sterile gloves. Take your sterile field from your

Figure 5
Cleaning the penis
prior to
catheterisation

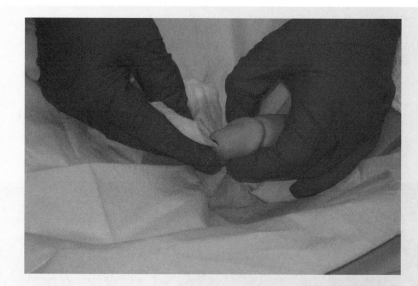

Figure 6
Administering the
lubricating
anaesthetic gel

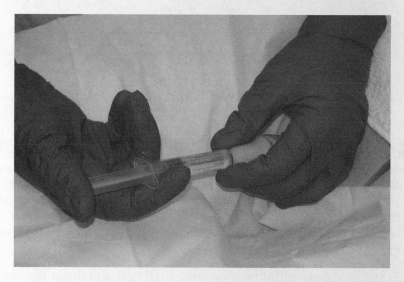

trolley, fold it twice and tear a hole at the folded corner. This will provide you with a hole through which to position the penis. Tear off the end of the inner wrapper enclosing the catheter, using the serrated edge. Place the catheter in the sterile receiver and bring it across to your sterile field. Hold the penis with your non-dominant hand and hold the catheter by the inner wrapper with your dominant hand. This ensures that the catheter itself is not touched (see Figure 7). Insert the catheter into the urethra, gradually withdrawing the inner wrapper, until urine flows into the receiver.

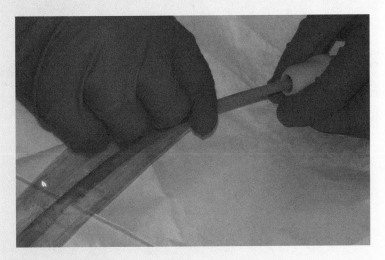

Figure 7
Inserting the
catheter

10. When you see urine flowing, insert the catheter further, almost to the bifurcation. This will ensure that the balloon portion of the catheter tip is inside the bladder.

11. Take your syringe of water for injection (amount dependant on manufacturer's instructions) and inject into the balloon port. This will inflate the balloon inside the bladder (see Figure 8).

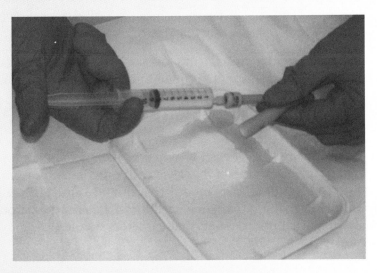

Figure 8
Inflating the
balloon

Figure 9
Connecting the
drainage bag

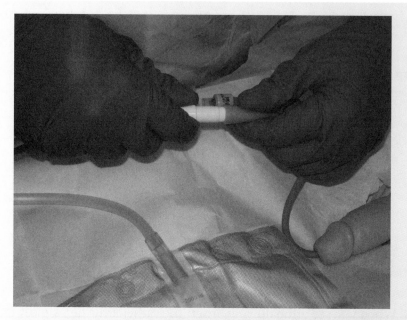

12. Once the balloon is inflated, gently withdraw the catheter until resistance is felt. This means that the balloon is correctly positioned in the neck of the bladder. Then connect the drainage bag to the outlet port of the catheter (see Figure 9).

13. Post-catheterisation:

    – position the catheter and drainage bag in a comfortable and secure position;

    – if you have retracted the patient's foreskin, make sure you replace it – failure to do this may result in a phimosis (swelling of the foreskin);

    – send a specimen of urine for microscopy and culture.

The above procedure will relieve Mr Akhtar of the discomfort caused by urinary retention. The catheter, however, will only remain *in situ* for a short time. The National Institute for Health and Clinical Excellence (NICE) stipulates that any patient's need for catheterisation should be reviewed at regular intervals, and that catheters should be removed as soon as possible (NICE, 2003).

Female catheterisation

The procedure for female catheterisation employs the same principles and procedures as for a male catheterisation, though there are some differences.

❑ The urethral meatus can sometimes be difficult to identify (see Figure 10.) If you are having problems locating the urethra and inadvertently insert the catheter into the vagina, leave it there and use a new catheter. This will prevent the same thing happening twice. Following successful catheterisation, the first catheter should, of course, be removed.

❑ Use a female-length catheter when catheterising women. This is due to the shorter length of the urethra compared with that of men. However, if your patient is obese, you may find that a male-length catheter is more comfortable for her.

❑ You will find that anaesthetic gel is not always used prior to female catheterisation and that sterile KY jelly is used instead. It is acceptable, however, to use anaesthetic gel, though 6 ml should be sufficient for the shorter urethra.

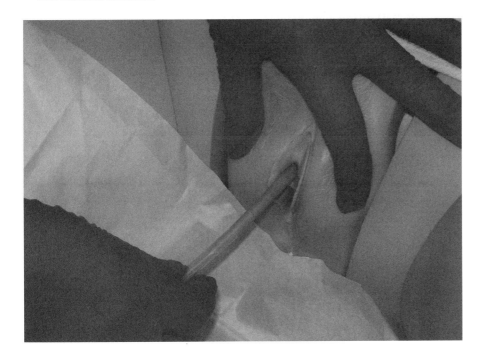

Figure 10
Inserting a urinary catheter into a female patient

Reflection

Many Trust policies around urinary catheterisation state that only male nurses may catheterise men and only female nurses may catheterise women. This does not, however, apply to doctors. What do you think about such policies in relation to:

❑ maintaining the dignity of patients?

❑ hierarchies that exist within health care settings?

Catheter care

With catheterised patients, it is vital to maintain a high standard of their personal hygiene in order to prevent urinary tract infections that, at the very least, would prolong their hospital admission. It is generally accepted that the cleansing of catheters should be carried out as part of the patient's daily washing routine.

❑ Female patients:

– The vulval area should be cleaned, using a disposable cloth, in a downward motion, using clean, warm soapy water.

– The catheter itself should be cleaned with a separate cloth, wiping in one direction, away from the patient.

– Ensure that the vulval area is dried thoroughly.

❑ Male patients:

– The foreskin (if present) should be retracted and the glans can then be cleaned using a disposable cloth and clean, warm, soapy water.

– The catheter can then be wiped with a clean disposable cloth in one direction, away from the patient.

– Ensure that the penis is dried thoroughly.

Removal of urinary catheters

Before removing any urinary catheter, ensure that the patient is passing faeces normally. This is because of the possibility of a distended colon or rectum putting pressure on the urethra and impeding the flow of urine during micturition.

Make sure you explain the procedure of catheter removal to your patient and obtain their consent to proceed. Some patients may be extremely anxious about having their catheter removed. These anxieties may be related to:

❑ fear of the pain associated with a recurrence of previous urine retention;

❑ fear of incontinence following catheter removal;

❑ fear of discomfort during the actual procedure.

When Mr Akhtar's catheter is removed, he may be concerned that he will not be able to pass urine. Reassurance should be given to the contrary, emphasising that a close eye will be kept on his bladder function. He will also require information regarding the possibility of becoming incontinent of urine due to his recent stroke. It may be useful to refer him to the local continence specialist nurse who will help Mr Akhtar to regain his bladder control. Before this can happen, however, Mr Akhtar's catheter needs to be removed, using the following procedure.

Urinary catheter removal

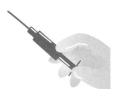

Equipment required

❑ Receiver

❑ Syringe (size dependent on amount of water in catheter balloon)

❑ Gloves and apron

❑ Specimen pot (if a urinary tract infection is suspected)

Procedure

1. Explain the procedure to the patient and obtain verbal consent.

2. Ensure that the patient is lying on the bed in a supine position. Place an absorbent pad under the buttocks and place the receiver between the legs.

3. Wash and dry hands using an appropriate technique.

4. Put on the apron and gloves.

5. Having checked how much water should be in the balloon, connect the syringe to the balloon port and withdraw the water from the balloon.

6. While reassuring your patient, pull out the catheter and place in the receiver.

Following the procedure:

❑ Make sure your patient is comfortable and has access to a nurse call bell in case assistance is required to the toilet.

❑ Encourage your patient to increase their oral fluid intake (if they are able to drink), or get the doctor to review their intravenous fluid regime.

❑ If a urinary tract infection (UTI) is suspected, send the catheter tip for microscopy and culture.

❑ Dispose of equipment appropriately.

Summary

❑ The decision to catheterise should not be taken lightly, and should be taken in consultation with the wider multidisciplinary team, based on clinical need.

❑ Urinary catheterisation is an undignified and embarrassing procedure. Bear this in mind when communicating with your patient during the process.

❑ The potential for the introduction of micro-organisms into the bladder during this procedure is high. Therefore a strict aseptic technique must be adhered to.

❑ Patients should be monitored post-procedure for early signs of urinary tract infection. Care should also be taken to keep the catheter clean.

References

National Institute for Clinical Excellence (2003) *Infection Control (No. 1) Standard Principles.* London, NICE

Nzarko, L. (2007) 'Continence problems following stroke'. *Nursing and Residential Care*, 9(4): 152–9

Chapter 8

BOWEL CARE, SUPPOSITORIES AND ENEMATA

Robin Richardson

The Nursing and Midwifery Council has set standards to measure your performance. The Essential Skills Clusters covered in this chapter include Sections 1, 3, 4, 5, 22, 26 and, specifically, **Section 2**:

Patients/clients can trust a newly registered nurse to:

i. Actively involve the patient/client in their assessment and care planning.
ii. Determine patient/client preferences to maximise comfort and dignity.
iii. Actively encourage patient/client to be involved in and/or ensure they are supported in own care/self care.
iv. Support a patient/client to identify their goals.
v. Assess a patient's/client's level of capability for self care.
vi. Provide care (or make provision) for those who are unable to maintain own personal care (e.g. mouth care, elimination, bathing, care of skin, cleaning teeth, hair washing, cleaning eyes and cleaning and cutting nails).

Introduction

As Mr Akhtar has had a stroke his mobility is drastically reduced. Initially he will be on bed rest but, even as his condition improves, his mobility will be impaired. This immobility can lead to several complications that may impede his recovery. These complications are as follows.

Chest infection

Lying down or sitting for long periods can decrease lung expansion during respirations and may lead to a chest infection. Patients should be encouraged to breathe deeply and to cough. They should also be referred to a physiotherapist.

Muscle wasting

Patients on prolonged bed rest are not working their muscles, particularly those in the lower limbs. This can, over a long period, lead to muscle wasting. To avoid this, patients should be encouraged to exercise in bed or while sitting. If they cannot do this for themselves, they will benefit from passive limb exercises, i.e. you move their limbs for them. A physiotherapist will be able to advise you about this.

Breakdown of skin integrity

See Chapter 9, page 195.

Pressure on the skin due to long periods of sitting or lying in the same position can cause the development of pressure ulcers (these used to be known as bedsores). If your patient cannot change their position unassisted, then you must help them. See Chapter 9 for further details.

Constipation

Normal daily exercise helps to stimulate peristalsis in the gastro-intestinal system. This natural gut mobility is what helps us to 'move our bowels', or pass faeces. If our mobility is reduced, for whatever reason, we are more likely to become constipated. Constipation, though initially a minor inconvenience, can, if left untreated, lead to much more serious complications such as intestinal obstruction.

See Chapter 10, page 223.

Mr Akhtar does have reduced mobility following his stroke. He is not able to eat and drink normally, due to the absence of a gag reflex. Having been referred to the hospital dieticians, Mr Akhtar is receiving nutrition and fluid via a nasogastric (NG) tube. (See Chapter 10 for more details on NG tubes.)

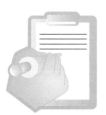

Activity 1.

1. Why might Mr Akhtar become constipated following his stroke?

2. How would you know if he was constipated?

3. What might you do to:

   – treat his constipation?

   – prevent it recurring?

Monitoring bowel function

The monitoring of bowel function in our patients is an extremely important part of a nurse's role. Constipation can become a serious complication in a patient's recovery and should not be underestimated. You must ask your patients the question, 'Have you had your bowels opened today'? While this may be embarrassing for the novice student nurse, it will soon become second nature. However, don't forget that such a question is also likely to be embarrassing for your patient, so it is, perhaps, not a good idea to bellow the question across the ward for all to hear. Be discreet!

If you are assisting someone in the toilet, have a good look at the faeces they have passed and make a note of:

❑ the amount they have passed;

❑ the consistency (is the stool hard, soft or diarrhoea?);

❑ colour: pale stools may indicate a problem in the billiary tract; very dark stools may indicate the presence of **occult blood**; any fresh blood may indicate haemorrhoids (piles) or bleeding in the intestines, and should be reported immediately.

Reflection

❑ If you were a patient in hospital, how would you feel about a nurse asking you about your bowel habits?

❑ As a nurse, how could you make this subject less embarrassing for your patients?

Promoting good, regular bowel habits in our patients

Promoting good and regular bowel habits in our patients will include:

❑ encouraging a good oral fluid intake of 2–3 litres per day;

❑ promoting a diet that is high in fibre;

❑ being aware of any constipating medications the patient might be taking, particularly opiate analgesia (such as: co-dydramol, dihydrocodeine and codeine phosphate);

❑ promoting regular exercise;

❑ use of oral aperients (laxatives) when constipation is noted, such as Lactulose or Sennakot.

Scenario review

It has been noted that Mr Akhtar has not passed faeces for several days and the doctor has prescribed two glycerol suppositories per rectum. The sister in charge of the ward has asked Helen, the student nurse, to administer them under the supervision of her mentor. How should this procedure be carried out?

Administration of suppositories

Suppositories are small 'torpedo'-shaped devices used to deliver a measured amount of a drug into the rectum where it may be absorbed. An example of a typical suppository can be seen in Figure 1. As you can see, the suppository has a tapered end and a blunt end.

Figure 1
A suppository

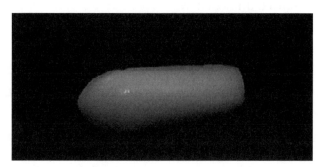

Suppositories may be used to deliver many types of systemic drugs, such as:

❏ antibiotics (e.g. metronidazole);

❏ anti-convulsive medication (e.g. carbemazepine);

❏ anti-inflammatory medication (e.g. diclofenac, aspirin);

❏ analgesics (e.g. paracetamol).

They can also be used to deliver topical preparations to the rectum, such as haemorrhoid preparations. They are also commonly used in hospitals to remedy constipation, as in the case of Mr Akhtar. Glycerol, when dissolved in the rectum, acts as a stimulant to the rectal wall, causing peristaltic waves and the passing of impacted faeces.

Suppository administration

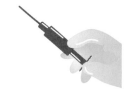

Before administering the suppositories, the patient should have the procedure explained to him and his verbal consent should be obtained.

Collect the necessary equipment:

❑ suppositories, as prescribed;

❑ prescription chart;

❑ receiver or disposable tray;

❑ lubricating gel;

❑ tissues.

Procedure

1. Wash and dry your hands. Put on a disposable apron and gloves.

2. Make sure you attend to the patient's dignity during this very undignified procedure. Do not expose the patient more than is required.

3. Position your patient on his left side, with his knees brought up toward his chest. This position is necessary due to the anatomical position of the rectum. Therefore, if you are a left-handed nurse, you will have to get used to administering suppositories with your non-dominant hand.

4. Remove packaging from around the suppository (see Figure 2) and cover the suppository with lubricant.

5. Using your left hand, part the patient's buttocks, exposing the anus. Warn the patient that you are about to insert the suppository – remember that they cannot see what you are doing.

6. Insert the suppository into the anus with your right index finger, blunt end first (see Figure 3). This particular positioning of the suppository helps the patient to retain it (Moppett, 2000).

7. If more than one suppository is to be administered, repeat the process.

Figure 2
Removing a
suppository from
its packaging

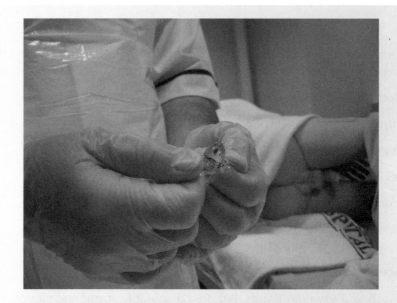

Figure 3
Inserting the
suppository

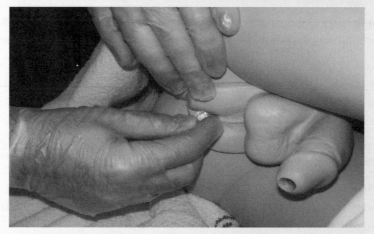

8. Using tissues, wipe away any lubricating gel from around the anus (see Figure 4).

9. Dispose of equipment.

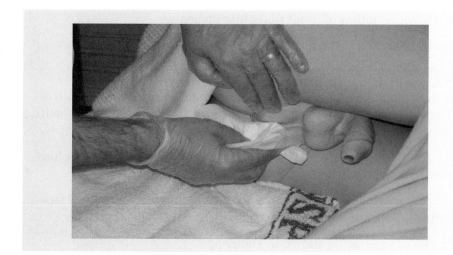

Figure 4
Wiping any
remaining lubricant
from the anus

Following the administration of suppositories

If the suppositories are to stimulate a bowel movement, the patient should be advised to retain the suppositories in his rectum for as long as possible. He should be warned, however, that the urge to defecate may become very powerful. Therefore you must ensure that the patient has access to a nurse call bell and/or a commode.

If the suppositories are drugs, they will need to be absorbed through the rectal wall. The patient should, therefore, be warned not to pass faeces for at least half an hour. Ideally, patients should be encouraged to empty their bowels prior to suppository administration.

Enemata

Introduction

Unfortunately, despite the administration of suppositories, Mr Akhtar is still not passing faeces. Therefore an enema is prescribed. An enema is a prescribed volume of fluid that is administered per rectum. Uses of enemata include:

❏ severe faecal impaction (where oral aperients and/or suppositories have been ineffective);

❏ the administration of drugs (retention enema);

❏ bowel cleansing.

Examples of enemas include:

❏ A phosphate enema (a 128 ml enema, used as an osmotic laxative). These powerful enemas should not be used on patients with inflammatory bowel conditions or those on a sodium restriction.

❏ A sodium citrate (Micralax™) enema. This contains a small volume (only 5 ml), allowing them to be administered more easily.

❏ Arachis oil (retention enema). This 130 ml enema is used as a faecal softener but should not be used on patients with a peanut allergy.

Examples of enemas are shown in Figure 5.

Figure 5
(a) Phosphate enema; (b) Sodium citrate enema

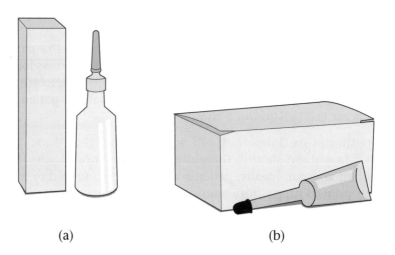

(a)   (b)

Administration of enemata

The administration of an enema, much like the administration of suppositories, is undignified and embarrassing for our patient. Therefore it is the role of the nurse to explain the procedure carefully, answer any questions the patient might have and obtain verbal consent. During the procedure, it is vital that the nurse is careful to maintain the patient's dignity and to provide reassurance.

Administering an enema

Equipment required

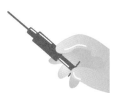

❑ Prescription chart. All enemas must be prescribed by a doctor or non-medical prescriber, prior to administration

❑ The correct enema, as required and prescribed. Note that some enemas, such as arachis oil retention enemas, should be warmed prior to administration. This can be achieved by removing the enema from its packaging and placing it in a jug of warm water for a few minutes

❑ Receiver

❑ Lubricating gel

❑ Tissues/toilet paper

❑ Commode or near access to a toilet

Procedure

1. Ensure privacy for the patient.

2. Wash your hands and put on gloves and an apron.

3. Place the patient on their left-hand side and ask them to bring their knees up toward their chest.

4. Remove packaging from the enema, including the cap on the end of the nozzle.

5. Lubricate the nozzle.

6. Encourage the patient to relax, perhaps by asking them to take some deep breaths in and out.

7. Use your left hand to part the patient's buttocks, exposing the anus. Inspect the anus for haemorrhoids.

8. Using your right hand, insert the nozzle of the enema carefully through the anus and into the rectum.

9. Squeeze the enema reservoir until all the contents have been delivered into the rectum.

10. While maintaining pressure on the enema reservoir, withdraw the nozzle carefully. Maintaining pressure as you do this prevents the enema fluid from re-entering the reservoir bag.

11. Clean the patient's anal area with tissues or toilet paper, and cover them with bedclothes.

Following enema administration

If you have administered a retention enema, you should encourage your patient to lie in the same position for half an hour to help absorption of the fluid in the rectum. You can help this process by elevating the end of the bed. If you have administered a phosphate enema or something similar to aid evacuation of impacted faeces, the effect is likely to be fairly rapid. However, you must advise your patient to hold onto it for as long as possible. Make sure that the patient has access to a commode or a toilet. If necessary, make yourself available to assist. Don't forget to offer the patient hand-washing facilities and wash your own hands thoroughly following this procedure. Document the effectiveness of the enema in the nursing notes and on the observation chart.

Summary

❑ Monitoring of bowel function is vital for all patients. Record bowel movements on the observation chart on a daily basis.

❑ Constipation can lead to serious complications if left untreated.

❑ With constipation, prevention is better than cure.

❑ Suppositories may be given to relieve constipation but may also be used to administer certain drugs.

❑ The administration of suppositories and enemata are extremely embarrassing procedures for our patients. Make sure you perform these procedures with sensitivity.

Reference

Moppett, S. (2000) 'Which way is up for a suppository?', *Nursing Times*, 96(19): 12.

Chapter 9

SKIN INTEGRITY ASSESSMENT AND PRESSURE AREA CARE

Ivan McGlen

To offer context to this chapter, it is important to consider the Essential Skills Clusters (Nursing and Midwifery Council, 2007) to which it relates. This chapter will be directly relevant to the Skill Clusters 'Care, Compassion and Communication' (Sections 1 and 3) and 'Organisational Aspects of Care' (Sections 9, 10, 18, 20).

Patients/clients can trust a newly registered nurse to:

Section 1   Provide care based on the highest standards, knowledge and competence.

Section 3   Treat them with dignity and respect them as individuals.

Section 9   Make a holistic and systematic assessment of their needs and develop a comprehensive plan of care that is in their best interests and which promotes their health and well-being and minimises the risk of harm.

Section 10   Deliver and evaluate care against the comprehensive assessment and care plan.

Section 18   Identify and safely manage risk in relation to the patient/client, the environment, self and others.

Section 20   Select and manage medical devices safely.

Introduction

In its most simplistic form, tissue viability can be considered the maintenance of effective cellular tissue function. In the case of Mr Akhtar, the role of the nurse is to undertake an appropriate assessment of his skin integrity and maintain appropriate pressure area care so as to minimise the risk of pressure ulcer development while he is unable to meet this need himself.

Pressure ulcers are an ever-present health care problem. The National Institute for Health and Clinical Excellence (2005a) considers there to be limited consensus within the published literature that seeks to identify the prevalence of pressure ulcers. This is due to often differing definitions/grading of ulcers and demographic factors. Vanderwee *et al.* (2007), seeking to develop a uniform data collection process to measure the prevalence of pressure ulcers within Europe (Belgium, Italy, Portugal, Sweden, the UK) identified the UK as having a prevalence of 21.9 per cent. The country with the lowest prevalence within their study was Italy (8.3 per cent).

From a financial perspective, Bennett *et al.* (2004) estimate (at 2000 prices) that the cost of treating a pressure ulcer ranges from £1,064 to £10,551 (for a Grade 1 to a Grade 4 pressure ulcer) and, if complications occur (e.g. **osteomyelitis**), the cost may reach £20,000 to £24,000. Bennett *et al.* (2004) further estimate that the cost to the NHS ranges from £1.43 bn to £2.14 bn, broadly equal to the total NHS expenditure on mental illness or community health services at the time of the study (1999/2000), and 4 per cent of the NHS budget expenditure at that time.

The cost of pressure ulcers cannot and should not only be measured from a monetary perspective. Work by Hopkins *et al.* (2006) sought to explore the lived experiences of patients suffering a pressure ulcer. The impact of a pressure ulcer was revealed by means of three major themes: pressure ulcers as a cause of endless pain, pressure ulcers as producing a restricted life and issues related to coping with a pressure ulcer (acceptance). Similar findings were identified by Spilsbury *et al.* (2007) who identified emotional, mental, physical and social affects of having a pressure ulcer. An association of pressure ulcers with pain, fluid leakage and smell were identified, as well as issues relating to limited mobility. Spilsbury *et al.* (2007) identified feelings of preoccupation with the pressure ulcer, clients '… hating their ulcer …' and clients attributing blame for their pressure ulcer development, citing their existing clinical condition, health status, weight loss, lack of knowledge or poor hygiene practices as causative factors. Blame was also directed at carers '… for failing to attach priority to their reports of an ulcer or delays in skin inspection'. The message is very clear:

❑ pressure ulcers are common;

❑ they pose a great expense to a health care service with finite resources;

❑ they have a profoundly negative effect on a person's entire well-being and their ability to return to their optimal level of wellness.

How and why do pressure ulcers develop?

To meet Mr Akhtar's needs within this area of care, it is important to consider how and why pressure ulcers develop. By understanding this, the nurse can apply appropriate nursing interventions to reduce the risk of pressure ulcer development.

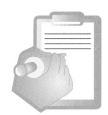

Activity 1.

Review what you already know about the skin and about pressure ulcers.

1.   How are the skin and underlying tissues structured?

2.   What are the functions of the skin?

3.   What is a pressure ulcer?

4.   What factors influence pressure ulcer development?

5.   What are the common sites for pressure ulcers to develop?

6.   How do you assess if a person is at risk of developing a pressure ulcer?

The structure and function of the skin

The skin is a protective covering to the body that is made up of three distinctive layers (see Figure 1):

❑ epidermis;

❑ dermis;

❑ subcutaneous (fatty) layer.

Functions of the skin

The functions of the skin are as follows.

❑ Protection of underlying tissues from the immediate environment and surroundings; some protection against ultraviolet light.

❑ Waterproof barrier.

❑ Thermoregulation – through peripheral **vasodilatation** and **vasoconstriction**. During peripheral vasodilatation blood flows to the surface of the skin and heat is lost through radiation and convection. During this process, sweat glands are also stimulated by the increased blood flow. Heat is lost through evaporation. When the body attempts to retain heat, vasoconstriction occurs resulting in a reduced blood flow to the dermis.

Figure 1
The structure of
the skin

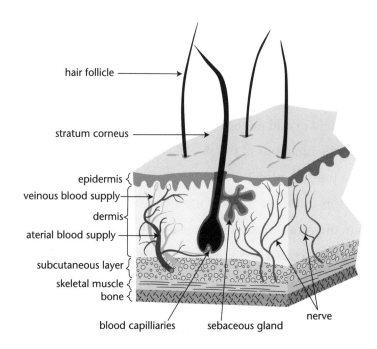

- hair follicle
- stratum corneus
- epidermis
- veinous blood supply
- dermis
- aterial blood supply
- subcutaneous layer
- skeletal muscle
- bone
- blood capilliaries
- sebaceous gland
- nerve

❏ Sensation – nerve endings within the skin alert the brain to the presence of pressure, pain or injury to a particular area of the body. A person should therefore be able to consciously or unconsciously withdraw from an unpleasant or dangerous sensation (if able).

Pressure ulcers: definition and classification

There appears to be broad consensus on how a pressure ulcer is defined. The most commonly used definition is that offered by the European Pressure Ulcer Advisory Panel (EPUAP) (1998a). The EPUAP define a pressure ulcer as '... an area of localised damage to the skin and underlying tissues caused by pressure, shear, friction or a combination of these'.

However, differing methods of grading or classifying pressure ulcers are offered in contemporary literature. The purpose of pressure ulcer classification, according to Nixon *et al.*, (2005), is to '... standardise record-keeping and provide a common description of the ulcer severity ...' Although, at first glance, differences in classification may appear minimal, it is important that all staff agree on a common method of assessing pressure ulcer formation. The method supported by the Royal College of Nursing and National Institute for Health and Clinical Excellence (2005a) is that offered by the European Pressure Ulcer Advisory Panel (1998a) (see Figure 2).

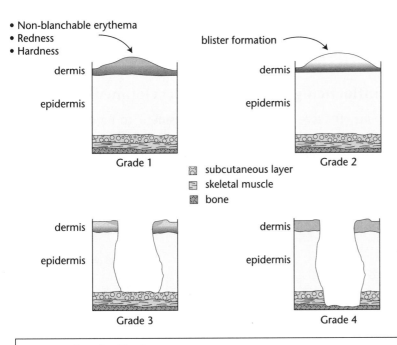

Figure 2
Pressure ulcer classification

Pressure ulcer classification

Grade 1: non-blanchable erythema of intact skin. Discolouration of the skin, warmth, oedema, induration or hardness may also be used as indicators, particularly on individuals with darker skin.

Grade 2: partial thickness skin loss involving epidermis, dermis, or both. The ulcer is superficial and presents clinically as an abrasion or blister.

Grade 3: full thickness skin loss invliving damage to, or necrosis of, subcutaneous tissue that my extend down to, but not through underlying fascia.

Grade 4: extensive destruction, tissue necrosis, or damage to muscle, bone, or supporting structures with or without full thickness skin loss.

European Pressure Ulcer Advisory Panel (1998)

Pressure ulcer assessment problems

While the EPUAP (1998a) classification system provides a method of identifying the key clinical features of the differing grades of pressure ulcer and offers a standardisation to such an assessment, it is important that nursing staff are consistent with their assessment classifications. In their investigation into consistency and reliability of pressure ulcer classification, Nixon *et al.* (2005) observed that ward nurses may make inaccurate assessments of the presence or grade of pressure ulcers (particularly with regard to Grade 1 and Grade 2 pressure ulcers). The implications of such inconsistencies can have far-reaching effects with regard to the nursing management. A possible solution offered by Nixon *et al.* (2005) is to use co-assessors or expert assessors when undertaking the assessment of pressure ulcers.

Factors influencing pressure ulcer development

To enable an effective pressure ulcer assessment to be undertaken, it is important that you are aware of the factors that influence pressure ulcer development. These factors may be considered as either intrinsic or extrinsic. The National Institute for Health and Clinical Excellence (2003, 2005b) identifies the following intrinsic and extrinsic risk factors (see Figure 3).

Figure 3
Intrinsic and extrinsic factors influencing pressure ulcer development

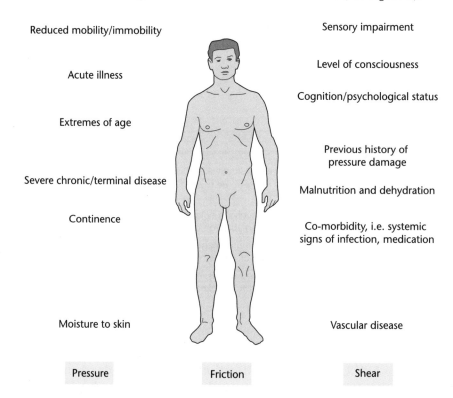

Reduced mobility/immobility

Acute illness

Extremes of age

Severe chronic/terminal disease

Continence

Moisture to skin

Sensory impairment

Level of consciousness

Cognition/psychological status

Previous history of pressure damage

Malnutrition and dehydration

Co-morbidity, i.e. systemic signs of infection, medication

Vascular disease

Pressure

Friction

Shear

Pressure

When prolonged pressure is applied to a particular area of skin, blood flow becomes decreased resulting in tissue damage (**necrosis**).

Friction

Friction, as stated by Grey *et al.* (2006), is the process whereby one surface opposes the movement of another. This results in blister formation within the epidermis, which can become skin lesions, and this accelerates pressure ulcer formation.

Shear forces

Grey *et al.* (2006) consider shear forces to be when bone and subcutaneous tissue move while the skin remains immobile or moves at a relatively reduced rate compared with that of the bone and subcutaneous tissue. In such circumstances, blood vessels become more easily occluded, thus increasing the risk of pressure ulcer development.

Common sites for pressure ulcer development

The European Pressure Ulcer Advisory Panel (1998b) highlights the body's bony prominences (see Figure 4) as being areas of particular focus during a

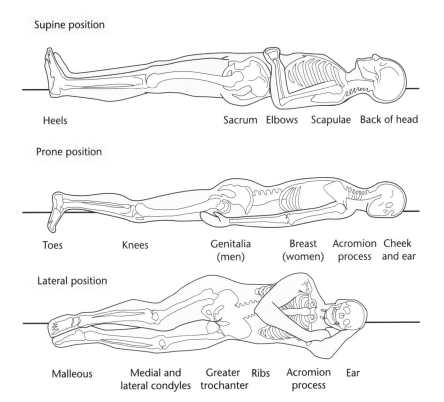

Figure 4
The body's bony prominences

Supine position

Heels   Sacrum Elbows   Scapulae Back of head

Prone position

Toes   Knees   Genitalia   Breast   Acromion Cheek
                            (men)   (women)   process   and ear

Lateral position

Malleous   Medial and   Greater Ribs   Acromion   Ear
              lateral condyles trochanter   process

pressure ulcer assessment. The majority of pressure ulcers occur on the lower half of the body, particularly the pelvis and lower limbs (Grey *et al.*, 2006). Such bony prominences may be more pronounced in a patient suffering significant weight and/or tissue loss (Defloor *et al.*, 2005), and this again increases the risk for pressure ulcer development. Careful consideration with regard to patient positioning and movement is required.

It is important to note that, however the patient is positioned, you should pay particular attention to the areas of direct pressure (see Table 1). This includes patient to bed/pressure aid contact or body surface to body surface contact.

Table 1 Areas of direct pressure

Prone position	Lateral position	Recovery position
❑ Ear	❑ Ear	❑ Ear
❑ Face – cheek/mandible	❑ Face – cheek/mandible	❑ Face – cheek/mandible
❑ Breast/sternum	❑ Shoulder	❑ Shoulder
❑ Shoulders – anterior	❑ Lateral border of chest wall	❑ Lateral border of chest wall
❑ Elbows and wrists	❑ Elbows and wrist	❑ Elbow
❑ Genitalia	❑ Pelvis	❑ Wrist
❑ Pelvis	❑ Knee – lateral aspect of knee	❑ Pelvis
❑ Knees	❑ Lateral maleolus	*Inferior leg*
❑ Dorsum of foot	❑ Lateral aspect of foot	❑ Inner thigh
❑ Toes		❑ Lateral aspect of knee
❑ Lateral maleolus – if ankles are inverted		❑ Lateral maleolus
		❑ Lateral aspect of foot
		Superior leg
		❑ Inner thigh
		❑ Medial aspect of knee
		❑ Medial maleolus
		❑ Medial aspect of foot

Defloor *et al.* (2005) note that moisture lesions, for instance within skin folds (due to a combination of pressure, friction and moisture), may be misinterpreted as pressure ulcers. They state that 'a wound not over a bony prominence is unlikely to be a pressure ulcer'. However, Defloor *et al.* (2005) point out that 'where soft tissue is compressed', by a urinary catheter for example, a pressure ulcer may develop. Therefore it is important that you are aware of all potential sites for pressure ulcer development and that you are able to differentiate between a pressure ulcer and a moisture lesion.

Pressure ulcer risk assessment

Although there are many approaches to a risk assessment process, the purpose of any risk assessment is to enable the identification, assessment, analysis and management of a potential risk, thus enabling appropriate interventions (National Patient Safety Agency, 2006). The National Institute for Health and Clinical Excellence (2005b) states that an initial pressure ulcer risk assessment should be undertaken within the first six hours of a patient's first care episode. This assessment will therefore form the basis for all future pressure ulcer risk assessments.

Risk assessment tools

The purpose of undertaking a pressure ulcer assessment is to identify those at risk of developing a pressure ulcer or, in those who already have developed one, to assess the risk of further development. Schoonhoven *et al.* (2005) note that there are approximately 40 risk assessment tools available, mostly reflecting expert opinion, empirical information or adaptations of existing models. Within any assessment, key areas are identified that enable the user to make a judgement about the risk of a patient developing a pressure ulcer. Given the availability of such a number of risk assessment tools, consistency of assessment is therefore difficult. Schoonhoven *et al.* (2005) point out that of the 40 or so risk assessment tools identified, only the Norton (Norton *et al.*, 1979, cited in Lindgren *et al.*, 2002) Waterlow (Waterlow, 2005) and Braden (Ayello and Braden, 2002) scales have been subject to any form of scientific scrutiny (the Braden scale being subject to the most), with many methodological inconsistencies noted.

It is therefore difficult to decide which is the most accurate method of undertaking an effective and appropriate risk assessment. All three scales offer a numerical assessment from which a level of risk may be identified, but all three differ in their choice of the key clinical areas on which the assessment is based (see Table 2).

Potential problems with the use of risk assessment tools

All three scales, collectively, appear to capture the risk factors which contribute to pressure ulcer development but, individually, a holistic assessment does not appear possible. Pancorbo-Hidalgo *et al.* (2006) consider risk assessment tools to be of value but there is no concrete evidence that their use reduces the occurrence of pressure ulcers. They further consider that the Braden scale and the Norton scale predict

Table 2
A comparison of the
Norton, Braden and
Waterlow scales

Norton scale	Braden scale	Waterlow scale
❏ Physical condition	❏ Sensory perception	❏ Build/weight
❏ Mental condition	❏ Moisture	❏ Gender
❏ Activity	❏ Activity	❏ Appetite
❏ Mobility	❏ Mobility	❏ Visual assessment of at-risk skin area
❏ Incontinent	❏ Nutrition	❏ Mobility
	❏ Friction and shear	❏ Continence
		❏ Tissue malnutrition
		❏ Neurological deficit
		❏ Major surgery/trauma
		❏ Medication

pressure ulcer risk more effectively than a nurse's own clinical judgement. The Royal College of Nursing and the National Institute for Health and Clinical Excellence (2005a) advocate the use of risk assessment tools as an adjunct (aid) to the assessment process but they think that such tools should not replace the individual clinical judgement of the nurse. As noted earlier, when discussing pressure ulcer grading, inconsistencies can occur with regard to the interpretation of a

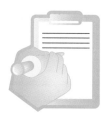

Activity 2.

Review what you already know about pressure ulcer risk assessment and the prevention of pressure ulcer development.

1.   What is the purpose of a baseline pressure ulcer risk assessment on admission?

     (a) When should it be undertaken and how often should an assessment be repeated?

     (b) What further issues should be considered when undertaking an initial assessment?

2.   What are the specific nursing interventions required to prevent the development of pressure ulcers?

3.   What are the types of pressure-relieving aids?

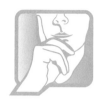

Reflection

Reflecting upon the previous section, consider how you have developed your understanding in relation to the development and assessment of pressure ulcers.

Having explored how pressure ulcers develop and how they are assessed, it is important to further consider the appropriate nursing interventions to reduce the risk of pressure ulcer development.

risk assessment tool and, in certain cases, in the appropriateness of a tool for particular patient groups. When undertaking a pressure ulcer assessment using any of the above tools, a level of underpinning technical knowledge must also be present to enable the user to more effectively interpret the meaning of the terms and choose the most appropriate numerical score within each section.

Baseline pressure ulcer risk assessment

As with any nursing intervention, the basis for an effective and structured approach to care is the initial assessment. An initial or baseline assessment provides a set of values or norms, establishing the standard from which all future care interventions (improvement/deterioration) will be measured. It is important therefore that an initial assessment is comprehensive, detailed and easy to interpret.

NICE (2005b) advocates that the initial assessment is undertaken within six hours of the first episode of care. The first episode of care may be interpreted as the admission to hospital or it may also begin at a change of care setting such as, for example, a change from a ward area to an intensive therapy unit or vice versa. Irrespective of the nature of care setting, given the multiplicity of reasons why a pressure ulcer can develop, it is advisable to undertake this initial assessment as soon as possible after the patient is admitted to a particular care setting.

As stated earlier in this chapter, there are many factors that contribute to the development of a pressure ulcer and specific tools are available to support an assessment of pressure ulcer risk. When undertaking an initial and ongoing assessment, the EPUAP (1998a) suggests that a pressure ulcer assessment should take the following issues into consideration:

❑ assessment of the pressure ulcer (if present) – location, grade, size, wound-bed, exudates, pain, status of surrounding tissue and identification of sinus formation;

❑ history and physical examination – a pressure ulcer should be assessed in the context of the patient's overall physical and psychosocial health and their identified needs addressed appropriately;

❑ assessment of complications:

– nutritional assessment and management

– pain assessment and management

– psychosocial assessment and management

❑ managing tissue loads:

– manual repositioning

– use of specialist equipment

❑ use of pressure ulcer prevention devices.

The EPUAP (1998a) suggests that further reassessments are undertaken daily or at least weekly. According to NICE (2005b), these assessments should be undertaken by a registered health care professional. As with any patient, should deterioration in any aspect of the patient's assessed condition be suspected or detected, a further reassessment should be undertaken (NICE, 2005b). By considering such factors in conjunction with a specific risk assessment tool, an effective baseline for future assessment and interventions is established.

Should a pressure ulcer be present, a further dimension to the assessment process is offered. The RCN and NICE (2005a) recommend that a baseline assessment should include the following:

Ulcer assessment:

❑ establish the severity of the pressure ulcer(s) in order to:

– generate a personal ulcer profile to develop a plan of care from which treatment interventions will be initiated;

– evaluate treatment interventions;

– assess for complications;

– communicate information about the pressure ulcer to those involved within care management.

Ongoing assessment should include:

❏ causes of ulcer;

❏ site/location;

❏ dimensions of ulcer;

❏ stage or grade;

❏ exudates – amount and type;

❏ local signs of infection;

❏ pain;

❏ wound appearance;

❏ surrounding skin;

❏ undermining/tracking (sinus or fistula);

❏ odour.

Assessment should be supported by photography/tracings (calibrated with a ruler).

(RCN and NICE, 2005a)

Preventing the development of pressure ulcers

The RCN and NICE (2005a) advocate that, where possible, all patients should be encouraged to independently mobilise irrespective of being in a bed, chair or wheelchair and that such intervention be determined by 'general health status, location of ulcer, general skin assessment, acceptability (comfort) to patient and carer'.

The focus of nursing management is to prevent the development of pressure ulcers and, at the most basic level, the avoidance of friction, pressure and shear forces, taking into consideration associated contributory factors. There is broad consensus that the patient's position should be altered regularly, usually at two-hourly intervals (Young and Clark, 2003). There is limited evidence to support this specific time-frame. However, there is recognition that positional changes should be undertaken far more frequently in light of individual patient risk factors and clinical need. Positioning a patient should also take into account other factors that may influence the range of positional changes/interventions. These factors may include:

❏ pre-existing breathing/respiratory problems;

❏ pre-existing pressure ulcers/wounds;

❏ skeletal injuries – i.e. spinal injury, upper/lower limb fractures;

❏ prolonged surgical procedures.

Types of pressure-relieving aids

To support the nursing intervention to minimise the risk of pressure ulcer development, pressure-relieving devices should be considered. The RCN and NICE (2005b) state that 'all individuals assessed as being vulnerable to pressure ulcers should, as a minimum provision, be placed on a high-specification foam mattress with pressure-relieving properties'. The RCN (2005, p.15) classifies pressure-relieving devices as 'low-tech' or 'high-tech':

❏ Low-tech (provides a support surface that distributes body weight over a large area):

– standard foam mattress;

– alternative foam mattress/overlay;

– gel-filled mattress/overlay;

– fluid-filled mattress/overlay;

– fibre-filled mattress/overlay;

– air-filled mattress/overlay.

❏ High-tech (dynamic systems):

– alternating pressure devices – patient lies on air-filled sacs which sequentially inflate and deflate relieving pressure for short periods;

– air-fluidised devices;

– low air loss devices;

– turning beds/frames.

As stated earlier, Mr Akhtar has suffered a stroke. He is unconscious on admission to the ward and has marked right-sided weakness. He is dependent on nursing staff to meet his complete care needs at this point.

Activity 3.

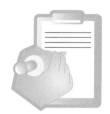

1. What are Mr Akhtar's risk factors for developing a pressure ulcer?

2. Which areas of his body are most susceptible to pressure ulcer formation?

3. What should the nurse consider when undertaking a pressure ulcer risk assessment?

4. What equipment is available to support the nurse in minimising the risk of pressure ulcer development?

5. How would you plan Mr Akhtar's care from the point of view of pressure ulcer prevention?

An aseptic dressing for a pressure ulcer

Mr Akhtar has developed a pressure ulcer and this has been dressed. The dressing now needs to be changed. The aim for undertaking an aseptic dressing is to reduce the risk of introducing pathogenic organisms into a wound or susceptible site, as well as to prevent the transfer of these organisms from the wound to other patients or staff (Wilson, 2006).

An aseptic dressing

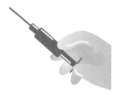

1. Review the patient's care plan. This allows for assessment of the wound when exposed and ensures you have identified the correct patient.

2. Identify the patient by checking the wrist band and ensure the right patient will receive the correct nursing intervention.

3. Explain to the patient what you are going to do and obtain verbal consent. This helps to reduce patient anxiety and encourages patient co-operation. It also prepares the patient for the dressing change.

4. The patient may experience pain when the dressing is changed so assess the patient for the need for analgesia before you change the wound dressing. With a qualified practitioner, administer with any analgesic medication required by the patient. Allow enough time for the analgesic medication to work.

5. Prepare the necessary equipment. Preparation is effective time management and allows for an organised approach to the change of dressing. Check expiry dates on all equipment to be used as out-of-date equipment is a danger to the patient. Clean the dressing trolley with detergent and soap (Thompson and Bullock, 1992).

See Chapter 21, page 455.

6. Wash hands using the procedure described in Chapter 21. Correct hand washing prevents the spread of micro-organisms and cross-contamination.

7. Close any curtains/doors around the patient to protect their privacy and dignity.

8. Ensure the bed is at an appropriate height. This will help to reduce your risk of back strain when you are carrying out the procedure.

9. Set the patient in a comfortable position that provides easy assess to the wound area.

10. Cover any exposed area on the patient, other than the wound area, to protect the patient's dignity. Loosen the existing dressing to reduce patient discomfort during dressing removal.

11. Wash hands using the procedure described in Chapter 21. In case of direct contact with bodily fluids or blood put on a clean plastic apron to prevent contamination of your uniform and the transfer of micro-organisms.

12. Open the necessary equipment and prepare a sterile field. Make sure equipment is within easy reach and that the sterile field is maintained.

13. Remove the soiled dressing carefully. If any part of the patient's skin is stuck to the dressing, use a small amount of sterile saline solution to help loosen and remove the dressing. The use of saline allows for easier removal while minimising tissue damage and pain for the patient. Do not reach over the wound.

14. Assess the soiled dressing for the colour, type or odour of any exudates on the dressing. If any exudate is present it should be documented. Place the soiled dressing in the correct waste receptacle and wash your hands.

15. Open cleaning solution and pour into a sterile container.

16. Put on sterile gloves.

17. Clean the wound from top to bottom, or from the centre to the outside of wound. Cleaning should be from the least to most contaminated area. Use a clean gauze square for each wipe, placing the used gauze in the waste receptacle. The clean gauze square for each wipe ensures a previously cleaned area is not contaminated again. Ensure no surfaces are touched with the gloves.

18. After the wound is clean, dry the area using clean gauze swabs. Drying the area is important because micro-organisms grow in a moist environment. Apply any treatment if prescribed.

19. Apply a dry sterile dressing over the wound. Dressings may reduce the growth of micro-organisms and promote the healing process. They also allow for any exudate to be absorbed.

20. Place a second sterile dressing over the wound site. A second layer allows for exudate to be absorbed and also allows for additional protection of the wound against micro-organisms.

21. Remove and dispose of gloves. Apply tape to secure the dressing. Tape is easier to apply after gloves have been removed.

22. Label dressing with date and time. This provides information for colleagues and demonstrates that the care plan has been followed.

23. Remove all equipment. Ensure the correct disposal of any sharps and waste materials. Ensure the patient is comfortable with the bed lowered to the lowest position for patient safety.

24. Clean the work surface, remove the protective clothing and wash hands using the procedure outlined in Chapter 21.

See Chapter 21, page 455.

25. Complete all relevant documentation and make sure the patient's care plan is updated and that any changes observed in the wound have been documented.

Further reading

Department of Health (2003) *Winning ways – working together to reduce health care associated infection in England*. London: DoH

National Institute for Health and Clinical Excellence (2003) *Infection control (Clinical Guideline 2)*. London: NICE

National Institute for Health and Clinical Excellence (2005) *The management of pressure ulcers in primary and secondary care*. London: NICE

Nursing and Midwifery Council (1998) *Guidelines for records and record keeping*. London: NMC

Royal College of Nursing (2004) *Good practice in infection control: guidance for nursing staff*. London: RCN

Royal College of Nursing (2005) *Wipe it out campaign*. London: RCN

Thompson, G. and Bullock, D. (1992) 'To clean or not to clean?' *Nursing Times*, 83(9): 71–5

Wilson, J. (2006) *Infection control in clinical practice*. London: Baillière Tindall

References

The list below also identifies electronic sources to aid your literature searches in relation to this subject area.

Ayello, E.A. and Braden, B. (2002) 'How and why to do pressure ulcer risk assessment'. *Advances in Skin and Wound Care*, 15(3): 125–31

Bennett, G., Dealey, C. and Posnett (2004) 'The cost of pressure ulcers in the UK'. *Age and Aging*, 33: 23–5

Defloor, T., Schoonhoven, L., Fletcher, J., Furtado, K., Heyman, H., Lubbers, M. *et al.* (2005) 'Statement of the European Pressure Ulcer Advisory Panel – pressure ulcer classification: differentiation between pressure ulcers and moisture lesions'. *European Pressure Ulcer Advisory Panel Reviews*, 6(3)

European Pressure Ulcer Advisory Panel (1998a) *Pressure ulcer treatment guidelines* [online at: **www.epuap.org/gltreatment.html**]

European Pressure Ulcer Advisory Panel (1998b) *Pressure ulcer prevention guidelines* [online at: **www.epuap.org/glprevention.html**]

Grey, J.S., Harding, K.G. and Enoch, S. (2006) 'ABC of wound healing: pressure ulcers'. *British Medical Journal*, 332: 472–5

Hopkins, A., Dealey, C., Bale, S., Defloor, T. and Worboys, F. (2006) 'Patient stories of living with a pressure ulcer'. *Journal of Advanced Nursing*, 56(4): 345–53

Lindgren, M., Unosson, M., Krantz, A.M. and Ek, A.C. (2002) 'A risk assessment scale for the prediction of pressure sore development: reliability and validity'. *Journal of Advanced Nursing*, 38(2): 190–9

National Institute for Health and Clinical Excellence (2003) *NICE guideline on pressure ulcer risk management and prevention (Guideline B)* [online at: **http://guidance.nice.org.uk/CGB/niceguidance/pdf/English**]

National Institute for Health and Clinical Excellence (2005a) *Pressure ulcer management – cost analysis of the new recommendations in the prevention and treatment of pressure ulcers quick reference guide. National cost-impact report: implementing NICE Clinical Guideline No. 29* [online at: **http://guidance.nice.org.uk/CG29/costreport/pdf/English**]

National Institute for Health and Clinical Excellence (2005b) CG29 *Pressure ulcer management: quick reference guide* [online at: **http://guidance.nice.org.uk/CG29/ quickrefguide/pdf/English**]

National Patient Safety Agency (2006) *Risk assessment programme: overview* [online at: **www.npsa.nhs.uk/site/media/documents/2128_0439_Overview.pdf**]

Nixon, J., Thorpe, H., Barrow, H., Phillips, A., Nelson, E.A., Mason, S.A. and Cullum, N. (2005) 'Reliability of pressure ulcer classification and diagnosis'. *Journal of Advanced Nursing*, 50(6): 613–23

Nursing and Midwifery Council (2007) 'Annexe 2 to NMC Circular 07/2007' [online at: **www.ukcc.org.uk/aFrameDisplay.aspx?DocumentID=2690**]

Pancorbo-Hidalgo, P.l., Garcia-Fernanadez, F.P., Lopez-Medina, I.M. and Alvarez-Nieto, C. (2006) 'Risk assessment scales for pressure ulcer prevention: a systematic review'. *Journal of Advanced Nursing*, 54(1): 94–110

Royal College of Nursing (2005) *The use of pressure-relieving devices (beds, mattresses and overlays) for the prevention of pressure ulcers in primary and secondary care* [online at: **www.rcn.org.uk/publications/pdf/guidelines/pressure-relieving-devices.pdf**]

Royal College of Nursing and National Institute for Health and Clinical Excellence (2005a) *The management of pressure ulcers in primary and secondary care. A clinical practice guideline.* [online at: **www.rcn.org.uk/publications/pdf/guidelines/rcn_guidelines.pdf**]

Royal College of Nursing and National Institute for Health and Clinical Excellence (2005b) *CG29 Pressure ulcer management: sources of recommendations used in the quick reference guide* [online at: **http://guidance.nice.org.uk/page.aspx?o=273131**]

Schoonhoven, L., Grobber, D.E., Bousema, M.T. and Buskens, E. (2005) 'Predicting pressure ulcers: cases missed using a new clinical prediction rule'. *Journal of Advanced Nursing*, 49(1): 16–22

Spilsbury, K., Nelson, A., Cullum, N., Igliss, C., Nixon, J. and Mason, S. (2007) 'Pressure ulcers and their treatment and effects on quality of life: hospital inpatient perspectives'. *Journal of Advanced Nursing*, 57(5): 494–504

Thompson, G. and Bullock, D. (1992) 'To clean or not to clean?' *Nursing Times*, 83(9): 71–5

Vanderwee, K., Clark, M., Dealey, C., Gunningberg, L. and Defloor, T. (2007) 'Pressure ulcer prevalence in Europe: a pilot study'. *Journal of Evaluation in Clinical Practice*, 13(2): 227–35

Waterlow, J. (2005) 'Waterlow pressure ulcer prevention/treatment policy'. *Waterlow Score Card*, available at Judy-Waterlow.co.uk [online at: **www.judy-waterlow.co.uk/the-waterlow-score-card.htm**]

Wilson, J. (2006) *Infection control in clinical practice.* London: Baillière Tindall

Young, T. and Clark, M. (2003) 'Re-positioning for pressure ulcer prevention (protocol)'. *The Cochrane Library*

3 CARE AND COMPASSION

This part includes the following chapters:

Scenario: Elsie Smith

Elsie Smith is a 76-year-old lady who has been living independently in warden controlled accommodation with her husband Walter. She also has a large extended family who see her on a regular basis.

Elsie is admitted to the medical ward via accident and emergency, having collapsed at home. She is diagnosed as having had a left-sided stroke. This has left her with a profound right-sided weakness and no gag reflex.

At this point, the text will consider Elsie in terms of her nursing problems that require intervention. These will include:

❑ moving and handling techniques;
   – positioning Elsie in bed
   – getting Elsie in and out of bed
❑ nutrition and hydration;
❑ intravenous infusion;
❑ nasogastric tube insertion.

Consideration will also be given to the role of the multidisciplinary team in Elsie's care: physiotherapist, dietician, speech and language therapist, doctor, pharmacist, etc.

After three weeks of rehabilitation, Elsie develops aspiration pneumonia leading to respiratory failure. At this stage, both Elsie and her relatives are told about Elsie's worsening condition and poor prognosis. Sadly, Elsie eventually dies.

At this stage, the skill of breaking bad news will be discussed, followed by details of performing last offices.

Thus, through the use of one running scenario, the skills identified within this section are covered.

10

NUTRITIONAL SUPPORT, HYDRATION AND FLUID BALANCE

Sam Pollitt

This chapter covers the following Nursing and Midwifery Council (NMC) Essential Skills Clusters (ESCs):

Patients/clients can trust a newly registered nurse to:

Section 27 Provide assistance with selecting a diet through which they will receive adequate nutritional and fluid intake.

Section 28 Assess and monitor nutritional status and formulate an effective care plan.

Section 29 Assess and monitor fluid status and formulate an effective care plan.

Section 30 Provide an environment conducive to eating and drinking.

Section 31 Ensure that those unable to take food by mouth receive adequate nutrition.

Section 32 Safely administer fluids when fluids cannot be taken independently.

Overview of nutrition issues

Nutritional issues have recently become a national obsession thanks to the influx of media nutrition gurus and diet doctors telling us what to eat and what not to eat. This nutritional revolution has resulted in better school meals, a wide range of organic options in supermarkets and innumerable nutrition self-help books. Yet even with this explosion of nutrition knowledge, media headlines such as 'Hospital starved our grandmother to death' (Sapsted, 2007) continue to haunt the National Health Service (NHS). This suggests dietary care received in hospital is still inadequate, often leading to incidences of malnutrition, morbidity and even mortality (McWhirter and Pennington, 1994; Söderhamn and Söderhamn, 2002; Green and Watson, 2005). The long-term consequences of poor nutrition are well documented. These include muscle atrophy, decreased healing, increased risk of infections, pressure sores and even heart failure (Clay, 2000). The significance of good nutritional care at a time when it is most needed is an important factor in achieving quality of life. In addition, the Nursing and Midwifery Council's (NMC) Essential Skills Clusters (ESCs), which are eventually to be integrated into all pre-registration nursing programmes, identify nutrition and fluid management as fundamental skills in which all practising and newly qualified nurses must be competent. Therefore the aim of this chapter is to discuss the nutritional requirements and the care of Elsie Smith following her admission to a general ward due to a stroke.

Nutritional assessment

In order to meet patients' nutritional needs we must first find out what those needs are. This can be achieved by carrying out a full nutritional assessment/screening of our patient. A nutritional assessment is simply a collection of information about their previous and current intake of diet and fluids, as well as their **anthropometrical measurements** – the scientific measurement of the body including the weight and height. There are many nutrition assessment/screening (nursing) audit tools to help us do that.

The Malnutrition Universal Screening Tool (MUST)

One such nutritional assessment tool commonly used in practice areas is the Malnutrition Universal Screening Tool (MUST) (British Association for Parental and Enteral Nutrition, 2000). This tool was designed as a simple and practical solution to screening, allowing health professionals across different care settings to quickly identify those already suffering from, or at risk of, malnutrition. MUST is a five-step tool requiring the user to calculate a patient's body mass index, percentage of unintentional weight loss and acute illness score in order to manage those people at risk of malnutrition most effectively.

The body mass index (BMI)

The body mass index (or the Quetelet index) calculates body weight in relation to height and determines whether a person's body weight is within the expected range for their particular height. The normal range is 20–25. A BMI value of less than 19 indicates that a person is underweight while 26 and over indicates a person is overweight to obese. Most clinical areas contain a BMI chart with the calculation done for you; all you need to do is plot where on the chart your patient sits.

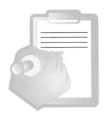

Activity 1.

Calculate BMI

1. Using a chart from your placement area, try calculating your own BMI value by weighing yourself and measuring your height. You can also find many BMI charts on the internet by typing in the search term 'body mass index'.

2. Now calculate Mrs Smith's BMI value and consider what you need to do for Mrs Smith in relation to this information. Her current weight is 47 kg and her height is 1.62 m.

Encouraging and supporting dietary intake

Assessing your patient and awarding them a score alone will not treat any underlying malnutrition. Sadly, many nurses feel referring an 'at risk' patient to a dietician is all their role requires. This is not the case. Good nutritional care requires the nurse to be proactive and provide the best dietary experience for each individual patient. The key aim is to encourage dietary intake. Therefore, if your patient can eat and shows no signs of **dysphagia** (inability to swallow) you must first find out what your patient likes and does not like to eat. You can then help the patient to pick out more favourable dishes from the menu but do not choose for them without their consent. Many studies have shown a link between appetite and food preference. Since pleasure plays a huge role in determining food choice, people tend to consume foods they enjoy and avoid those they don't (Ottley, 2000). In addition, you can assess the availability of appropriate food for the patient and, where necessary, communicate with catering services about an individual patient's needs. In addition, ensure the environment is conducive to the patient eating. This simply means you must check if the setting enables the patient to feel relaxed enough to enjoy their meal.

A good eating environment

Before the meal arrives ensure:

❑ the patient is sitting in a comfortable upright position;

❑ if requested they can wash their hands;

❑ they have a fresh cold drink available to help wash down their food;

❑ all bedpans, commodes and other offensive equipment have been removed from the general area;

❑ you have washed your hands according to the universal hand washing guidelines (see Chapter 21, page 455) and changed your apron.

See Chapter 21 page 455.

Once the meal has arrived ensure you;

❑ place it within your patient's reach;

❑ remove any difficult covers and open any packages;

❑ assess whether your patient needs assistance cutting the food up into manageable pieces;

❑ assess if they are able to feed themselves or whether they will need assistance from a nurse.

Some older patients can feel 'overfaced' with large meal portions or all of their meal being served at once. Would you want to eat at a restaurant that served your starter, main and pudding all at the same time? If this is the case then serve one course at a time, leaving the remaining courses to one side until your patient is ready for them. Always remember to go back and serve them their next course.

Food intake charts

When used properly food intake charts are a useful way of assessing exactly what your patient has been eating while under your care. Each clinical area will have its own version of a food intake chart, but they all contain very similar information. The chart will require you to document what the patient has eaten, how much and when. Other information such as the position of the patient, whether any assistance was required and any changes in their intake may also be requested. They must be completed after each meal or snack and not as you place the meal in front of your patient as, at this point, you can only guess or estimate what your patient might eat. This is false information and can lead to an incorrect judgement about that patient's actual dietary intake.

Nutritional support

Some patients may need assistance with feeding. Often they need help with all of their meal. At other times they may be able to start feeding themselves but tire very quickly requiring you to step in and help them finish their meal. Knowing how to help someone else to eat can cause anxiety for those undertaking this task for the first time. However, once this skill is mastered, it can be the most rewarding and, equally, the most important thing you can do for your patient.

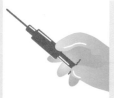

Feeding a patient

When feeding a patient you must:

❑ Ensure your patient is sitting in a comfortable semi-upright/upright position.

❑ Sit beside your patient, rather than in front of them, so that they can see their environment, and do not feel they are being watched while they are eating (see Figure 1). Some people suggest that you sit in front of your patient like you would a baby, but this can feel obtrusive

Figure 1
Feeding a patient

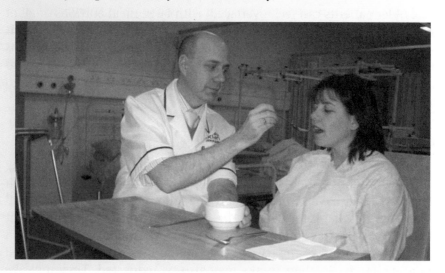

and embarrassing for your patient, as the proximity can feel too intimate. Do not stand hovering above your patient as this will make them feel you are in a rush and begrudge helping them.

❑ Bring the spoon or fork towards their mouth; don't expect them to strain towards the spoon or fork.

❑ Give small amounts at a time.

❑ Wait for your patient to finishing chewing and swallowing before introducing the next mouthful.

❑ Leave a small pause between mouthfuls so your patient does not feel rushed.

❑ Offer frequent sips of fluid to keep their mouth moist.

❑ Tell the patient what they are eating. If they are expecting peas and mash but find themselves with a mouth full of rhubarb and custard this could be distressing. This is especially important when feeding a patient a puree diet as they are then able to picture the flavour before they taste it.

❑ Relax and talk to your patient; if you are tense they will be too.

❑ Make a mental note of any changes or difficulty with feeding. For instance, was there any difficulty with chewing or swallowing, was there excess dribbling of salvia, did they become unusually drowsy during the meal? Make sure you then document and report your comments.

Supplements

Other ways of supporting patients nutritionally is through the use of supplements. These supplements come in several forms such as those detailed below:

❑ milk-based sip feeds such as Ensure Plus and Fortisip;

❑ yoghurt style such as Fortifresh;

❑ juice-based supplements such as Enlive and Provide Extra;

❑ high-fat emulsions such as Calogen;

❑ powders such as Scandishake, Calshake, Procal, Maxijul and Quickcal.

In addition, a patient may be encouraged to consume a high-protein or high-calorie diet. This would include selected fortified dishes such as fortified soups and milk puddings, full cream milk, extra butter and frequent meals and snacks throughout the day. Small changes like this to the diet can be enough to prevent further weight loss and promote weight gain.

Enteral nutrition

Elsie Smith's stroke has left her with no gag reflex, which means any food she swallows may go straight into her lungs (aspirate) leading to aspiration pneumonia and possibly even death. Therefore Elsie will need a referral to the dietician and the speech and language therapists (SALT). In addition, her diet will need to be administered through enteral nutrition (also called tube feeding), either in the short term or on a more permanent basis. Enteral nutrition delivers a liquid formula through a tube placed in the patient's stomach (gastric feeding) or intestine (duodenal or jejunal feeding). Gastric enteral nutrition is typically prescribed for:

❏ patients who cannot eat normally due to dysphagia (difficulty swallowing);

❏ patients who are unconscious or intubated;

❏ patients who are recovering from gastrointestinal (GI) surgery;

❏ patients in a hyper-metabolic state (due to burns, sepsis, multiple trauma and cancer).

The location of a feeding tube and type of tube used for enteral nutrition depends on the length of time the enteral feeding is expected to be administered (whether short term or long term), the condition of the patient's gastrointestinal tract and their aspiration risk as well as their overall condition. The different locations of feeding tubes are as follows:

❏ nasogastric (NG) (through the nose);

❏ orogastric (through the mouth);

❏ gastrostomy (through a surgical opening);

❏ percutaneous endoscopic gastrostomy (PEG) (through the abdomen);

❏ nasojejunal (through the nose).

In the case of Elsie Smith she will require the insertion of an NG tube.

Nasogastric tube insertion

NG tubes come in two different widths, wide bore and fine bore. The particular size you choose is based on the condition of your patient, the duration of the feeding programme and type of feed to be administered (see Figure 2).

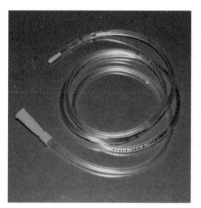
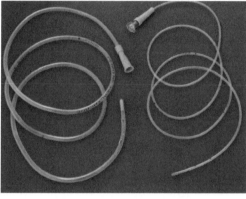

Figure 2
Wide bore and fine bore nasogastric tubing

An advantage of using a wide bore feeding tube is its easy access and, in addition, it is less likely to block than other tubes. However, the disadvantages of wide bore feeding tubes include discomfort and intolerance, rhinitis, pharyngitis, oesophageal erosions/haemorrhage, oesophageal sphincter incompetence/aspiration and respiratory difficulties. Advantages of fine bore tubes are that they allow normal swallowing to continue while they are in place, they are more comfortable, and there is a reduced chance of pharyngitis, rhinitis, lower oesophageal incompetence and mucosal erosions. The disadvantages of fine bore tubes include oesophageal or pulmonary perforation, abdominal distension, vomiting and tube blockage.

Passing a nasogastric tube

Equipment required

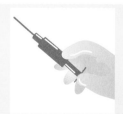

❑ A clinically clean tray/trolley

❑ A nasogastric tube (of the appropriate size)

❑ A sterile receiver

- ❏ Lubricating jelly/sterile water
- ❏ Indicator strips
- ❏ Hypoallergenic tape
- ❏ A 20 ml syringe
- ❏ A spigot
- ❏ A glass of water and a straw
- ❏ A towel or protective pad

Procedure

1. Introduce yourself and ensure you have the correct patient for the procedure.

2. Tell the patient what you are planning to do and the reason for the procedure. Gain the patient's consent – this is to make sure the patient fully understands what is going to happen and is therefore able to give valid consent before the NG tube is passed.

3. Assist the patient into a comfortable semi-upright position either in the bed or a chair, making sure their head is supported by a pillow. This position aids optimal neck/stomach alignment making swallowing easier and ensuring the epiglottis is not obstructing the oesophagus.

4. Place a protective pad or towel across the patient's chest to minimise contact with any gastric content.

5. Arrange a signal – for example raising their hand or tapping the bed/chair – by which the patient can communicate if they want the procedure to be stopped for any reason. This can be a very frightening and uncomfortable process for the patient so ensuring that they have some control over the procedure can reduce their anxiety.

See Chapter 21, page 455.

6. Wash hands according to the universal hand washing guidelines (see Chapter 21, page 455), put on a clean apron and assemble the required equipment. Although this is not an aseptic procedure it is an invasive procedure, therefore it is important to minimise cross-infection.

7. Measure and mark the distance the tube is to be passed. To get the right length of tube, start at the patient's earlobe and measure to the bridge of the nose, and then to the xiphisternum – this ensures the correct length of tube enters into the stomach.

8. Examine the patient's nostrils for deformity/obstructions to determine the best side for insertion. You can check for the most patent nostril by asking the patient to sniff with one nostril closed and then repeat with other nostril. Chose the clearest nostril for NG tube insertion.

9. Lubricate at least 15–20 cm of the tube with a thin coat of lubricating jelly or sterile water (check the protocol of the clinical area). This will reduce friction between the mucous membrane and the tube, making it easier and more comfortable to pass.

10. Insert the end of the tube into the clearest nostril and slide it backwards and inwards along the floor of the nose, past the pharynx and into the oesophagus. This will help the tube pass into the oesophagus by following the natural anatomy of the nose.

11. If there is some resistance you can try rotating the tube slowly and gently as you advance the tube, or withdraw the tube and try again in a slightly different direction and, if necessary, use the other nostril.

12. As the tube passes down into the back of the throat ask the patient to start swallowing or sipping water through a straw. The swallowing action both closes the glottis, enabling the tube to pass into the oesophagus, and focuses the patient's attention on something other than the tube.

13. Withdraw the tube immediately if the patient's respiratory status changes significantly, if the patient begins to cough or turns blue or if the tube coils in the patient's mouth.

14. Advance the tube as the patient swallows until the mark you made on the tube is reached. Again, if, at this point, the patient shows signs of distress remove the tube immediately as this could mean the tube is in the bronchus.

15. Check the tube is in the correct position by aspirating (withdrawing) 0.5 ml/1 ml of gastric content using a 20 ml syringe and testing the aspirate with pH testing paper. Note that it is now not regarded as

good practice to test gastric content with Litmus paper. This is because lung secretions can also give an 'acidic' reading. Using pH paper will give a lower pH reading with gastric contents than it will with lung secretions. An X-ray can also be used to check correct positioning. If you are in any doubt about the position of the tube do not commence feeding. Note, you must always refer to the Trust protocol for your individual areas. Confirming the correct position of NG feeding tubes in adults is essential prior to commencing each feed, before administering medication via the NG tube, following an episode of vomiting or coughing and if you suspect the NG tube has been moved for any reason. Failure to do so could result in the patient aspirating the feed.

16. Secure the tube to the nostril with hypoallergenic dressing tape. In addition, the tube can be secured to the cheek and behind the ear. This is to hold the tube securely in place and to ensure patient comfort.

17. Document:

    – the date and time of procedure;

    – the type of tube used;

    – the length of the tube;

    – the pH and nature of the aspirate;

    – the reason for the NG tube insertion; and

    – the condition of the patient during and after the procedure.

Percutaneous endoscopic gastrostomy (PEG) feeding

Gastrostomy feeding may be recommended if the digestive system is still working well but nutritional support is likely to be needed for more than a few weeks. Gastrostomy feeding involves surgically creating an opening, known as a **fistula**, through the abdominal wall. A feeding tube is then passed through the opening and into the stomach. The feeding tube is held in place with either a stitch, a small inflated balloon around the tube just under the skin, or a flange around the tube just under the skin. Caring for a PEG involves cleaning the area around the tube daily with soap and water and making sure it is thoroughly dried. The tube must be flushed with 30 ml of water before and after each feed.

Hydration and fluid balance

All humans have a basic need for a continuous supply of fluid to maintain the healthy functioning of their bodies. Water intake must match water output to retain balance (**homeostasis**). Water is lost through insensible losses, such as the skin (perspiration) and lungs (respiration), and sensible losses such as urine and stools (elimination). A healthy adult needs an average of 1 ml to 1.5 ml of water per calorie intake consumed. Therefore, if 2,000 calories are consumed in one day, between 2,000 ml (2 litres) and 3,000 ml (3 litres) of fluid must also be consumed (Stockslager *et al.* 2003). Fluid balance is shown in Table 1 (Williams, 2001).

Approximate daily intake	Approximate daily output
1,500 ml in liquid	1,500 ml urine
700 ml in food	150 ml faeces
300 ml metabolism	850 ml insensible losses

Table 1 Fluid balance

Dehydration

When too much fluid is lost and not enough fluid consumed, dehydration will occur. Early signs of mild dehydration include having a dry mouth and feeling thirsty; when thirst becomes noticeable dehydration is already present. At this stage it is important to offer the patient a fresh cold or warm drink immediately. If left untreated at the mild stage dehydration increases, with more signs and symptoms developing. Signs of moderate to severe dehydration include:

❑ sunken eyes;

❑ reduced skin turgor (skin loses its firmness);

❑ reduced urine output (due to the kidneys' attempt to conserve body fluids);

❑ rapid and deep breathing (due to electrolyte imbalance);

❑ tachycardia (fast, weak pulse);

❑ low blood pressure (due to reduced blood volume);

❑ fainting (due to reduced blood supply to vital organs such as the brain);

❑ convulsions.

Signs of severe dehydration are:

❏ cold extremities (hands and feet);

❏ peripheral cyanosis (bluish discoloration of the skin caused by lack of oxygen in the blood);

❏ rapid pulse;

❏ very low or even undetectable blood pressure;

❏ death.

Assessment of dehydration

If you suspect your patient is becoming dehydrated it is important to complete a thorough nursing assessment and commence treatment immediately. This assessment includes obtaining a recent and accurate history of fluid and diet intake.

Thirst

Feeling thirsty is an important sign of fluid depletion. Those suffering fluid loss due to **pyrexia** (high temperature), diarrhoea, vomiting and **hyperglycaemia** experience this sensation of thirst most. Thirst is a natural response to fluid depletion and normally causes people to increase their fluid intake, thereby restoring fluid balance or homeostasis.

The nail-blanch test

The nail-blanch test (or the capillary nail refill test) is performed on the nail beds to test the amount of blood flow to the tissues. The nurse briefly applies pressure to the patient's nail bed using her/his thumb and finger. Once pressure is released the nurse checks how quickly colour returns to the patient's nail bed. If colour returns quickly (after approximately 2 seconds) this would suggest the heart is pumping blood around the body (cardiac function) sufficiently. However, a delayed capillary refill response (approximately 6 seconds or more) would be a sign of poor cardiac function and a reduced circulatory blood volume.

The skin turgor test

The skin turgor test involves gently pinching the skin on the back of the hand and observing how quickly the skin recoils once released. When pinched up, the skin of a healthy person returns immediately to its normal position once released. However, when skin turgor is reduced it can take several seconds longer to recoil and, in the severely dehydrated, it will stay in the pinched position (see Figure 3). This suggests the patient has a fluid volume deficit and that may result in a patient becoming more susceptible to developing pressure sores.

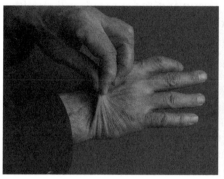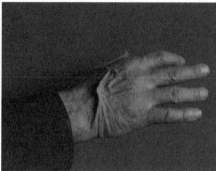

Figure 3
Skin turgor test – note the inelasticity of dehydrated skin

Blood pressure

A low blood pressure often accompanies fluid volume dehydration, resulting in inadequate blood flow to the heart, brain and other vital organs. Symptoms such as dizziness and light-headedness will be experienced. **Postural hypotension** may occur. This can be assessed by the nurse firstly recording the patient's blood pressure while the patient is lying down and then immediately rechecking the patient's blood pressure while they are standing up. A sustained decrease in blood pressure when the patient is standing is known as postural hypotension. In more severe cases of dehydration, hypotension occurs even when the patient is lying flat.

Pulse

A fast pulse, or **tachycardia**, indicates that the heart is beating more rapidly than is normal. The average heart beats at around 80 beats per minute (bpm); a heart rate above 100 bpm is considered tachycardic. There can be lots of causes of tachycardia but, when assessing for dehydration, you not only consider the rate per minute but also the strength and rhythm of the pulse (see Chapter 17). Tachycardia accompanied by a weak thready pulse can be a sign of a decreased intravascular volume caused by dehydration.

See Chapter 17, page 351.

Respiration

See Chapter 17, page 353.

The respiratory rate should be recorded while the patient is at rest and is done by counting the number of breaths taken in by the patient in 1 minute (see Chapter 17). Abnormalities or alteration from the patient's normal (baseline) respiratory rate may indicate an underlying disorder of fluid, electrolyte or acid–base balance. When dehydrated a patient's respiration rate will often increase, becoming more rapid and shallow. This is to compensate for the reduced oxygen supply to both the extremities and the body's organs as a result of the decreased blood volume and blood pressure.

Urine output

See Chapter 21, page 463.

Measuring urine output is important in a patient you suspect is dehydrated. Urine output of less then 500 ml daily is called **oliguria** and may develop as a result of the reduced circulating fluid. The volume, colour and specific gravity of urine can also provide important information about abnormalities and you therefore may be required to do a urinalysis (see Chapter 21).

Other tests for dehydration include:

❑ blood chemistries (electrolytes);

❑ full blood count (FBC);

❑ creatinine;

❑ blood urea nitrogen (BUN).

However, the above blood tests will only be carried out by those specifically trained and qualified to do so.

Dehydration assessment checklist

Using the dehydration assessment checklist shown in Figure 4, we discover that, following her stroke, Elsie Smith has:

❑ a reduced diet and fluid intake;

❑ BP 80/50 mm;

❑ a pulse of 112 bpm;

❑ a respiration rate of 28 breaths per minute;

❑ a urinalysis shows an increase in specific gravity.

Dehydration Assessment Checklist	
Assessment	Check
1. Diet and fluid history	
2. Thirst	
3. Skin/nail blanch test	
4. Skin turgor test	
5. Blood pressure	
6. Pulse	
7. Respirations	
8. Neurological test	
9. Urinalysis	

Figure 4
Dehydration assessment checklist

In addition, Elsie's extremities are cold with poor perforation to her nail bed and she is complaining of dizziness, a headache and feeling thirsty. Elsie is moderately to severely dehydrated and intravenous fluid therapy is prescribed and commenced immediately.

Intravenous fluid therapy

Intravenous (IV) fluid therapy is the administration of sterile liquids directly into a vein to provide volume replacement, to restore and maintain fluid and electrolyte balance, and, in some instances, for nutritional purposes (**parenteral nutrition**) and for the administration of drugs (see also Chapter 5). IV fluids are classed as one of two groups, either **crystalloids** or **colloids**.

See Chapter 5, page 115.

Crystalloids

Crystalloids include normal saline, dextrose solutions and Hartmann's solution, and are so called because they are aqueous in nature, containing water soluble molecules which enable them to pass freely through a semi-permeable membrane.

Colloids

Colloids are more concentrated substances containing larger insoluble molecules which do not pass easily through a semi-permeable membrane and therefore remain in the intravascular compartment for longer. Colloids include Dextran, gelatin (Gelofusine, Haemaccel) and blood.

Both crystalloids and colloids must be prescribed before they can be administered and under no circumstances is a student nurse allowed to connect/reconnect or commence/recommence an IV infusion of any kind. Instead, your role is to observe and report on the condition of the patient receiving the IV infusion and ensure the IV site is free from infection or phlebitis.

Maintaining fluid balance charts

Fluid balance charts provide a record of all fluid intake and output for a 24-hour period. It is of diagnostic significance and maintaining an accurate chart is an important nursing responsibility. Fluid balance charts should not be estimated but must be an accurate record of a patient's actual fluid intake and output. To record the intake you must include fluid gained from all sources, such as drinks or an IV infusion. Similarly, when recording fluid output you must include all sources such as urine, vomit, gastric aspirate, losses from wound or drainage tubes and from diarrhoea. It is important to inform the patient and relatives when a fluid balance chart is in place so they can also record their own fluid input and output where possible. Once the input and output have been totalled there may be a negative or positive balance. A negative balance arises when more fluid has been lost than taken in. In this instance, the negative balance must be reported and acted on. A positive balance means that more fluid has been taken in than lost and is the aim when managing dehydration and fluid volume deficit. Elsie Smith is prescribed 2 litres of normal saline daily and her fluid intake and output is documented on a fluid balance chart. A positive balance is achieved.

Summary

Elsie Smith was at great risk of developing malnutrition and dehydration due to the stroke, which had left her with an inability to swallow. This risk was quickly picked up on following a nutritional assessment and the completion of a dehydration assessment checklist. An IV infusion was commenced to prevent further dehydration, and an NG tube was passed to retain dietary intake. For all patients admitted under our care it is important to establish their nutritional status and individual requirements. This can be achieved by completing a nutritional assessment, including obtaining a dietary history and list of likes and dislikes. Next, we must aim to meet individual needs by assisting to make meal times a pleasant occasion even while in hospital. However, the most important aspect of nutritional care is listening to your patient, respecting their wishes and being patient with them at all times.

Hints

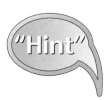

❑ Make sure the food you serve is appetising i.e., that it looks good, smells good and tastes good. If you wouldn't eat it, why should they?

❑ Fifteen minutes before the food arrives remind your patients that it is nearly meal time and get them to talk about what they have ordered. This causes a physiological response where the body begins to prepare itself for eating. Without this process we are unable to consume as much as we may need to. It is funny how we are not hungry until somebody mentions food.

❑ Play music quietly in the background. Research by Ragneskog *et al.* (1996) showed that patients ate twice as much when music was played during mealtimes compared with periods when no music was played. Think about your own experiences in restaurants with background music and restaurants with no music. As a rule we are more self-conscious of the noises we make and conversations that can be overheard when there is no background music, which is not a very relaxing atmosphere to eat in.

❑ Provide condiments for those patients that request it (although not for patients prescribed a low salt or renal diet). In these health-conscious times we are constantly telling our patients what they can and cannot do but, if this results in patients not eating because the food tastes too bland, we are doing them a disservice. This could result in a loss of appetite and weight loss, eventually leading to malnutrition, and all because they wanted salt on their chips.

Further reading

Best, C. (2001) 'Improving practice with a nurse nutrition team'. *Nursing Standard*, 15(19): 41–4

Green, S.M. and Watson, R. (2006) 'Nutritional screening and assessment tools for older adults: literature review'. *Journal of Advanced Nursing*, 54(4): 477–90

Pancorbo-Hidalgo, P.L., Garcia-Fernandez, F.P. and Ramirez, C. (2001) 'Complications associated with enteral nutrition by naso-gastric tube in an internal medicine unit'. *Journal of Clinical Nursing*, 10(4): 482–90

Sargent, C., Murphy, D. and Shelton, B. (2002) 'Nutrition in critical care'. *Clinical Journal of Oncology Nursing*, 6(5): 287–9

Stockslager, J.L., Mayer, B.H., Munden, J., Munson, C. and Theodore, R. (2003) *Nutrition made incredibly easy*. London: Lippincott Williams & Wilkins

References

British Association for Parenteral and Enteral Nutrition (2000) *Malnutrition Universal Screening Tool 'MUST'*. Essex: BAPEN

Clay, M. (2000) 'Nutritious, enjoyable food in nursing homes'. *Elderly Care*, 12(3): 11–15

Green, S.M. and Watson, R. (2005) 'Nutritional screening and assessment tools for use by nurses: literature review'. *Journal of Advanced Nursing*, 50(1): 69–83

McWhirter, J.P. and Pennington, C.P. (1994) 'Incidence and recognition of malnutrition in hospital'. *British Medical Journal*, 308: 945–8

Nursing and Midwifery Council (2007) *Essential Skills Clusters (ESCs) for student nurses*. London: NMC

Ottley, C. (2000) 'Food and mood'. *Nursing Standard*, 15(2): 46–52

Ragneskog, H., Brane, G., Karlsson, I. and Kihlgren, M. (1996) 'Influence of dinner music on food intake and symptoms common in dementia'. *Scandinavian Journal of Caring Science*, 10(1): 11–17

Sapsted, D. (2007) 'Hospital starved our grandmother to death, a family tells inquest'. See: **www.telegraph.co.uk**

Söderhamn, U. and Söderhamn, O. (2002) 'Reliability and validity of the nutritional form for the elderly (NUFFE)'. *Journal of Advanced Nursing*, 37(1): 28–34

Stockslager, J.L., Mayer, B.H., Munden, J., Munson, C. and Theodore, R. (2003) *Nutrition made incredibly easy*. London: Lippincott Williams & Wilkins

Williams, S.R. (2001) *Basic nutrition and diet therapy*, 11th edn. St Louis, MI: Mosby.

MOVING AND HANDLING

Paul Cairns

The Nursing and Midwifery Council has set standards to measure your performance. The Essential Skills Clusters covered in this chapter include Sections 1, 3, 5, 6, 8, 9, 17, 18, 20 and, specifically, **Section 2**:

Patients/clients can trust a newly registered nurse to:

i. Actively involve the patient/client in their assessment and care planning.
ii. Determine patient/client preferences to maximise comfort and dignity.
iii. Actively encourage patient/client to be involved in and/or ensure they are supported in own care/self care.
iv. Support a patient/client to identify their goals.
v. Assess a patient's/client's level of capability for self care.

Overview of manual handling practice

The public and private health services are among the largest employers in the United Kingdom (Heath and Safety Executive) (HSE, 2006). The moving and handling of patients and clients is associated with the greatest risk of musculoskeletal injury for those involved in the direct care of patients and clients (HSE, 2006). Similarly, the HSE reports that more than a third of all over-three-day injuries reported each year involve a musculoskeletal injury as a direct consequence of moving and handling (HSE, 2006). The Department of Health (DoH) (2004) states that more than 11 million working days are lost each year due to back pain and this painful condition costs industry £5 billion. While these figures relate to the overall working population, Retsas and Pinikahana (2000) state that nursing has a higher incidence of back injury than other professions. The Royal College of Nursing (RCN) (2000) illustrates that manual handling injuries affect some 80,000 nurses. In the most recent survey of self-reported work-related illness the HSE (2006) estimated that, in 2001/02, 1.1 million people in Great Britain suffered from musculoskeletal disorders (MSDs) caused or made worse by their current or past workplace situation. In a survey of their members, UNISON (2000) revealed that 32 per cent of respondents in a caring role reported that they regularly experienced back pain. However, more concerning is the fact that the UNISON survey later suggests that 53 per cent of respondents expose themselves to physically lifting loads. This is despite professional nursing guidance that physical lifting should be avoided except in exceptional circumstances (RCN, 2000), and the introduction of manual handling legislation (Manual Handling Operations Regulations – MHOR 1992) which highlights the need for training on a regular basis for those involved in the caring professions.

Reflection

> Despite legislation, patient handling inadequacies remain in place and nurses in particular expect and accept manual handling injuries as part of their role. (Kneafsey, 2000)

Consider the above statement and relate it to your clinical practice. If you have had previous experience of moving and handling, reflect upon those experiences and consider reasons why nurses and caring staff may expose themselves to risk.

The application of the principles of manual handling does not just apply in your professional life. In order to protect our backs we must approach back care holistically. Now consider the activities you do every day of your life and reflect upon how you may actually sustain a back injury. You may be surprised that a lot of your activities involve stooping, twisting and bending. Remember: we don't always see the risk.

Legislative and professional aspects of manual handling practice

The introduction of legislation was intended to reduce the risk of back injury for those in the care sector. However, Lloyd (1997) reports that the introduction of the MHOR 1992 has not had a dramatic impact on the reduction of nurses' back injuries. The key piece of legislation that governs our overall health and safety in the workplace is the Health and Safety at Work Act (HASAWA) 1974. The key component of this legislation is to ensure, so far as is reasonably practicable, the health, safety and welfare at work of all employees. A number of elements are highlighted. These include:

❑ provision of safe systems of work;

❑ ensuring health and safety in the use of these systems;

❑ provision of information, instruction, training and supervision necessary to ensure health and safety.

The HASAWA 1974 provides guidance not only for the employer but also for the employee. As an employee you would, under the legislation, be expected to:

❑ take reasonable care of your own and others' health and safety, where others may be affected by your own acts or omissions;

❑ to co-operate with the employer in performing their duties.

The key elements highlighted relate to the theory and practice of manual handling. In order that manual handling risks are reduced the employer must put in place a system whereby the safety of the employee is protected. Therefore the Management of Workplace Regulations 1999 requires that the employer make a suitable and sufficient assessment of the risks to the employee. Following this assessment, if any possibility should exist that the employee may be exposed to a manual handling risk of injury, then the MHOR 1992 as amended in 2002 would come into force. These regulations govern a wide range of manual handling activities, including lifting, lowering, pushing, pulling or carrying. The load may be either inanimate – such as a box or a trolley – or animate – a person. Specifically the employer must ensure that as a handler you adopt the following approach.

❑ **Avoid** – manual handling so far as is reasonably practicable.

❑ **Assess** – unfortunately it is difficult to avoid manual handling when dealing with people. Assessment would involve assessing the use of resources (carers and equipment), the task and the load.

❑ **Reduce** – reduce the risks of injury where reasonably practicable.

Consideration of the manual handling activities that Mrs Smith requires

Transfer from bed to wheelchair

Having had her nasogastric tube inserted, Mrs Smith now requires an X-ray examination to check its position. In order for the X-ray to take place, Mrs Smith requires assistance to transfer from her bed to the wheelchair. Prior to any manual handling task, Dougherty *et al.* (2004) suggest that the following points should be considered as a means to minimise the risk of injury during manual handling manoeuvres:

❑ the physical aspects of the patient, for example weight, body size and shape, physical fitness and strength;

❑ the psychological aspects, for example cognitive ability, apathy or disinterest.

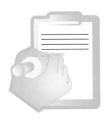

Activity 1.

Prior to carrying out the action on Mrs Smith, what physical and psychological aspects do you need to assess and consider when planning this manoeuvre?

Physical aspects

❑ Weight assessment - this is a fundamental element of manual handling guidance. You must be aware of the loads and weight that you, as a carer, can comfortably manage (MHOR, 1992).

❑ Physical fitness – Mrs Smith is dehydrated and malnourished. Therefore maintaining skin integrity is vital during manual handling manoeuvres.

❑ Physical capabilities – these will be reduced in Mrs Smith; her ability to assist with manoeuvres will be affected by her nasogastric tube and intravenous infusion. Despite this the RCN (2000) suggest that, where appropriate, the patient should be encouraged to be as independent as possible.

❑ Preparing Mrs Smith physically – for example, her clothing and footwear. Do not forget her privacy and dignity.

❑ Communication – are glasses and/or a hearing aid required?

Psychological aspects

❑ Mrs Smith may appear distressed and disinterested, tired and lethargic.

❑ Fear – she may be apprehensive about her future.

❏ Comprehension – this may be impaired due to the effects of hospitalisation and news of her diagnosis.

❏ Communication – consider how you are going to instruct and assist Mrs Smith in the manoeuvre.

Risk factors

In addition to the patient assessment, as a carer you must also consider a number of risk factors in your planning and preparation. Johnson (2005) suggests that the following elements of risk assessment must be included in the overall assessment prior to manual handling activities:

❏ task;

❏ load;

❏ individual capability;

❏ environment;

❏ other factors.

What is the task?

Using our patient Mrs Smith as our example, we have to consider the manual handling activities that are involved in transferring her from bed to wheelchair (this is the task element of risk assessment).

As Mrs Smith has had a stroke we need to consider how this affects the manual handling task. When establishing the elements of risk under the task heading we need to consider the following factors in the assessment and ask ourselves whether the task involves:

❏ holding or manipulating loads away from the body;

❏ twisting, stooping or reaching upwards;

❏ excessive lifting or lowering distances;

❏ excessive carrying distances;

❏ excessive pulling or pushing;

❏ risk of sudden movement of loads;

❏ frequent or prolonged physical effort;

❏ insufficient rest or recovery periods;

❏ a rate of work imposed by a process.

When caring for adult patients you are immediately exposed to handling loads which exceed the guidelines for lifting and lowering as suggested by the manual handling guidelines (MHOR, 1992). Having considered the history and problems that Mrs Smith has, the task of moving her potentially exposes you as a carer to risk of injury as many of the responses to the above issues would be 'yes'.

The load (as a person – Mrs Smith)

While we do not view our patients as loads we must take into account their weight and handling characteristics prior to moving and handling them. You must remember that loads may also be inanimate. However, for the purposes of this assessment, we are concentrating on animate objects, i.e. live patients. Under this heading we must consider the following:

❏ How much help does the person need?

❏ What are the patient's expectations/wishes?

❏ Is the patient able to weight bear?

❏ Is the patient experiencing pain/or on any medication?

❏ Are there tissue viability/wound care issues?

❏ Is the patient able to communicate with others?

❏ What about the level of predictability?

❏ Is the person a vulnerable adult?

❏ Any behavioural issues?

❏ Any cultural issues?

❏ Any physical inabilities due to operations/investigations?

❏ The patient's comfort?

❏ Influencing factors due to body shape?

❏ Height and weight of the person?

❏ History of falls?

Individual capability

This relates to your capability as a handler. This element of risk assessment is vitally important as you must recognise your limitations when you are about to undertake any manual handling activities. You may have previously been exposed to generic manual handling manoeuvres which, for a large variety of your practice, will be suitable. However, in specialist areas of health care, for example spinal injuries and specialist orthopaedic surgery, you may require specific manual handling training. This will include the use of any specialist handling equipment that will be utilised in specialist manual handling techniques.

When considering your own capabilities for manual handling procedures the following is a checklist of questions that you should ask yourself prior to commencing any manual handling activity. By conducting this self-assessment you will ensure you remain fit for purpose in your duties and that patient safety is maintained. Therefore, does the manual handling task require any of the following considerations?

❑ Does it require unusual strength or height?

❑ Does it create a hazard to those who have a health problem, for example a pre-existing back problem or pregnancy?

❑ Is it to be undertaken by someone who doesn't normally take part in manual handling activities, for example occasional visitors or allied health professionals such as a speech therapist?

❑ Does it require specialist information or training – do you have the necessary level of skill, knowledge and competence?

Environment

The environmental considerations are a vital element of the manual handling risk assessment process. Each clinical area or working environment will be unique. Working within a client's home will pose many problems for you during manual handling activities. However, despite the clinical/working environment, it is vitally important that you apply the correct principles of manual handling in all environments. When assessing the environment do any of the following apply?

❑ Are there space constraints on posture? For example, if you are in a client's home when undertaking a dressing to a foot, do you adopt the correct position to avoid stooping?

❑ Are there uneven, slippery or unstable floors? For example, is the floor wet, are you moving from carpeted to smooth flooring surfaces, or are you assisting with a manoeuvre outside, say in a car park from wheelchair into a car?

❑ Are there variations in working levels of floors or surfaces?

❑ Are there extremes of temperature or humidity? Consider the season of year, the time of day.

❑ Are there ventilation problems, for example environmental control measures such as air-conditioning?

❑ Is there poor lighting? Is there sufficient lighting in order to complete the manual handling task?

Equipment

Another important aspect of manual handling is the utilisation of equipment during manual handling activity. While equipment is not required in all manual handling activities we must remember that an important aspect of safer moving and handling is the avoidance of hazardous manual handling. If the patient is unable to manoeuvre themselves independently then you as a carer will need to intervene with the physical aspects of manual handling. The use of equipment may reduce the likelihood of injury to both the client and the carers. However, equipment can introduce positive and negative aspects and the user should be fully aware of the implications of the drawbacks and the benefits of using any handling aid (Johnson, 2005). In Mrs Smith's case we are using a mechanical hoist to facilitate the manoeuvre. Prior to the manoeuvre, consider the following points:

❑ the need for, and use of, handling equipment;

❑ the environment in which the manoeuvre is to take place – consider light, temperature, flooring and obstacles;

❑ the task itself – will it require prolonged effort, or will it require you to potentially adopt an abnormal posture?

❑ the capabilities of you and your team of handlers – are you trained for the task? Are there enough carers to carry out the task?

❑ planning and organisation of the manual handling task – is there teamwork and communication in operation? If used effectively, these assist in eliminating handling injuries.

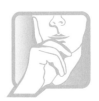

Reflection

Are you now ready to transfer Mrs Smith, based on your assessment?

At this point you may want to consider how you or others have conducted this type of transfer in clinical practice. Patients and clients require assistance with transfer from bed to chair on a regular basis. Reflect on a patient you have looked after during your clinical placement. Consider how many times a day they needed to be moved or have their position changed. As an example, a hospital in-patient would move from bed to chair, or chair to commode/toilet, numerous times each day. Again, reflect on your current/last clinical placement area and consider how many times in one day you were involved in assisting one patient with this manoeuvre.

Perhaps count the number of times that the patient required to use the toilet, got in and out of bed, went for interventions, etc. Now consider how many patients you assisted that day. You may find that the total amount of manual handling manoeuvres in one day or period of duty is quite high, and the greater the number of occasions, the greater the risk of exposure to manual handling injuries.

Moving Mrs Smith

You should bear in mind that Mrs Smith has a right-sided weakness, so she will require additional assistance on her right side. Where possible you should encourage Mrs Smith to use her left arm to help support her during her transfer from the bed to the wheelchair. The manoeuvre should involve two carers: one to support the right side, while the other carer may assist with verbal commands and positive encouragement. Similarly, as the right leg may be weak, the second carer may be required to support this limb during the manoeuvre.

When executing manual handling manoeuvres all carers must remember to protect themselves and apply safe principles of manual handling. For example, carers should keep their spine in a natural posture, not bent or twisted, maintain a stable base, and make sure the load is kept close at all times (Adams and Dolan, 2005). Due to the nature of Mrs Smith's condition it is more appropriate to use mechanical equipment because, as a consequence of her stroke, her ability to weight bear is impaired and you will be dealing with a load which has an unequal weight distribution. Therefore, for the safety of all involved, a hoist will minimise the risk of injury.

Using a hoist

Each clinical area will have a differing range of manufacturers' hoists. As such, it should be a key learning objective for you to understand how to use this vital piece of manual handling equipment in each new clinical area in which you work. The discussion of hoists within this chapter is based upon general principles of hoist usage. Bear in mind that each individual piece of equipment will have unique operating features and you, as the user, must be aware of these prior to use with patients and clients.

When using the hoist in Mrs Smith's situation it will facilitate the movement from bed to chair and maintain safety for both Mrs Smith and the carers involved in the manoeuvre. Orchard (2005) suggests that the use of a hoist and sling can maintain both safety during patient transfer and the dignity of the user. In addition, the use of mechanical equipment may reduce the risk of injury due to back pain experienced by carers (Orchard, 2005). Moreover, Hignett *et al.* (2003) say that mechanical hoists are a component of the equipment that should be available when moving patients and clients on a regular basis. Mechanical equipment also leads to decrease in fatigue, improved comfort during manual handling activities for colleagues and an increased perception of safety among staff (Yassi *et al.*, 2001).

Communication

When assisting Mrs Smith ensure that clear authoritative commands are provided by the lead carer. This ensures that everyone works in unison and therefore reduces the risk of manual handling injury to carers. Johnson (2005) highlights the importance of communication in manual handling activities for both patients and carers. However, no matter how much you plan and prepare you must always remember that patients can be highly unpredictable. Risk assessment is vital to protect both patient and carers, particularly when caring for someone who has a hemiplegia (Crumpton and Hignett, 2005).

A safe environment

Also, in your planning, consider the ergonomics of the working environment that affect manual handling procedures. Can you physically change the environment to promote safety? For example, is the bed height adjustable? Can the bed be moved to accommodate carers, equipment and the patient?

Preparation for hoist transfer

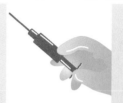

1. Explain the full manual handling procedure to Mrs Smith and gain her consent and co-operation.

2. As a fundamental element of the risk assessment process decide on the number of carers required to complete the manoeuvre. While some hoists can be used by one carer it is safer practice to have two carers – one to support the patient and the second carer to operate and manoeuvre the hoist.

3. Carry out any self-preparation prior to the manoeuvre, for example handwashing. Consider if you are fit for purpose. Prior to using any hoist or mechanical equipment consider the individual capability of risk assessment (see above, page 241). Are you and your colleague proficient, confident and competent in its use? If the answer is 'no' then you must stop and consider alternative ways of moving Mrs Smith. You must not use the hoist until you have received an appropriate level of supervision, instruction and training in the equipment's use.

See this Chapter, page 241.

4. Preparation of the equipment – collect the hoist and ensure it is fit for purpose:

   - Has it sufficient stability to take the load/weight of Mrs Smith? Has it been maintained and serviced regularly in line with the manufacturer's and legislative guidelines (Lifting Operations and Lifting Equipment Regulations 1998; Provision and Use of Workplace Equipment Regulaions 1998).

   - The maximum weight and the date of the last service should be clearly labelled and visible on the hoist.

   - Despite the hoist having regular servicing, it is still an essential element of good practice to ensure the hoist is in good working order prior to each use. The following are points to consider:

❑ Are key parts in working order? For example, ensure the rising and lowering mechanisms and all four brakes are functional and easy to apply and release.

❑ If electrical, has the hoist has been fully charged?

❑ Is the hoist in a clean state?

❑ Do the wheels and the hoist move freely in all directions?

❑ Ensure none of the lubricating fluid is leaking.

5. Sling selection – when selecting the sling for any patient it is important to consider the following general principles:

   – Is it fit for purpose?

   – Are there any rips, holes or tears in the fabric – does it have good integrity?

   – Is it clean – no blood, urine, faeces?

   – Is the label evident? This highlights maximum weight and care instructions.

   – Is it suitable for your patient's physical condition or do you need an adapted sling, for example for toileting, amputees, etc.?

   – Are hooks, straps and clips all in good order, with no cracks or breaks? Is everything in good condition?

Figure 1
A typical hoist sling

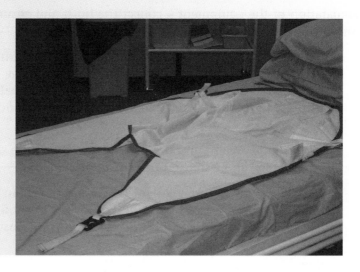

Chapter 11   MOVING AND HANDLING

Figure 1 illustrates a typical hoist sling.

6. Environmental preparation:

– Prepare the working area around the bed to ensure there is enough safe manoeuvring space for the patient, you, your colleague(s) and the equipment that you intend to use.

– You may need to move or reposition the bed and the chair that Mrs Smith is to be transferred into.

– Can the bed locker and bed table be moved temporarily?

– Can the bed mechanisms accommodate the legs/base of the hoist?

– Can you manoeuvre Mrs Smith without detriment to her privacy and dignity? For example, will the curtains close around the bed effectively when you are undertaking the manoeuvre in the hoist?

– Is the floor safe to manoeuvre the hoist? For example, make sure there are no spillages or recent domestic activities.

– Make sure there are no electrical cables in the way, from fans, beds or equipment for example.

Once you have established that the environment is safe you can proceed with manoeuvring Mrs Smith into the sling and hoist.

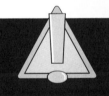

Be aware that all hoists are different in clinical practice. This section provides general principles of hoist and sling usage. Prior to using any mechanical equipment you will need specific training in the use of that particular handling device.

Planning

7. Plan with your colleagues how you intend to position Mrs Smith in the sling. Remember the fundamental principles of manual handling practice. Consider your working height when manoeuvring patients on the bed. As a manual handling team you and your colleague(s) must decide if the working height eliminates or reduces the need for twisting, stooping or bending during the positioning or handling.

8. When you are planning how to roll Mrs Smith, consider which side you are intending to roll her onto. If you choose to roll her on the affected side (right-sided weakness), decide how many carers this may take. If Mrs Smith can assist with this manoeuvre then you are avoiding manual handling or reducing the risk of injury to you as a carer. Mrs Smith can utilise the bed rails or cot sides which would promote independence and assist you as a carer in positioning the hoisting sling. If utilising cot sides in any manual handling procedure ensure that they are positioned correctly and are safely secured to prevent accidental injuries.

9. Patients who may have some ability to assist in the manoeuvre mean that you can effectively avoid some physical manual handling. However, it is important that you provide clear and direct instructions prior to any proposed manoeuvre that the patient is expected to undertake themselves. To facilitate the manoeuvring of Mrs Smith you should instruct her to reposition her left leg by crossing it over her right leg. Similarly her left arm should be crossed over her torso and she should be encouraged to reach for and hold onto the cot side to assist with rolling. In addition her head should be positioned to look to the right. All these small manoeuvres help to raise the left side of the body which will make the manoeuvring and positioning much easier for Mrs Smith to do with a degree of independence (see Figure 2(a)–(e)).

Figure 2 (a)–(e)
A patient repositioning himself onto his right side

(a)

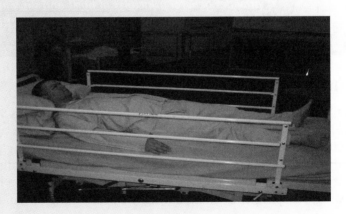

(b)

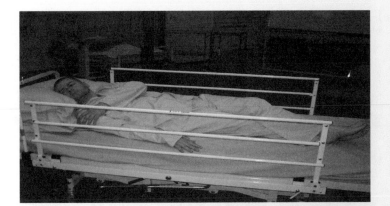

Figure 2
continued

(c)

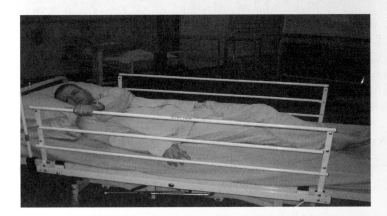

(d)

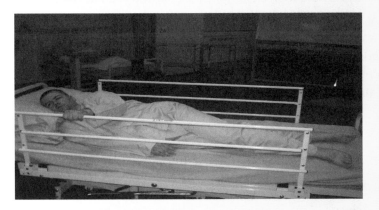

Figure 2 (e)
continued

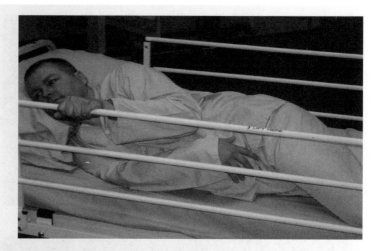

10. If, following assessment, Mrs Smith is not able to assist you with repositioning herself onto her right-hand side then you and your colleague will need to intervene. Bear in mind that, if you do intervene, you must never work over the cot side as this will cause you undue musculoskeletal stresses and strains. In addition, your working base may be affected – for example, will your feet remain flat on the floor in this situation?

11. Positioning to the right-hand side may involve two or more carers. However, always base this on your assessment of load – the size, shape, actual weight of the patient and their ability to assist. Prior to assisting always ensure that the opposite side of the bed has the cot side in place in order to avoid the risk of falling from bed during the procedure.

12. When rolling Mrs Smith onto the left-hand side you will need to position her weakened limbs on the right side. When doing so consider the risk factors involved and the physical comfort of the patient.

    – Don't bend or twist unnecessarily – consider your posture throughout.

    – Remember that weakened limbs will be heavy and, as such, holding them and positioning them means that you are handling a load away from the body. Therefore, in order to remain safe, always keep loads close to your centre of gravity. In this case this will mean the arm and leg of the affected side.

- When positioning the right arm ensure it is placed so that it will not be crushed during rolling – i.e. place Mrs Smith's right arm on her left shoulder to avoid the right arm being crushed by the abdomen during rolling.

- When positioning the lower limbs, position the right leg over the left leg.

- Also position the head of Mrs Smith to look to the left.

13. At this stage you and your colleague should be ready to assist Mrs Smith in the manoeuvre. Ensure that you work as a team and decide on your instructional commands during the manual handling procedure. Always ensure that commands are clear – for example, when using the commands 'ready', 'steady', 'roll', are you both moving on the 'roll' command? Also ensure that Mrs Smith is aware of this too. Ensuring that everyone in the team is moving at the same time will reduce the risk of injury.

14. Prior to the manoeuvre ensure:

    - The working height is still safe for both carers.

    - Your working base is safe;

        ❏ Your feet are hip width apart;
        ❏ Your knees and hips are slightly flexed;
        ❏ One foot is slightly in front of the other in a walking position;
        ❏ In terms of spinal awareness your posture is natural and upright.

    If these factors are observed then your safety should be maintained.

15. When undertaking the manoeuvre one of the carers should assume the lead co-ordinating role. This facilitates communication for the carers and the patient.

Positioning the sling

16. Once Mrs Smith is positioned on her side the sling can be rolled into position under her left side. When positioning the sling ensure, as far as possible, that it is evenly placed, crease free and that you have enough room to position her safely with an equal

amount of sling distributed across the mattress so that she is positioned centrally on the sling. When the sling has been positioned encourage Mrs Smith to roll onto her back. Advise her that this may be temporarily uncomfortable, depending on the thickness of the sling.

Bed manoeuvres

While the hoist can be used for the transfer of patients from bed to chair, when moving patients in bed other pieces of manual handling equipment can be utilised. These include the use of electric profiling beds. These beds can assist in the movement of patients with decreased mobility (Orchard, 2005) as they eliminate some of the handling tasks that the carer normally performs – for example, moving a patient from a lying to a sitting position – as the profiling bed will do this mechanically. The beds can be operated by the patient, if they are able, and this promotes independence. In our situation the controller unit would need to be placed at the non-weak side of Mrs Smith. In addition, other pieces of equipment could be used to help patients move in bed. These include rope ladders, bed rails and trapeze (monkey pole) (see Figure 3).

Figure 3
Some moving and handling equipment

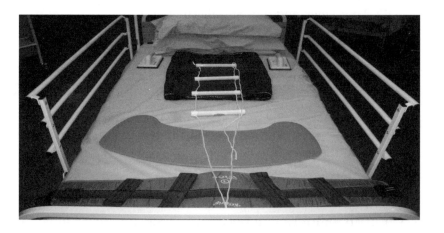

Reflection

Think about how you will react if your clinical mentor asks you to assist her with a moving and handling procedure that contravenes the safe guidelines. What would be your rationale for your reaction? Reflect on this honestly.

Summary

Throughout this chapter we have discussed the principles and practices related to safe, effective moving and handling procedures. During your clinical placements as a student nurse you will, unfortunately, witness nurses and other health care professionals performing unsafe, ritualistic practices that will conflict with what you have been taught in your higher education institution. This may be due to a variety of reasons, such as:

❏ lack of physical resources, such as hoists and other moving and handling equipment;

❏ lack of time – have you ever heard the line: 'We are too busy to do it properly'?

❏ lack of training.

These excuses are invalid because, as we have learned, employers are obliged by law to provide the resources required to move and handle loads safely. However, despite this, as a student nurse you may be invited to participate in these outdated and unsafe practices. You are now faced with a dilemma. You can either:

❏ collude with the perpetrator and participate in the unsafe or outlawed practice, jeopardising both the patient's safety and your own back; or

❏ politely refuse to participate and insist that the correct moving and handling techniques are employed.

The latter alternative will require some assertion and, perhaps, bravery on your part, but will ultimately make you a better and more professional nurse. It is your choice but remember the following points.

❏ If you injure your back, you will find it extremely difficult to work as a nurse. This may have short-term implications for your economic situation and, perhaps, even graver long-term implications for your career.

❑ If you injure yourself, or one of your patients, while using the correct techniques as stipulated in the Trust's policies and procedures manual, you will be covered by the Trust's insurers through vicarious liability. If you work outside these guidelines, however, say by cutting corners to save time, you may find yourself accused of the civil offence of negligence.

❑ As a student you are not yet accountable to your profession. However, you do have responsibilities to work within the scope of your own capabilities, using the methods you have been taught.

In short, if you are ever tempted, or asked, to contravene the Code of Conduct – don't do it.

References and further reading

Adams, M. and Dolan, P. (2005) 'Biomechanics of low back pain'. In Smith, J. (ed.), *The guide to the handling of people*, 5th edn. Teddington, Middlesex: Backcare/RCN, pp. 45–56

Crumpton, E. and Hignett, S. (2005) 'Evidence-based practice'. In Smith, J. (ed.), *The guide to the handling of people*, 5th edn. Teddington, Middlesex: Backcare, pp. 111–16

Department of Health (2004) *The prevalence of back pain in Great Britain*. London: DoH

Dougherty, L., Lister, S.E., Lee, S.J. and Otunbade, E. (2004) 'Moving and handling of patients'. In *The Royal Marsden Hospital manual of clinical nursing procedures*, 6th edn. Oxford: Blackwell

Health and Safety Executive (2006) *Health and safety in health and social care services*. London: HSE [online at: **www.hse.gov.uk/healthservices/index.htm** (last accessed 5 July 2007)]

Hignett, S., Crumpton, E., Ruszala, S., Alexander, P., Fray, M. and Fletcher, B. (2003) 'Evidence-based patient handling: systematic review'. *Nursing Standard*, 17(33): 33–6

Johnson, C. (2005) 'Manual handling risk assessment – theory and practice'. In Smith, J. (ed.), *The guide to the handling of people*, 5th edn. Teddington, Middlesex: Backcare/RCN, pp. 89–110

Kneafsey, R. (2000) 'The effect of occupational socialisation on nurses' patient handling practices'. *Journal of Clinical Nursing*, 9(4): 585–93

Lloyd, P. (ed.) (1997) *The guide to the handling of patients: introducing a safer handling policy*, 4th edn. Middlesex: NBPA/RCN

Orchard, S. (2005) 'Lying to sitting'. In Smith, J. (ed.), *The guide to the handling of people*, 5th edn. Teddington, Middlesex: Backcare/RCN, pp. 189–222

Retsas, A. and Pinikahana, J. (2000) 'Manual handling activities and injuries among nurses: an Australian hospital study'. *Journal of Advanced Nursing*, 31(4): 875–83

Royal College of Nursing (2000) *Introducing a safer handling policy*. London: RCN

UNISON (2000) *Manual handling and back pain in the public sector: a survey for UNISON by the Labour Research Department*. London: UNISON

Yassi, A., Cooper, J.E., Tate, R.B., Gerlach, S., Muir, M., Trottier, J. and Massey, K. (2001) 'A randomised controlled trial to prevent patient lift and transfer injuries of health care workers'. *Spine*, 26(16): 1739–46

BREAKING BAD NEWS

Chapter 12

Sam Pollitt

The Nursing and Midwifery Council (NMC) Essential Skills Cluster (ESC) most relevant to breaking bad news is 'Care, Compassion and Communication'.

Patients/clients can trust a newly registered nurse to:

Section 1	Provide care based on the highest standards, knowledge and competence.
Section 2	Engage them as partners in care. Should they be unable to meet their own needs then the nurse will ensure that these are addressed in accordance with the known wishes of the patient/client or in their best interests.
Section 3	Treat them with dignity and respect them as individuals.
Section 4	Care for them in an environment and manner that is culturally competent and free from discrimination, harassment and exploitation.
Section 5	Provide care that is delivered in a warm, sensitive and compassionate way.
Section 6	Listen, and provide information that is clear, accurate and meaningful at a level at which the patient/client can understand.
Section 7	Protect and treat as confidential all information relating to themselves and their care.
Section 8	Ensure that their consent will be sought prior to care or treatment being given and that their rights will be respected.

Introduction

Breaking bad news is considered one of the most difficult and anxiety-provoking activities that nurses may have to undertake. If handled poorly by the health care professional it can have far-reaching consequences for all involved. Although previously considered a predominantly medical task, with the increase in nurse specialist posts and an increased awareness by patients of their own symptoms and diagnosis, it can fall to the qualified nurse to break bad news either to the patients or relatives. It requires highly skilled communication and interpersonal skills, which the Nursing and Midwifery Council (NMC) Essential Skills Clusters (ESCs) (2007) identify as a fundamental skill. Therefore the aim of this chapter is to discuss the breaking of bad news to Elsie Smith who, following her admission to a general ward with a stroke, has developed **aspiration pneumonia** that is not responding to treatment. The prognosis (expected outcome) is poor as her condition deteriorates daily.

What is bad news?

Buckman (1992, p.15) defines bad news as 'any information which adversely and seriously affects an individual's view of his or her future'. Therefore anything can be classed as bad news if it is negatively significant to an individual. What may be considered bad news to one person may be immaterial to another. However, whatever the bad news is, it is always difficult to give and always more stressful to receive.

Reflection

Reflect on the last time you received bad news.

1. Think about who gave you the news

2. How did they break the news to you?

3. What did they say to you?

4. How did you feel?

5. How would you prefer to have been told the news?

How to break bad news

There is no prescriptive way to break bad news as the words and approach you use with one patient may not be appropriate with another. As with all care, the breaking of bad news must be individualised to the needs and wishes of each particular patient. However, the way bad news is given can impact on how a patient copes with and adjusts to the news (Chauban and Long, 2000). Therefore, the following action plan can be used as a guide for breaking bad news.

Breaking bad news action plan

Preparation	Action	Reason
1. Information	Make sure you have all the facts before you break bad news.	To enable you to be clear about what you need to say and plan how you are going to say it. You may use both verbal and written information and even diagrams to ensure full comprehension.
2. Environment	Ensure you and your patient have comfort and privacy (free from interruptions).	To ensure sensitivity to your patient's reaction to potentially devastating news, and to facilitate communication and openness.
3. Support	Arrange for the patient to have someone with them at their request.	This may be a relative, a friend or another member of the health care team who acts as an advocate, spokesperson or even just a support for the patient.
4. Awareness	Ask your patient what they already know and understand about their illness.	To assess and clarify the patient's current understanding of their illness and to identify at what level to deliver the new information.
5. Request	Find out how much information your patient wants to know about their illness, diagnosis, treatment or prognosis.	Not all patients want to know, or feel able to cope with, the details of their condition or prognosis. Therefore it is important to establish how much your patient really wants to know before you disclose this information. Remember they can request more information at a later date.
6. Dialogue	Provide the information in clear manageable amounts at the patient's own pace and avoid using medical jargon.	To enable absorption of the information just received and ensure clear understanding.
7. Clarification	Check the patient has received information correctly by repeating key points and asking them to tell you what they understand about what you have just told them.	Continuously checking understanding throughout your discussion with the patient allows you to assess how much of the information they have taken in and what may need repeating.
8. Empathy	Allow your patient to express their feelings and emotions openly. Recognise and validate their responses.	Empathising with a patient demonstrates to the patient that you understand how they feel.
9. Comfort	Spend time with your patient after you have broken the news.	To enable the patient to work through their early emotions to a point where you can plan their next step together. Even if their prognosis is poor you must still discuss their options in relation to managing their illness, care, any pain and even their social and financial responsibilities.
10. Debrief	Once you are safely able to leave your patient in the care of another member of staff or their relatives, reflect on this experience with your mentor, clinical supervisor or manager.	Breaking bad news is a stressful and emotional responsibility. Therefore it is important for you to debrief as soon as is practical after the event. Taking care of yourself is as important as taking care of your patient.

In addition, there are other useful guidelines on breaking bad news you can refer to such as the Baile *et al.* (2000) six-step protocol for delivering bad news.

In relation to Elsie Smith, a time was arranged when the consultant and a staff nurse could meet with Elsie to discuss her worsening condition. Permission was gained from Elsie for her husband Walter to attend the meeting. At this time Elsie was feeling too weak to be manoeuvred in and out of her bed so she was transferred into a side room for privacy and comfort. The consultant broke the news to Elsie and her husband ensuring they both understood the information clearly and answering any questions they had empathetically. After a while, Elsie and Walter were left alone for a few minutes while the staff nurse arranged for some tea to be brought to their room. Then the staff nurse went back to Elsie and Walter and spent time answering any further questions they had and discussing their concerns.

Answering difficult questions

It can be a useful technique to reflect a patient's questions back in an empathetic way. It can clarify why the patient is asking the question. Many questions may not be answerable due to the uncertainty of health, life and death. Therefore it is more beneficial to explore the patient's own feelings, concerns and wishes as appropriate.

Avoiding bad practice

❏ Do not – give news to relatives before the patient.

❏ Do not – agree to a relative's demands to withhold information from the patient (this is collusion).

❏ Do not – use euphemisms such as 'little lump' instead of 'cancer', 'gone to sleep' instead of 'died' (this is commonly used when speaking to children but can cause serious misunderstanding).

❏ Do not – make assumptions about the patient's understanding.

The dying person

According to the National Hospice Organisation (NHO) Gallup survey (1992), 90 per cent of all respondents want to die in their own home, surrounded by their own things and their loved ones. In reality, 74 per cent of all deaths occur in institutions; 57 per cent of these are in hospitals and 17 per cent are in nursing homes, 20 per cent are at home and 6 per cent occur in other places. This means you will encounter dying patients at some point in your nursing career. Although a student nurse will not be the person required to break bad news to a patient you will be required to care for and communicate with terminally ill or dying patients. Because of this, many student nurses worry about issues such as: who is responsible for telling a patient they are dying; what do I say to a dying patient and what should I do if they ask me directly if they are dying? The following section aims to address some of these key issues and suggest ways to respond to a dying patient.

Who is responsible for telling a patient they are dying?

A consultant, doctor or delegated other such as a qualified nurse, never a student nurse, is responsible for telling a patient that they are dying. Although a student nurse should never be responsible for officially telling a patient their prognosis, you can still have a conversation about their illness, death and dying and how they feel about it.

What if they ask me directly 'am I dying?'

Avoid poor responses: never lie and say 'no, you are not' if you know they *are* dying. Never accuse them of being silly by saying such a thing. Never ignore their question or change the subject and never walk away, leaving the question hanging in the air, claiming you are going to get someone to come back and talk to them – your actions will have already answered the question for them. Instead, stop whatever you were doing, sit down and ask the patient why they think they might be dying. This demonstrates that you are taking their concerns seriously and allowing them to explore their own understanding of and feelings about the situation. After listening to your patient you may find they have decided they do not want to know if they are dying. In this instance you must respect their wishes. However, you must still report what happened to the nurse in charge. Alternatively, the patient may still be indicating that they do want to know if they are dying, in which case you can now suggest you will go and get someone qualified to come and talk to them. Always make sure that someone does go back to the patient.

What do I say to a dying patient?

The most important words a nurse can say to a dying patient are: 'How can I help you the most?' In addition, you can share other patients' experiences. For example, you can say things such as 'when I've nursed previous patients who were dying they've found this (music therapy, back rubbing, reading the Bible, etc.) very comforting, helpful or useful'. Comments like this make the dying patient aware they are not alone, that many people have been through this experience and that you are there to help them through it.

What if they ask me to put them out of their misery?

Do not ignore them or pretend you did not hear the request. Instead, ask them directly why they have asked you to do that. This turns the focus back to them as they now need to respond to your question. Your role is to listen. This question may be linked to the stage of grief they are in and/or the fear or unbearable pain they are experiencing. In particular, people say things like this when they feel like they are not in control. You can help them get back that control in other areas such as giving them control over their pain, and giving them practical control over what time they get up or go to bed, what they eat and some of their treatment, etc.

What if they say 'why me, why now?'

Tell them the truth and answer that you don't know 'why them and why now', then turn your response into an empathetic statement such as 'it's hard, isn't it'. This will enable the patient to open up to you about how they are really feeling. Questions such as this may indicate that the patient could be in the anger phase of the grieving process and should be allowed to express that anger safely and with support.

What if they say to me 'how would you feel?'

Be honest and sincere. How would you really feel if it was you?

Summary

Due to her swallowing difficulties Elsie Smith developed aspiration pneumonia after inhaling food and fluids. She was commenced on antibiotics but did not respond to treatment. Elsie's condition began to worsen and it became clear she would eventually develop respiratory failure and the prognosis was poor. It was decided by the consultant to break this news to Elsie and her husband so they could prepare for the worst. Following a breaking bad news action plan enabled the news to be broken in a caring manner, ensuring privacy, clarity and empathy.

Hints for practice

"Hint"

❏ Be sensitive. You may have nursed many dying patients, but if you become insensitive to their needs and feelings you are failing to care.

❏ Be there. Avoiding a dying patient out of fear of what to say to them is the worst thing you can do. Better to have the company of someone with nothing to say than to be alone at the point of death.

❏ Be honest. Although a student nurse will not be the person required to break bad news to a patient or tell them they are dying, you must never lie about their diagnosis or prognosis.

❏ Be realistic. Never give your patient false hope.

Further reading

Kubler-Ross, E. and Kessler, D. (2005) *On grief and grieving: finding the meaning of grief through the five stages of loss*. New York: Simon & Schuster

References

Baile, W.F., Buckman, R., Lenzi, R., Glober, G., Beale, E.A. and Kudelka, A.P. (2000) 'SPIKES – a six-step protocol for delivering bad news: application to the patient with cancer'. *Oncologist*, 5: 302–11

Buckman, R. (1992) *Breaking bad news: a guide for health care professionals*. Baltimore, MD: Johns Hopkins University Press

Chauhan, G. and Long, A. (2000) 'Communication is the essence of nursing care 1: breaking bad news'. *British Journal of Nursing*, 9(14): 931–8

National Hospice Organization Gallup Survey (1992) *Gallup poll reveals first American attitudes about terminal illness and hospice care*, Press Release. Arlington, VA: National Hospice Organization, 29 July.

Chapter 13

LAST OFFICES

Angela Wilton

The Nursing and Midwifery Council (NMC) Essential Skill Cluster (ESC) most relevant to this chapter is 'Care, Compassion and Communication'.

Patients/clients can trust a newly registered nurse to:

Section 1   Provide care based on the highest standards, knowledge and competence.

Section 2   Engage them as partners in care. Should they be unable to meet their own needs then the nurse will ensure that these are addressed in accordance with the known wishes of the patient/client or in their best interests.

Section 3   Treat them with dignity and respect them as individuals.

Section 4   Care for them in an environment and manner that is culturally competent and free from discrimination, harassment and exploitation.

Section 5   Provide care that is delivered in a warm, sensitive and compassionate way.

Section 6   Listen, and provide information that is clear, accurate and meaningful at a level at which the patient/client can understand.

Section 7   Protect and treat as confidential all information relating to themselves and their care.

Section 8   Ensure that their consent will be sought prior to care or treatment being given and that their rights will be respected.

Introduction

Mrs Smith's relatives have been called and asked to come to the hospital. She is not for resuscitation due to her poor prognosis. However, before her relatives arrive, you check on her and it appears that she has stopped breathing and you think she has died. What is it you need to do now?

Last offices

The term 'last offices' relates to the care given to a deceased person. Respect, dignity, communication skills with relatives, staff and patients, cultural and religious beliefs, knowledge of local policies and procedures are all issues health care professionals must consider when dealing with a deceased individual.

Death remains a taboo subject for many and, although policies and procedures may prescribe the necessary actions required by staff dealing with the transition from a living person to a dead body, all nurses need to consider their own personal views, values and culture surrounding the handling of patients after death.

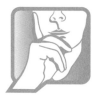

Reflection

Ask yourself the following questions:

- ❑ What experience of death and dying have you had in your own life?

- ❑ How might this affect you in your professional role?

- ❑ How would you like nurses to deal with your loved ones when they die?

- ❑ What are the important issues for relatives when a loved one dies?

- ❑ How can we accommodate both patients' and relatives' needs during this important time?

- ❑ If you were unsure of any religious practices peculiar to a particular religion where would you go for advice/help?

Religious and cultural beliefs

As a health care professional you will come into contact with a variety of religious or cultural beliefs – for example, Catholic, Church of England, Muslim, Sikh, Jehovah's Witness – so it is advisable to become familiar with those most prevalent in your area of practice. Here is a brief summary of the last offices practices of some UK religions.

Catholicism

When death is imminent, Roman Catholics may wish for a priest to carry out the sacrament of the 'Anointing of the Sick', which is also known as the Last Rites or Extreme Unction. If appropriate to their state of health, the patient may also wish to receive Holy Communion and confess their sins to a Catholic priest or chaplain.

There are no particular rituals associated with last offices for Roman Catholics, and this also applies to other forms of Christianity.

Hinduism

Death in hospital can cause considerable religious distress to a Hindu patient and their family and they should, if at all possible, be allowed to die at home. If they are to die in hospital, they will need to be in a situation in which they can be surrounded by their family. The family will want to read passages from holy texts, say prayers with their dying relative and perform certain required ceremonies.

After death, real distress may be caused if a non-Hindu touches the body without wearing disposable gloves, so this should be avoided at all costs. Unless otherwise advised by the family, close the eyes and straighten the legs. Do not attempt to cut any hair, nails or beards. Hands should be placed on the chest with the palms together and fingers under the chin. Religious objects or jewellery should not be removed. The body should be wrapped in a plain white sheet.

Judaism

A Jew who is dying may wish to hear or recite special psalms (particularly Psalm 23). After death the body should be touched by care staff as little as possible and disposable gloves should be worn at all times. Contact should be made with either the next of kin or the Rabbi as soon as possible as they will arrange for the preparation of the body. The face should be covered with a clean cloth or sheet, arms should not be crossed but left at the side of the body with palms facing inwards. Any catheters, drains and tubes should be left in place, as should any wound dressings. Open wounds should be covered. If the patient dies at night the light should be left on when there is no one in the room or bed space. Female bodies should be attended to by female care staff and, if at all possible, male bodies by male care staff.

Islam

As death approaches, a Muslim patient will expect to have their family and friends around them, which sometimes amount to a considerable number of people visiting at any one time. If this happens, caring for the patient in a side room may be preferable. If members of the family are not in attendance when death occurs, health care staff should wear disposable gloves so that they do not directly touch the body. The person's head should be turned towards Mecca (usually south-east in the UK), the arms and legs straightened, eyes and mouth closed and the body covered entirely with a clean white sheet. Female bodies should be attended to by female care staff and, if at all possible, male bodies by male care staff. The remaining preparation of the body will be carried out by a member of the family, who should be contacted immediately.

Sikhism

Sikhs have five 'signs' which they should wear at all times, known as the 'five Ks'. They are the:

❑ kesh – uncut beard and hair;

❑ kangha – wooden comb;

❑ kara – a steel bracelet worn on the right wrist;

❑ kirpan – sharp knife with a double-edged blade (often now in the UK in the form of a badge/brooch);

❑ kaccha – long underpants/trousers.

If a member of the family is not available when death occurs, health care staff should wear disposable gloves to avoid direct contact with the patient. Do not undress the body, wash the body or remove any of the five Ks, as that is something the family would wish to carry out themselves. Drains and other tubes can be removed. The body should then be wrapped in a clean white cloth/sheet ready for the family to care for.

Buddhism

A Buddhist who knows that they are dying will probably wish to have their family and friends with them to meditate and chant mantras as death approaches. They will need as much peace and quiet as possible to allow this to happen. After death, do not touch or move the body of a Buddhist patient until advice has been sought from an appropriate source (for example, the family, friends or the hospital chaplain).

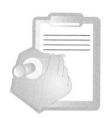

Activity 1.

Find out more about the most common religious and cultural ideologies in your area of the United Kingdom and familiarise yourself with any specific beliefs, rituals or preferences when handling deceased members of their communities.

Policies and procedures

Last offices policies can vary across the country so it is therefore important to familiarise yourself with your own Trust policy, preferably before you encounter a death on the ward. Ideally, last offices policies should be addressed in initial orientation packages for all new staff and students. The policy should also be easily accessible and visible in case deaths in that particular clinical area are not commonplace. Therefore information that you may not remember from your training should be available at the time you experience and/or are required to manage a death on the ward. Also, health and safety, infection control and legal requirements must always be considered. These might include requirements for dealing with MRSA patients, the certification of death, removal of tubes and IV lines, safe manual handling practices, etc. The following is a general guide to some of the actions required when conducting last offices. These are examples of the actions required but this is by no means comprehensive, and consideration of the deceased as an individual within a particular social community must be respected at all times.

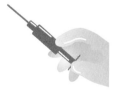

❑ Ensure privacy and dignity by drawing curtains securely.

❑ Contact the appropriate member of the nursing or medical team to certify or verify the death. Check in the deceased's medical notes for any information regarding tissue donation, religion, culture, etc., as it is important to know these things prior to any discussion with relatives.

❑ Inform relatives/next of kin. See Chapter 12 for the way in which this delicate communication should be handled.

See Chapter 12, page 256.

❑ This is a good time to ask, if you are not sure (or there is nothing documented in the medical notes), about organ donation, religious or cultural preferences. Ask the relatives if they wish to see the hospital chaplain or any other appropriate religious leader.

❏ Ask if relatives wish to view the patient on the ward or in the chapel of rest at a later date. Check your local policy regarding this, as some Trusts have a specific time limit for relatives to attend on the ward, while others may prefer relatives to visit the deceased in the mortuary or chapel of rest. Ensure you have all the details the relatives will need to arrange this and give directions to find the appropriate hospital entrance if the relatives are not being accompanied by staff. Also, be clear about any particular arrangements for night-time and weekend visits.

❏ If the patient has been transferred from a nursing or residential home, ask the next of kin for permission to inform relevant staff and do so as soon as possible.

Patient handling

Again, local policies differ but most Trusts stipulate that the deceased person's personal hygiene should be attended to prior to relatives viewing (if appropriate) and before moving to the mortuary. However, relatives may wish to attend to this, which is why it is important to check for religious and cultural preferences and to ask. If relatives are attending to the body then nursing staff should be present throughout to ensure correct procedures regarding property and valuables are carried out. If last offices are performed by staff there should always be two people present to witness and sign all appropriate documentation.

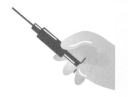

The procedure for performing last offices

❏ Wear gloves and aprons (as per infection control policy).

❏ If the death is to be referred to the coroner (if, for example the death has been unexpected or the cause of death is unknown), then all tubes, IV cannulae, catheters, etc., must be left in position. However, remember to seal these with spigots or leakage will occur and this may be distressing for relatives. If you are in any doubt about tubes, etc. then leave them in place.

❏ Leakage from orifices should be attended to and pads or pants used to absorb this. Remember to warn relatives or inexperienced staff about this and about the potential for air to be released when moving the body while it is being washed.

❏ Male patients may be shaved (using wet or electric shavers). Apply E45 cream to the skin to prevent brown streaks occurring.

❏ Attend to mouth care and hair care as appropriate. Dentures should be replaced in the mouth if possible. If this is not possible, then they must be placed in a plastic pot clearly labelled with patient's name and hospital number, and then the dentures in the pot should be placed in property bags so that staff in the mortuary can retrieve them quickly and easily. Record this in patient property records.

❏ Dress the patient in their own nightwear, a hospital gown or a shroud, depending on Trust policy. If there is a risk of a communicable disease or infection, adhere to the relevant policy. Please note that if you dress your patient in their own nightwear, this should be recorded in the property book. Remove jewellery (although wedding rings are usually left in place, often taped securely to the finger). If relatives request jewellery to be left in place then do so. Again, record this clearly in the property book and ensure all property is collected and documented safely. If there is any property held within the ward safe ensure that this is also accurately recorded.

❏ No property or valuables should be given to relatives, unless they have signed for it first. Often Trusts and clinical departments have a specific patient property procedure that should be followed. This procedure will include the way in which property should be handled and delivered safely to the Patient Affairs Office, etc. (For example ward clerks or porters may be responsible for collecting property, notes and X-rays, which may need to be put into a zipped bag for confidentiality).

❏ Once the patient is clean, dry and dressed appropriately, place them in a neutral supine position. Close the eyelids. Apply gentle pressure for approximately 30 seconds if necessary.

❏ A pillow under the jaw may be required to support jaw closure but remember to remove this before relatives enter to view.

❏ Ensure identity bracelets are in place (often two are required, one on the wrist and one on the ankle). Cover the patient with a clean sheet and perhaps a counterpane, allowing the arms and face to be exposed for relatives to touch and say goodbye.

❑ Clear the room and bed area of all medical equipment and subdue the lighting. This helps to create a peaceful environment in which the bereaved relatives can spend some time saying goodbye to their loved one.

❑ Remember, people deal with grief in very many ways, and it is part of your job as a nurse to support them through this distressing period. This may make you feel extremely awkward at first, but as your career and experience moves forward, you will become more confident in this type of situation.

Transfer

Prior to escorting the deceased patient to the mortuary with the porters, ensure that the 'Notice of Death' forms are attached at the appropriate places. Commonly, they are secured with tape to the patient's nightwear, with another taped to the top sheet, which is ultimately used to wrap the patient in. A final copy is stapled to the front of patient's notes. Check your local Trust policy for more details. Request transfer from the ward to the mortuary and ensure privacy, dignity and respect during this journey. Use appropriate moving and handling techniques to ensure staff and patient safety.

Informing all appropriate individuals

Ensure the appropriate office (for example, the Patient Affairs Office) has been informed of the patient's death and any ward database system is updated according to hospital policy. The Patient Affairs Office will always inform the patient's GP but the medical or nursing team may consider it appropriate to inform the patient's GP immediately and this should be documented. Ensure any other agencies are also informed, for example palliative care, district nurses, social services, etc. Again, you should document this in the notes.

Consider other patients' feelings and ensure they are informed individually that the death has occurred. Be prepared to deal with their particular issues concerning either the deceased's death or perhaps their own. Also consider issues for all the staff and ensure either debriefing or counselling sessions are arranged as appropriate. This is often difficult due to workload pressures but should be a priority to ensure the staff's own mental health issues. Specific teams are often available to accommodate this important activity.

Part

4 MEDICINES MANAGEMENT

This part includes the following chapters:

Scenario: James Roper

James Roper, known as Jim, is a 65-year-old gentleman who, until quite recently, has been living at home with his wife. Over the past four years he has been becoming increasingly forgetful, with progressive memory loss and increasing periods of confusion. He has become increasingly irritable and loses his temper easily. He has been admitted to the older people's mental health unit under the relevant mental health legislation following a diagnosis of Alzheimer's disease.

Jim refuses to take his medication and so staff decide to disguise his medication in his morning porridge.

Chapter 14

THE LEGAL, ETHICAL AND PROFESSIONAL ASPECTS OF MEDICINES MANAGEMENT

Susan Ramsdale

The chapter has been written to relate to the Nursing and Midwifery Council (NMC) Essential Skills Clusters (ESCs) for pre-registration nursing programmes (NMC, 2007a) for medicines management (skills 33–42).

Patients/clients can trust a newly registered nurse to:

Section 33 Correctly and safely undertake medicines calculations.
Section 34 Work within the legal and ethical framework that underpins safe and effective medicines management.
Section 35 Work as part of a team to offer a range of treatment options of which medicines may form a part.
Section 36 Ensure safe and effective practice through comprehensive knowledge of medicines, their actions, risks and benefits.
Section 37 Order, receive, store and dispose of medicines safely in any setting (including controlled drugs).
Section 38 Administer medicines safely in a timely manner, including controlled drugs.
Section 39 Keep and maintain accurate records within a multidisciplinary framework and as part of a team.
Section 40 Work in partnership with patients/clients and carers in relation to concordance and managing their medicines.
Section 41 Use and evaluate up-to-date information on medicines management and work within national and local policies.
Section 42 Demonstrate understanding and knowledge to supply and administer via a Patient Group Direction (PGD).

Introduction

In this chapter we are going to look at the legal, ethical and professional aspects of the management of medicines. We will examine the principles pertaining to these aspects, which will enable you to think through the issues and apply your professional judgement in any decisions that you make with and on behalf of your patients. We will look at national policies and legislation but it will also be necessary for you to refer to local policies and protocols to ensure currency within your locality. The key learning goals for this chapter are for you to:

❑ work within the legal and ethical framework that underpins safe and effective medicines management;

❑ understand the need for the recording and maintenance of accurate records;

❑ identify the issues for patients and carers in relation to concordance and medicines management;

❑ work within the guidelines of national and local policies;

❑ understand what is meant by consent and how this is achieved.

The management of medicines does not merely relate to giving out tablets and administering injections. It involves working with your patient to ensure that their needs are being met and that they are involved in and consenting to the treatments offered. Drug therapy is a major part of health care provision in Britain and, although much is written about medication, major studies are completed and trials carried out, the man in the street still tends to rely on what he is told by the local GP or the nurse on the ward. Practitioners have a duty of care to their patients and this includes acting in their best interests in relation to any kind of treatment administered. To be able to do this successfully and confidently, the practitioner must have skills and knowledge in the area in question, in this case medication.

The legal aspects of medicines management

When working with medication it is essential that you have an understanding of the relevant legislation and that you comply with this. Legislation exists in relation to the prescribing, supply, storage and administration of medication. The first comprehensive piece of legislation on medicines in the United Kingdom was the Medicines Act 1968 (primary legislation). This has been further developed via various statutory instruments (secondary legislation) and now provides the legal framework for the manufacture, licensing, prescription, supply and administration of medicines. The Medicines Act 1968 classifies medicines into the following categories:

❑ prescription only medicines (POMs) – supplied or administered to a patient on the instruction of an appropriate practitioner (doctor or dentist) and from an approved list for a nurse prescriber;

❑ pharmacy only medicines – these can be purchased from a registered primary care pharmacy, provided that the sale is supervised by a pharmacist;

❑ general sale list medicines (GSLs) – these do not need a prescription or the supervision of a pharmacist and can be obtained from retail outlets.

The Misuse of Drugs Act 1971 prohibits the possession, supply and manufacture of medicinal and other products, except where such possession, supply and manufacture has been made legal by the Misuse of Drugs Regulations 1985. This legislation deals with what are known as controlled drugs. It categorises these into five schedules. In health care it is mainly the schedule two medicines that we need to know about – medicines such as morphine, diamorphine and pethidine – and schedule three drugs such as barbiturates.

Most medicines are licensed to treat certain conditions. An unlicensed medicine is the term used to refer to a medicine that does not have a product licence. If an unlicensed medicine is administered to a patient, the manufacturer will have no liability for any harm that may befall the patient. The liability will fall to the prescriber but there could be implications for you if you are involved in obtaining informed consent. We will look at informed consent later in the chapter.

Professional practice

The NMC *Guidelines for the administration of medicines* state:

> The administration of medicines is an important aspect of the professional practice of persons whose names are on the Council's register. It is not solely a mechanistic task to be performed in strict compliance with the written prescription of a medical practitioner. It requires thought and the exercise of professional judgement … (Nursing and Midwifery Council, 2004b)

If this is the case, how can you exercise your professional judgement about a written prescription? What factors would you need to consider and what might prompt you to question the prescription at that time?

Reflection

Take a few minutes to reflect on any instances you have been involved in where there have been concerns about administering a prescribed medication to a patient. What were the reasons? If you have not experienced this ask your fellow students if they have had this experience and, if they have, discuss it with them.

When administering medicines you must know the patient and what is in their care plan. You must also know the therapeutic uses of the medication, its normal dosage, side effects, precautions and contra-indications. You should also take into account the condition of the patient at the time of administration and alert the prescriber or other authorised prescriber if you have concerns about contra-indications, allergic reactions or, if after assessment, you believe that the medication is no longer needed. This is exercising your professional judgement and accountability in the best interests of your patient.

Concordance

Sometimes, even though you have explained all the facts and reasons to your patient, it can be difficult to get them to accept medication. There could be many reasons why this is happening.

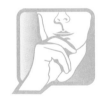

Reflection

Can you think of a time when this happened with one of your patients? What was the reason for it? How was it resolved? Were you and the patient happy with the outcome? If you have not experienced this ask your fellow students if they have had this experience and, if they have, discuss it with them.

Until quite recently the term non-compliance was used to describe the refusal of medication and/or treatments. This has now been changed to non-concordance. Why do you think that is? Compliance has been defined as 'the extent to which the patient takes the medication as prescribed' (Fawcett, 1995). Concordance takes things one step further: you are involving the client and obtaining their agreement to take the medication rather than coercing them. Establishing a good relationship with your client and improving their knowledge about their medication can really help. Many people stop taking medication because they are unsure about it. They are frightened of side effects or the regime is too complicated for them. If you work with your client on these issues you can help promote concordance.

The capacity to consent

If we look at Jim's case, what are the reasons he is refusing his medication? Does he understand the consequences of this and is he capable of making an informed decision about this? This is a very different scenario to that of a patient who has weighed up the benefits and disadvantages of taking medication and made an informed choice. Jim lacks the capacity to consent and a clear distinction should be made between those patients who have the capacity to refuse medication and whose refusal should be respected and those who lack this capacity. So what does it mean to lack capacity to consent?

Every adult must be presumed to have the mental capacity to consent to or refuse treatment, including medication, unless he or she:

❏ is unable to take in and retain the information provided about the medication by the treating staff, particularly as to the likely consequences of refusal; or

❏ is unable to understand that information; or

❏ is unable to weigh up the information as part of the process of arriving at a decision.

Although the actual responsibility for the assessment for capacity lies with the treating clinician, other practitioners retain a responsibility to participate in discussions about the assessment.

If a patient is capable of giving or withholding consent, no medication should be given without their agreement, even if refusal could adversely affect their health or shorten their life. The patient should be provided with adequate information about the nature, purpose, risks and viable alternatives to the proposed medication. Registered nurses, midwives and health visitors must respect a competent adult's refusal as much as they would his or her consent. The consequences of failing to do so can be severe, amounting to criminal battery or civil trespass and also a breach of their human rights. There is an exception to this principle which is concerned with treatment authorised under the relevant mental health legislation which will be discussed later in the chapter.

Reflection

This is a very difficult situation for both the nurse and the patient. Take a few minutes to think about any situations like this in which you were involved. Did they involve lack of capacity or was it an informed refusal? If you have not been involved in a situation like Jim's, discuss the circumstances with fellow students and identify key issues, your feelings and your reactions.

Who makes the decision?

If a patient is deemed to be incapable of providing consent, or the wishes of a mentally incapacitated patient appear to be contrary to the best interests of that person, then someone has to make a decision. Should this be the doctor in charge or do you think there is a more collaborative way of reaching a decision? It is the registered practitioner's responsibility to provide an objective assessment of the patient's needs and the type of treatment that has been suggested. This shouldn't, however, be done in isolation. There are many people involved in the care and treatment of patients and the following people could be consulted:

❑ relatives;

❑ carers;

❑ members of the multidisciplinary team.

If any previous instructions have been given by the patient while still competent, these should also be respected. This could be in the form of a living will or advance statement. These wishes should be respected provided that they are clearly applicable to the present circumstances and there is no evidence to suggest that the patient has changed their mind.

Imagine that you are the spouse of a patient who is unable to give consent and the doctor asks you to give consent for treatment. What do you think your position is? Can the doctor do this? The views of people close to the patient can be helpful in clarifying a patient's wishes and establishing their best interest but no one, not even a spouse, can consent for someone else. We must remember that people can be incapable of giving consent for many reasons and this may only be temporary. They might be in a coma or unconscious or mentally ill or just suffering from the sedative effects of medication. None of these need be a permanent state and so it is important to remember that capacity to consent may change and therefore needs to be addressed on a regular basis by the team involved with the patient.

Consent and mental illness

If, like Jim, the patient is detained under the relevant mental health legislation, the principles of consent still apply to any medication that is not related to the mental disorder for which they have been detained. It is essential to continue to assess their capacity to consent to, or refuse, such medication. The same principle applies to people with a learning disability who are not suffering from a mental illness. The position is very different, however, with regard to medication for the mental disorder for which the patient has been detained. Medication can be given against the patient's wishes for the first three months of the treatment order or after this if sanctioned by a second opinion approved doctor (SOAD). A SOAD is appointed by the appropriate statutory mental health commission to provide second opinions on treatment.

Children and consent

We have been discussing capacity to consent at length but only in relation to adults. Can a child give consent? We shouldn't assume that they can't. The same principles governing consent apply equally to everyone but with some restrictions. If a child is under the age of 16 they are generally considered to lack the capacity to consent to or refuse treatment, including medication. The parents (or those with parental responsibility) retain this right unless the child is considered to have significant understanding and intelligence to make up their own mind. You can find out more about this by reading the Fraser Guidelines, which were the result of the court case *Gillick* v. *West Norfolk and Wisbech Area*

Health Authority (1985) in which a mother argued against a doctor's decision to prescribe contraception to her daughter, who was under the age of 16, without consulting the mother. A child of 16 or 17 is presumed to be able to consent for themselves. The refusal of a child of any age can be overridden by the parents or those with parental responsibility. In exceptional circumstances, this may involve seeking an order from the court or making the child a ward of the court. In Scotland the law is slightly different. The parents' consent cannot override a refusal of consent by a competent child, regardless of age.

The covert administration of medication

The act of disguising medication in someone's food or drink is referred to as the covert administration of medication. It is a widely debated subject involving the basic principles of client autonomy and consent to treatment. Under common law we have the right to make our own decisions and this has been further strengthened by the Human Rights Act 1998. Although disguising medication in this way may be seen as a way of helping a patient get the right medication and thus helping them get well, it is an act of deception. The Nursing and Midwifery Council's Code of Professional Conduct requires each registered nurse, midwife and health visitor to act at all times in such a manner as to justify public trust and confidence. They must also work co-operatively with patients and families and respect their involvement in the planning and delivery of care.

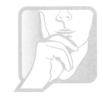

Reflection

Spend a few minutes thinking about the consequences of disguising medication. Have you come across this in practice? When, if ever, could you do this?

Generally speaking, if you disguise medication in food or drink, you are leading the patient to believe that they are not receiving any medication, when in reality they are. If, as a registered nurse, midwife or health visitor, you decide to do this you must be sure that you are doing it in the best interests of your patient and you will be accountable for the decision. In every case, the best interests of the patient are what is most important, and not the interests of the team or organisation. The best interests of the patient relates to interventions that would save life or prevent deterioration or ensure an improvement in the patient's physical or mental health. However, the right of the patient to give or withhold consent should always be fully recognised. Any decisions made regarding the administration of covert medication should be clearly documented in the current care plan.

Record-keeping

Record-keeping is an integral part of health care. It is a tool that, if used correctly, can benefit both the patient and the practitioner. If done badly, the effects can be devastating. Good record-keeping in relation to the administration of medication is of equal importance to that of any other type of medical record.

The prescription chart

You are, as a registered practitioner, accountable for your actions and omissions. You have to use your professional judgement and apply your knowledge and skills in any given situation, including the administration of medication. The prescription chart itself should contain at least the following information:

❑ patient's name;

❑ generic/brand name of substance to be administered;

❑ the form of the drug, e.g. tablet;

❑ strength;

❑ dosage;

❑ timing;

❑ frequency of administration;

❑ route of administration;

❑ start and finish dates;

❑ authorised prescriber's signature with date;

❑ any known allergies.

You should be able to read the entries on the chart. Many drugs have long complicated names and these can be very similar to the names of other drugs. It can be easy to make mistakes. This has led to the Department of Health publishing the document *Building a safer NHS for patients: improving medication safety* (2004).

What can you do to reduce such errors? Never give a drug if you are unsure of what is actually written on the prescription. Always know about your patient's illness/condition and the types of medication prescribed for this. A useful aid to have with you whenever you are administering any medication is the *British National Formulary* (BNF). The BNF is a book that is published by the British Medical Association (BMA) and the Royal Pharmaceutical Society of Great Britain (RPS) twice a year and lists all the drugs available to the health service in Britain. There is also a version of the BNF for children (see Chapter 15), and both publications are available online at **http://bnf.org/bnf** and **http://bnfc.org/bnfc**. The BNF provides a comprehensive breakdown on the use, dosages, side effects and indications and contra-indications of these medications. It is provided to pharmacists and doctors and is always available in the NHS where medication is administered.

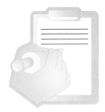

Activity 1.

Find a copy of the BNF – there will be one on your clinical placement – and look up some of the drugs currently being prescribed for your patients.

Changes to a prescription

Sometimes you can find yourself in a dilemma. Changes to a prescription have been suggested or found necessary but haven't been written on the chart. Do you think you could accept a telephone instruction to administer a previously unprescribed substance? No. This is not acceptable. Under exceptional circumstances, if the medication had been previously prescribed and changes to the dose are considered necessary but the prescriber is unable to issue a new prescription, then a fax, email or text could be used (NMC, 2007b). This should be followed up by a new prescription confirming the changes within a time period agreed within the organisation. The NMC suggests a maximum of 24 hours.

The importance of good record-keeping

Good record-keeping should help to deliver care to patients that is of a consistently high standard. If accurate records are maintained then teams can offer continuity of care and all members of the team can be fully informed of progress and changes. Poor record-keeping can be an indicator of problems with an individual's practice, whereas good record-keeping is seen as the mark of a skilled and safe practitioner.

It is not unusual for patient records to be called in evidence, either at a local level to investigate a complaint or even in a court of law. This is when the standard of record-keeping is really tested. The courts adopt a very straightforward view of record-keeping – 'if it is not recorded, it has not been done'. You must be very clear when recording drug administration on prescriptions. If the drug is given then the appropriate time slot should be completed and the signature of the person administering it entered. If, as student nurse, you are being supervised in drug administration then your signature should be countersigned by the registered nurse. If, for any reason, the drug is omitted then the reason for omission should be clearly recorded. It is just as important to know why something was not done.

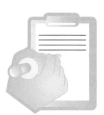

Activity 2.

Obtain the policies and procedures relating to the administration and storage of medicines in your locality and make yourself familiar with their requirements.

Summary

In this chapter you have been given an overview of the professional, legal and ethical aspects of medicines management and you must always administer any medicines with these in mind. We have considered the need to adhere to and be up to date with both national and local policies and to work collaboratively with our patients to gain both consent and concordance. We have considered the need for accurate and current record-keeping and your accountability in the whole process. We have looked closely at the requirements of the prescription chart and learned how to use the BNF. Continue to work in this way and you should become a safe and competent practitioner.

References

British Medical Association and Royal Pharmaceutical Society of Great Britain (2007) *British National Formulary*. London: BMJ Publishing and RPS Publishing

Department of Health (2004) *Building a safer NHS for patients: improving medication safety*. London: DoH

Fawcett, J. (1995) 'Compliance: definitions and key issues'. *Journal of Clinical Psychiatry*, 56: 4–8

Gillick v. West Norfolk and Wisbech Area Health Authority (1985) AC 112

Nursing and Midwifery Council (2004a) *Code of professional conduct: standards for conduct, performance and ethics*. London: NMC

Nursing and Midwifery Council (2004b) *Guidelines for the administration of medicines*. London: NMC

Nursing and Midwifery Council (2007a) *Essential Skills Clusters (ESCs) for pre-registration nursing programmes*, Annexe 2 to NMC Circular 07/2007. London: NMC

Nursing and Midwifery Council (2007b) *Standards for medicines management*. London: NMC

Chapter 15

THE ADMINISTRATION OF MEDICINES

Julie Cummings

This chapter will provide the reader with a broad introduction to the administration of medicines and covers essential aspects of the Nursing and Midwifery Council (NMC) Essential Skills Clusters (ESCs) in relation to 'Medicines Management' (Sections 33–42).

Patients/clients can trust a newly registered nurse to:

Section 33 Correctly and safely undertake medicines calculations.

Section 34 Work within the legal and ethical framework that underpins safe and effective medicines management.

Section 35 Work as part of a team to offer a range of treatment options of which medicines may form a part.

Section 36 Ensure safe and effective practice through comprehensive knowledge of medicines, their actions, risks and benefits.

Section 37 Order, receive, store and dispose of medicines safely in any setting (including controlled drugs).

Section 38 Administer medicines safely in a timely manner, including controlled drugs.

Section 39 Keep and maintain accurate records within a multidisciplinary framework and as part of a team.

Section 40 Work in partnership with patients/clients and carers in relation to concordance and managing their medicines.

Section 41 Use and evaluate up-to-date information on medicines management and work within national and local policies.

Section 42 Demonstrate understanding and knowledge to supply and administer via a Patient Group Direction (PGD).

Introduction

At the end of this chapter you should be able to:

❑ identify the importance of administering medicines safely;

❑ enhance your understanding of basic pharmacology;

❑ describe the various routes for the administration of medicines;

❑ describe how to prepare selected drugs for injection;

❑ identify sites used for intradermal, subcutaneous, intramuscular and intravenous injections;

❏ describe suitable techniques for the administration of medicines via various routes;

❏ correctly and safely calculate drug dosages using recognised formulae;

❏ work within the legal and ethical framework that underpins safe and effective medicines management in practice;

❏ extend your range of skills in drug administration.

See Chapter 14, page 273.

Throughout this chapter consider the professional and legal issues relating to drug administration (see Chapter 14) and reflect on the following documentation, all of which can be downloaded from the NMC website at **www.nmc-uk.org**:

❏ the *Standards for medicines management* (2007);

❏ the *Code of professional conduct: standards for conduct, performance and ethics* (2004);

❏ the *UKCC position statement on the covert administration of medicines – disguising medicine in food and drink* (2001).

General safety issues

The Department of Health (DoH) (2004) has made recommendations for the safer administration of medicines which includes the following points:

❏ Right Patient, Right Drug, Right Dose, Right Route, Right Time:

- **Right Patient** – check name bands, taking particular care with children if siblings are present;

- **Right Drug** – clarity of prescription;

- **Right Dose** – calculations: grams, milligrams, micrograms, nanograms;

- **Right Route** – for example, oral, rectal, intramuscular, intravenous, etc.

- **Right Time** – for example, once every four hours;

- And don't forget to check the **expiry date**.

These are often referred to as the 5Rs of medicines administration.

❏ You should have access to appropriate reference sources while administering drugs to support safe administration (i.e. the *British National Formulary* and the *British National Formulary for Children*);

❑ You should confirm the accuracy of complex dose calculations.

❑ Staff should be trained and assessed as competent before administering drugs.

❑ Patients with allergies should wear readily distinguishable wrist bands.

❑ Serious administration errors and 'near misses' should be reported to the National Patient Safety Agency (NPSA). The NPSA advises health care organisations on safety issues following incidents occurring in the NHS. New recommendations to improve medication safety and reduce the number of medication errors in the NHS were published in March 2007. For more information visit **www.npsa.nhs.uk**.

See Chapter 21, page 455.

Whatever the route of administration you should remember to wash your hands (see Chapter 21) and consider the following principles:

❑ wash and dry hands prior to administration and after administration of medicines;

❑ use gloves where appropriate and remember hand washing is still just as important when wearing gloves;

❑ explain and gain consent from the patient and ensure that they are comfortable following any procedure;

❑ check the medicine against the prescription chart – ensure the right patient, right medication, right dose, right time and that the medicine is within the expiry date;

❑ use a non-touch technique – do not handle key parts.

Basic pharmacology

To be effective, a drug must reach the desired concentration in the part of the body where it is required to act and, ideally, it must be maintained at this concentration for the appropriate period of time. This goal is influenced by the key interactions that take place between the drug and the body after the drug has been administered. All substances carry risks and can be toxic. Before administering any unfamiliar medication always take time to familiarise yourself with the correct dose and the possible side effects of that medication.

Medical pharmacology is the science of drugs and how they interact with the body. These chemical interactions are referred to as:

❑ **pharmacokinetics** – the study of the action of drugs in the body and the way in which the body handles a drug; and

❑ **pharmacodynamics** – the study of the action of drugs on the human body and the way in which a drug works.

For further reading visit **www.druginfozone.nhs.uk**.

Pharmacokinetics

The therapeutic effect of a drug is also referred to as the desired effect of the drug. A side effect is an effect that is unintended and may range from mild and harmless to severe and harmful. Allergic reactions may be either mild or severe. A mild reaction may include a variety of symptoms such as a skin rash or loose stools. It is important to ask your patients about, and observe them for, side effects. If we consider our patient Jim in this regard, he might not be able to tell you that he had developed a rash but you might see him scratching his arm and then consider the effects of medication as a possible cause.

A severe allergic reaction, usually occurring immediately after the administration of a drug, is referred to as an **anaphylactic reaction**. This requires immediate treatment of symptoms and can, in some instances, be fatal if not treated promptly (Berman *et al.*, 2007). For more information on anaphylaxis visit **www.anaphylaxis.org.uk** (Anaphylaxis Campaign) and **www.resus.org.uk** (UK Resuscitation Council).

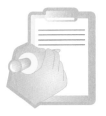

Activity 1.

Pharmacokinetics

Match the following words to the appropriate descriptions given below:

METABOLISM, EXCRETION, ABSORPTION, DISTRIBUTION

1.   The process by which fluids, nutrients and drugs are taken up by the body tissues. The major site for this process is the small intestine which is lined with villi, which increase the surface area of the intestine. The rate at which this happens is determined by the route of administration and the solubility of the drug – that is, whether the drug is water or fat soluble.

2. When a drug enters the bloodstream it is rapidly diluted and transported through the body. Drugs then bind to plasma proteins in the blood. The unbound part is free to move from the blood stream to apply its pharmacological effect.

3. The first stage of drug clearance, the means by which a drug is chemically altered to aid elimination from the body. The primary site where this occurs is the liver. Other organs and tissues where this process occurs to a minor extent include the lungs, kidneys, blood and intestine.

4. The metabolites of a drug leave the body. The primary routes for this are through the gastrointestinal system (faeces) or the renal system (urine). Other routes include evaporation, exhalation, saliva, breast milk.

Pharmacodynamics

Most drugs produce their effects by acting on proteins known as receptors in the following ways:

❑ They replace chemicals that are deficient in the body – for example, vitamins.

❑ They interfere with the function of receptor sites by enhancing the response – for example, metformin which increases receptor sensitivity to insulin in patients with type 2 diabetes mellitus. (This is known as an **agonist drug**.)

❑ They interfere with the function of receptor sites by preventing usual responses – for example, tamoxifen which binds to the receptor site and blocks normal cell function and activity. This in turn prevents cell growth stimulation in oestrogen-dependent breast tumours. (This is known as an **antagonist drug**.)

❑ They act against invading cells in the body – for example, antibiotics.

❑ They act against abnormal cells in the body – for example, anti-cancer drugs.

❑ They interfere with cell functions and metabolic pathways by either stimulating or inhibiting normal levels of activity in, for example, hormone disorders.

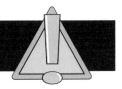

Children differ both anatomically and developmentally from adults and this should be taken into consideration when administering drugs.

Children and pharmacology

Children are different. Here are some important points in relation to medication calculation and administration when treating children:

❑ From birth to adolescence the child is undergoing dramatic changes in physical growth, psychosocial development and sensitivity to drugs. As the body's composition changes with development so does the rate and extent of drug distribution.

❑ Plasma protein levels are lower in children. Variable plasma protein levels can increase drug toxicity or speed up the elimination process.

❑ Total body water composition is greater in children under two years including the proportion that is extracellular fluid. As water-soluble drugs are distributed mainly in the extracellular fluid a greater mg to kg dose of water-soluble drugs is needed in young children. As a result, if the child is dehydrated, the response to drugs will vary and the dose of drug may become a toxic dose. If doses are repeated before the dehydration is corrected there is a greater risk of toxicity occurring.

❑ Drug metabolising enzymes are limited in infants. However, as maturity progresses, the liver is able to metabolise most drugs. Immature organ systems are sensitive to toxic effects and have limited compensatory mechanisms.

❑ Changes in pharmacokinetics are likely to occur at times of change – for example at puberty.

If you would like to know more about pharmacology in relation to children read the articles by Kanneh (2002a, 2002b, 2002c)and/or consult a textbook on paediatric pharmacology.

Drug calculations

A major part of the nurse's role involves preparing, checking and administering medicines, monitoring the effectiveness of the treatment, reporting adverse reactions and teaching their patients about their drugs.

During your nursing experience you will frequently be called upon to administer or supervise the administration of all types of medicines. This requires the development of a certain degree of mathematical skill to make you a safe and efficient practitioner. The most common type of medication error is administering the wrong dose (Pentin and Smith, 2006).

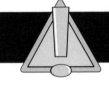

Note that when administering medicine to children two registered nurses must always check and administer.

Some drug administrations can require complex calculations to ensure that the correct volume or quantity of medication is administered. In these situations it may be necessary for a second registrant to check the calculation in order to minimise the risk of error. The use of calculators to determine the volume or quantity of medication should not act as a substitute for arithmetical knowledge and skill. (NMC, 2007)

All drug calculations are based on an understanding of arithmetic and the metric system.

Standard measurements

1 kilogram (kg)	=	1,000 grams (g)
1 gram	=	1,000 milligrams (mg)
1 milligram (mg)	=	1,000 micrograms (mcg)
1 litre	=	1,000 millilitres (ml)
1 millilitre (ml)	=	1,000 microlitres
1 pint	=	568 ml

Some standard accepted common medical abbreviations used in prescriptions

Latin abbreviation	Instruction
p.o.	by mouth
s.c.	subcutaneous
i.m.	intramuscular
i.v.	intravenous
b.d.	twice a day
t.d.s.	three times a day

p.r.n.	given as necessary
q.d.s.	four times a day
a.c.	before food
p.c.	after food
stat	given immediately
e.c.	enteric coated
caps	capsules
elix	elixir
guttae	drops
neb	nebuliser
kg	kilograms
g	gram
mcg	microgram
mg	milligram
l	litre
ml	millilitre

Activity 2.

Examine a prescription chart for its legibility and accuracy. Have any of the abbreviations in the table above been used? Discuss the 5Rs with your mentor and talk about the importance of administering medicines via the prescribed route.

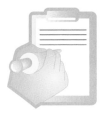

Medication in tablet form

In many instances dosage calculations can be carried out using mental arithmetic, but it is important to understand the principles involved and have a working knowledge of the formulas (based on proportions) for more complex calculations (Downie *et al.*, 2006). On a drug administration chart you may be given the total dose a patient is to receive. Your task will be to calculate the correct amount of tablets required to make up the prescribed dosage.

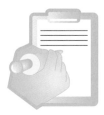

Example

A patient is prescribed 120 mg of a drug but the tablets are available as 40 mg tablets only. The solution is to find out how many 40 mg tablets there are in 120 mg, or in other words 120 divided by 40. The formula is:

$$\text{Number of tablets} = \frac{\textbf{Amount prescribed}}{\textbf{Amount in each tablet}}$$

In other words, the prescription is the total quantity you are asked to administer – 'what you want'. The availability is the quantity in each tablet – 'what you've got'.

$$\text{Number of tablets} = \frac{\textbf{What you want}}{\textbf{What you've got}}$$

In this case the answer is: 120 mg (what you want) divided by 40 mg (what you've got) which equals three – so three tablets should be given. If in doubt, always check answer back thus:

3 × 40 mg = 120 mg

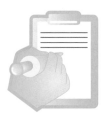

Activity 3.

1.   1 mg of a drug is prescribed and the tablets are 500 micrograms each. How many tablets will you give?

2.   625 mg of a drug is prescribed and the tablets are 1.25 g each. How many tablets will you give?

Medication in liquid form

When drugs are in liquid form, the availability is given in terms of the concentration of the solution or suspension. As an example, pethidine hydrochloride is available as 50 mg/ml. This means that 50 milligrams of pethidine hydrochloride are dissolved in every millilitre of liquid. If the quantity of drug to be given is known, and the concentration of the drug in solution is known, we can calculate the volume of liquid required. This is necessary for drugs in liquid form as prescriptions are usually by weight, whereas the drugs are labelled by concentration. Note that drugs administered to children are calculated according to body weight.

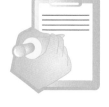

Example

A patient is prescribed 400 mg of a syrup. The syrup is available as 500 mg of the drug in 5 ml. The formula is:

$$\text{Dose required (mg)} \times \frac{\text{Available volume dose (ml)}}{\text{Dose available (mg)}}$$

or:

$$\frac{\text{What you want}}{\text{What you got}} \times \text{Dilution (ml)}$$

$$\frac{400 \text{ mg}}{500 \text{ mg}} \times 5 \text{ ml} = 4 \text{ ml}$$

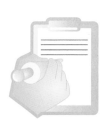

Activity 4.

1. A patient is prescribed a drug that is requested in milligrams per kilogram. If we require 3 mg per kg and the patient weighs 70 kg how much of the drug would we administer?

2. Jon is five years old and he weighs 20 kg. He needs a dose of Ibuprofen. The doctor has prescribed 400 mg four times daily. You suspect this dose is too high and decide to check a paediatric formulary. The formulary states that Ibuprofen is 20 mg/kg in four divided doses. What is the correct dose for Jon?

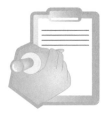

Activity 5.

1.   The drug is available as 10 mg/2 ml and the prescription is for 5 mg. How many ml will be given?

2.   The drug is available as 20 mg/5 ml and the prescription is for 40 mg. How many ml will be given?

3.   The drug available as 20 mg/5 ml. How many mg will be in 7.5 ml?

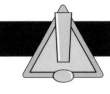

Remember – if in doubt, consult experienced colleagues.

Routes of drug administration

The doctor will usually prescribe both the medication and the route by which medication is to be administered. Most drugs are available in preparations for one or two specific routes of administration. Not all drugs can be administered by all the possible routes. The doctor will prescribe the most appropriate route and this will depend on a number of factors, for example the patient's general condition, potential side effects of the drug, speed of onset and rate of absorption required.

Each route of administration has both advantages and disadvantages. For example, the patient with chronic asthmatic bronchitis who is having breathing difficulties may be prescribed the drug Ventolin™ (salbutamol) for symptom relief. Rather than being given the drug orally the prescriber would prescribe an inhalation to give rapid localised relief by introducing the drug directly into the respiratory tract. Drugs can be administered in many ways, as shown in the following table:

Oral – by mouth

Sublingual – under the tongue

Rectal – into the rectum

Vaginal – into the vagina

Inhalation – via the respiratory tract

Nasal – into the nose

Topical – onto the skin or mucous membranes

Optic – into the eye

Aural – into the ear

Injection – intramuscular, subcutaneous, intradermal and intravenous

Intraosseous – into the substance of the bone (in resuscitation situations)

Intra-articular – into the cavity of a joint

Intracardiac – into the heart

Intrathecal – into the spinal fluid

Epidural – into the epidural space

The oral administration of drugs

Important points relating to the oral administration of drugs include the following:

❏ This is considered the most convenient and safest route.

❏ Medicines will have a lower therapeutic effect if administered orally. Therefore there is more time to react if side effects occur.

❏ Efficacy depends on the rate and extent of absorption, how well the drug dissolves in physiological solutions (for example gastric juices) and the chemical properties of the drug.

❏ Absorption of drugs can only take place when the drug has dissolved/disintegrated into the gastric juices. With liquid medicines or pre-dissolved tablets this has already been accomplished and thus speeds up the process so drugs are absorbed more rapidly.

❏ The appearance, smell and taste of the medicine may pose issues for some patients, particularly children.

❏ Oral medications may be in the form of tablets, capsules, lozenges/pastilles and linctus, elixir or syrups. There are also sublingual preparations – medications that are placed under the tongue (in spray form or tablets).

Such issues would have to be considered in relation to Jim in our scenario. Perhaps liquid medication would be easier to administer than medication in tablet form?

Rectal administration

See also Chapter 8, page 185.

Drugs that are given rectally are presented in the form of suppositories (solid torpedo-shaped formulation) or enemas (liquid form). Enemas are generally used as a treatment for constipation or to prepare the bowel for investigations or surgery. The absorptive surface area of the rectum is small but the good blood supply ensures rapid absorption (Downie *et al.*, 2006). Please note that faecal impaction will delay the absorption of the drug and, as such, would be a contra-indication, as would recent colorectal or gynaecological surgery.

Advantages and disadvantages of rectal administration

Advantages	Disadvantages
❑ Can be given if the patient is nauseous or vomiting.	❑ Anal or rectal irritation can occur.
❑ Can be used in patients with swallowing difficulties and unconscious patients.	❑ They are made to melt at body temperature so need to be kept refrigerated.
❑ Avoids destruction of the drug by gastric acid and irritation of the upper gastrointestinal tract.	❑ Side effects can include inflammation and even perforation of the colonic mucosa.
	❑ Aesthetic considerations.

Remember that many patients may be unwilling to have drugs administered via this route and a careful assessment should be made of the appropriateness of this route of choice.

Examples of drugs administered via this route are:

❑ diclofenac (analgesia);

❑ paracetamol (anti-pyretic);

❑ diazepam (given to stop a seizure);

❑ aminophylline (bronchodilator);

❑ prochlorperazine (anti-emetic).

See Chapter 8 for the administration procedure. Please note that when giving a suppository to an infant or young child, the child may lie on his/her back with the legs flexed. For children under three years the little finger should be used.

See Chapter 8, page 189.

Topical administration

The topical route consists of drug administration via the epidermis (the outer layer of the skin) and external mucous membranes. It therefore includes administration into the eyes and ears (optic and aural administration).

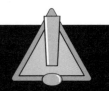

As with any procedure performed on a patient it is important to remember the important issues of hand washing and infection control. When handling creams and ointments you are advised to wear gloves to prevent absorption and cross-infection.

Form of topical (on-the-skin) preparations

- ❑ **Creams** – oil-based preparations, which are easier to apply, for example hydrocortisone cream for inflammatory skin disorders. It is advisable to apply creams and ointments to the skin with a gauze swab.

- ❑ **Ointments** – water or oil-based, semi-solid and usually dispensed in tubes. Eye ointment should be applied to the inside of the lower lid, usually at night.

- ❑ **Pastes** – thick in texture and therefore need to be 'spread', for example zinc and coal tar paste for psoriasis. It will be necessary to use a wooden or plastic spatula to aid application.

- ❑ **Local anaesthetic** – for example, Ametop gel and EMLA cream used to block superficial pain from venepuncture and cannulation, particularly used with children. Follow the manufacturer's instructions for use.

- ❑ **Transdermal patch** – comes as a small patch that adheres to the skin. Most are attached to the chest, abdomen or upper arm, and the site should be changed each time. For example, hyoscine to prevent motion sickness and oestrogens for hormone replacement come as patches.

Optic administration

❏ **Eye drops** – presented in solution in either single-use containers or in a larger bottle with a dropper. They are for single patient use only and also, if used in both eyes, there should be a separate bottle for each eye that is labelled 'left' and 'right'. Avoid touching the eye with the dropper end as this would contaminate it, and drop vertically inside the lower lid. Ask the patient to blink between drops.

❏ **Eye ointment** – using your forefinger, gently pull the lower lid downwards to form a small pocket for the ointment. Squeeze the ointment tube until the ointment forms a ribbon and apply inside the lid margin.

Aural administration

❏ **Ear drops** – ask the patient to sit upright with their head leaning slightly away from the affected ear. Pull the pinna of the ear upwards and backwards and instil ear drops as prescribed.

For further reading on topical administration visit the British Association of Dermatology website at **www.bad.org.uk**.

Drug administration via inhalation

Inhalation therapy is the most effective way to administer preventative and symptom-relieving drugs. Through inhalation the drug will reach the lungs directly, requiring a lower dose and minimising systemic side effects.

Inhaler devices

There are a number of different inhaler devices with different operating methods (see Figure 1). It is important that nurses learn the correct technique for each type of inhaler in order to check and review client technique. A regular review of client technique improves treatment adherence and symptom control, and also reduces the incidence of acute episodes (O'Connor, 2001; Roberts, 2002).

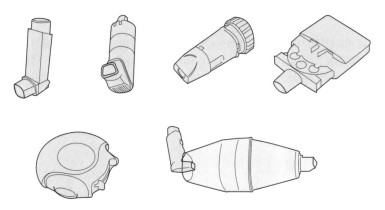

Figure 1 Various inhaler devices

For each design or type, the patient will be inhaling an aerosol (a mixture of air and medication), and the speed of inhalation (the inspiratory flow) will influence where the medication contained within the device will be deposited or absorbed. Inhaler devices are designed to deliver drug particles of a certain size to the small airways during inhalation. The particles are either in aerosol (in a suspension or a solution) or dry powder form.

Metered dose inhalers (MDIs)

The most commonly used inhaler, the MDI consists of a plastic housing and a metal aerosol canister (see Figure 2). The canister contains a mix of propellant and medication. When pressed, a precise quantity of this mixture is released. With most MDIs, the aerosol is delivered under pressure at high speed. The inhalation should be timed with actuation of the device and should be slow and steady. Inhaling too fast may cause a greater proportion of the aerosol to impact at the back of the throat and be subsequently swallowed, thus reducing the beneficial clinical effect and increasing the potential for local and systemic side effects.

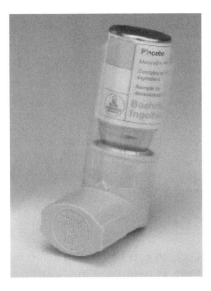

Figure 2
A metered dose inhaler (MDI) device

MDIs with holding chamber/spacer

A container that holds the aerosol cloud produced by an MDI is known as a spacer or chamber. There are different types of these MDIs. They remove the need to co-ordinate inhaling and pressing the canister (many people find this difficult), and they also help to reduce the number of large particles in the aerosol cloud (which are too big to reach the parts of the lung that would benefit).

Dry powder inhalers (DPIs)

Drug delivery from DPIs is triggered by inhaling through the device (see Figure 3). While each design of dry powder is very different, the basic principle remains the same. A metered quantity of powdered medication is drawn into the airflow and follows a specific route within the inhaler towards the mouth of the patient.

Figure 3
Dry powder devices

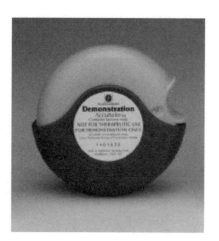 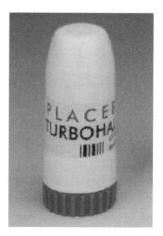

Different designs of inhalers

The internal resistance of the inhaler has a significant effect on how fast a patient can inhale through it, which, in turn, affects the quantity and quality of medication the patient receives and where in the respiratory tract it is deposited.

Nebulisers

Oxygen can be administered via bottled or piped gas supply at the same time as nebulised medication to treat acute respiratory problems in the hospital setting. Alternatively a compressor can be used. Each method requires a nebuliser pot and mask or mouthpiece (see Figure 4). A nebuliser is a device which is used to administer a solution of drug in the form of a fine mist for a patient to inhale. The pump (compressor unit) forces air through the liquid (drug solution) in the drug chamber (nebuliser chamber). This changes the liquid into a fine mist which the patient breathes in through a mask or mouthpiece.

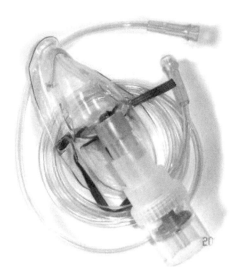

Figure 4
A nebuliser

The prescription and preparation of injectable medicines

A good injection technique is fundamental to nursing care and it is essential that you possess the necessary knowledge and skill to undertake this safely.

Drawing up drugs for injection – remember safety and the 5Rs

The complexities associated with the prescription, preparation and administration of injectable medicines means that there are greater potential risks for patients than for other routes of administration. The National Patient Safety Agency (NPSA) has produced a standard template for prescribing, preparing and administering injectable medicines in clinical areas, which incorporates the following guidelines:

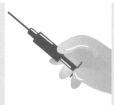

Prescribing

1. All prescriptions for injectable medicines must specify the following:
   - the patient's name;
   - the prescriber's signature;
   - the approved medicine name;
   - the dose and frequency of administration;
   - the date and route of administration;
   - the allergy status of the patient.

2. Where relevant, the prescription, or a readily available local protocol, must specify the following:
   - the brand name and formulation of the medicine;
   - the concentration or total quantity of medicine in the final infusion container or syringe;
   - the name and volume of diluent and/or infusion fluid;
   - the rate and duration of administration;
   - stability information to determine the expiry date of the final product;
   - type of rate-control pump or device(s) to be used;
   - the age and weight of any patient under 16 years of age, where relevant;
   - the date on which treatment should be reviewed;
   - arrangements for fluid balance or clinical monitoring – these should be made on an individual patient basis and according to local protocol and clinical need.

Preparation

General

3. Read all prescription details carefully and confirm that they relate to the patient to be treated.

4. Ensure that the area in which the medicine is to be prepared is as clean, uncluttered and free from interruption and distraction as possible. Ideally, preparation should take place in an area dedicated to this process.

5. Assemble all materials and equipment: sharps bin for waste disposal, medicine ampoule(s)/vial(s), diluent, syringe(s), needle(s), alcohol wipes, disposable protective gloves, clean re-usable plastic tray.

   Check the following:

   – expiry dates;

   – damage to containers, vials or packaging;

   – that medicines were stored as recommended, for example in the refrigerator. Beware of the risk of confusion between similar looking medicine packs, names and strengths. Read all labels carefully.

   Check that:

   – the formulation, dose, diluent, infusion fluid and rate of administration correspond to the prescription and product information;

   – the patient has no known allergy to the medicine;

   – you understand the method of preparation. Calculate the volume of medicine solution needed to give the prescribed dose. Write the calculation down and obtain an independent check by another qualified health care professional.

6. Prepare the label for the prepared medicine.

7. Cleanse your hands according to local policy. Put on a pair of disposable protective gloves.

8. Use a 70 per cent alcohol wipe or spray to disinfect the surface of the plastic tray.

9. Assemble the syringe(s) and needle(s). Peel open wrappers carefully and arrange all ampoules/vials, syringes and needles neatly in the tray.

10. Use a 'non-touch' technique, i.e. avoid touching areas where bacterial contamination may be introduced, for example syringe tips, needles, vial tops. Never put down a syringe attached to an unsheathed needle.

11. Prepare the injection by following the manufacturer's product information or local guidelines.

Withdrawing solution from an ampoule (glass or plastic) into a syringe

12. Tap the ampoule gently to dislodge any medicine in the neck.

13. Snap open the neck of glass ampoules, using an ampoule snapper if required.

14. Attach a needle to a syringe and draw the required volume of solution into the syringe. Tilt the ampoule if necessary.

15. Invert the syringe and tap lightly to aggregate the air bubbles at the needle end. Expel the air carefully.

16. Remove the needle from the syringe and fit a new needle or sterile blind hub.

17. Label the syringe.

18. Keep the ampoule and any unused medicine until administration to the patient is complete to enable further checking procedures to be undertaken.

19. If the ampoule contains a suspension rather than solution, it should be gently swirled to mix the contents immediately before they are drawn into the syringe.

20. The neck of some plastic ampoules is designed to connect directly to a syringe without use of a needle, after the top of the ampoule has been twisted off.

Withdrawing a solution or suspension from a vial into a syringe

21. Remove the tamper-evident seal from the vial and wipe the rubber septum with an alcohol wipe. Allow to dry for at least 30 seconds.

22. With the needle sheathed, draw into the syringe a volume of air equivalent to the required volume of solution to be drawn up.

23. Remove the needle cover and insert the needle into the vial through the rubber septum. Invert the vial. Keep the needle in the solution and slowly depress the plunger to push air into the vial.

24. Release the plunger so that solution flows back into the syringe.

25. If a large volume of solution is to be withdrawn, use a push-pull technique.

26. Repeatedly inject small volumes of air and draw up an equal volume of solution until the required total is reached. This 'equilibrium method' helps to minimise the build-up of pressure in the vial.

27. Alternatively, the rubber septum may be pierced with a second needle to let air into the vial as solution is withdrawn. The tip of the vent needle must always be kept above the solution to prevent leakage.

28. With the vial still attached, invert the syringe. With the needle and vial uppermost, tap the syringe lightly to aggregate the air bubbles at the needle end. Push the air back into the vial.

29. Fill the syringe with the required volume of solution then draw in a small volume of air. Withdraw the needle from the vial.

30. Expel excess air from the syringe. Remove the needle and exchange it for a new needle or a sterile blind hub.

31. The vial(s) and any unused medicine should be kept until administration to the patient is complete.

32. If the vial contains a suspension rather than solution, it should be gently swirled to mix the contents, immediately before they are drawn into the syringe.

Reconstituting powder in a vial and drawing the resulting solution or suspension into a syringe

33. Remove the tamper-evident seal from the vial and wipe the rubber septum with an alcohol wipe. Allow to dry for at least 30 seconds.

34. Withdraw the required volume of diluent (for example, water for injections or sodium chloride 0.9 per cent) from ampoule(s) into the syringe.

35. Inject the diluent into the vial. Keeping the tip of the needle above the level of the solution in the vial, release the plunger. The syringe will fill with the air which has been displaced by the solution. (If the contents of the vial were packed under a vacuum, solution will be drawn into the vial and no air will be displaced.) If a large volume of diluent is to be added, use a push-pull technique.

36. With the syringe and needle still in place, gently swirl the vial(s) to dissolve all the powder, unless otherwise indicated by the product information. This may take several minutes.

37. Withdraw the required volume of solution from the vial into the syringe. Alternatively, the rubber septum may be pierced with a second needle to let air into the vial as solution is withdrawn. The tip of the vent needle must always be kept above the solution to prevent leakage.

38. If a purpose-designed reconstitution device is used, the manufacturer's instructions should be read carefully and followed closely.

Labelling injection and infusion containers

39. All injections should be labelled immediately after preparation, except for syringes intended for immediate push (bolus) administration by the person who prepared them. Under no circumstances should an operator be in possession of more than one unlabelled syringe at any one time, nor must an unlabelled syringe be fitted to a syringe driver or similar device.

40. Labels used on injectable medicines prepared in clinical areas should contain the following information:

    – the name of the medicine;

    – strength;

- the route of administration;

- the diluent and final volume;

- the patient's name;

- the expiry date and time;

- the name of the practitioner preparing the medicine.

41. Place the final syringe or infusion and the empty ampoule(s)/vials(s) in a clean plastic tray with the prescription for taking to the patient for administration.

(NPSA, 2007)

The NMC has produced the following position statement on the preparation of medicines for administration.

It is unacceptable to prepare substances for injection in advance of their immediate use or to administer medication drawn into a syringe or container by another registrant when not in their presence. An exception to this is an already established infusion which has been instigated by another registrant following the principles set out above, or medication prepared under the direction of a pharmacist from a central intravenous additive service and clearly labelled for that patient/client.

You may be required in an emergency to prepare substances for professionals. In this instance the direction must be signed by a doctor or dentist and a pharmacist who should have been involved in developing the direction, and who must be approved by the appropriate health care body. (NMC, 2007)

Injection technique

Note that although skin cleansing before an injection is routinely carried out in many hospitals there is evidence to suggest that, as long as the patient is physically clean and the nurse maintains a high standard of hand hygiene and employs a non-touch technique, skin disinfection is unnecessary (Little, 2000). If skin disinfection is undertaken then skin should be cleaned with an alcohol swab for 30 seconds and then allowed to dry for 30 seconds (Mallet and Doherty, 2000).

Suggested needle size for different types of injection (not including intravenous)

Type of injection	Needle gauge	
	Adult	Child
Intradermal	26 G × 10 mm	26 G × 10 mm
Subcutaneous	25/26 G × 16 mm	26 G × 16 mm
Intramuscular	21 G × 40 mm	23 G × 30 mm

Intradermal injection technique

The injection is placed between the layers of the skin, just below the epidermis. Small amounts of medication, no more than 0.5 ml, are administered via this route. The most common site is the central forearm.

Subcutaneous injection technique

The subcutaneous route is used for slow, sustained absorption of medicine. The sites for subcutaneous administration are illustrated in Figure 5.

Figure 5
Recommended
subcutaneous
injection sites

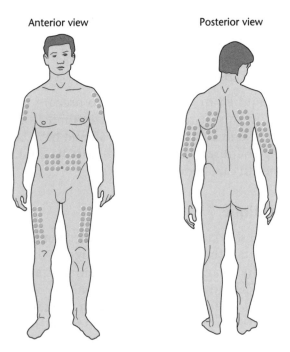

Anterior view   Posterior view

Traditionally, subcutaneous injections have been given at a 45 degree angle into a raised skin fold. However, if using one of the shorter insulin needles, 5, 6 or 8 mm, the angle should be 90 degrees. Regular injections such as insulin should have the site rotated. It is not necessary to aspirate after needle insertion and before injecting subcutaneously as piercing a blood vessel with this type of injection is very rare (Peragallo-Dittko, 1997). The depth and angle of introduction of the needle is demonstrated in Figure 6 for the different injection techniques.

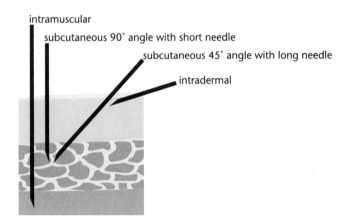

intramuscular

subcutaneous 90° angle with short needle

subcutaneous 45° angle with long needle

intradermal

Figure 6
Depth and angle for different injection techniques

Intramuscular injections

Intramuscular injections deliver medication into well-perfused muscle, providing rapid systemic action and absorbing relatively large doses. There are several sites used for injection but, wherever is chosen, it is important to inspect the site for signs of inflammation, infection or skin lesions. The site should also be assessed for muscle mass, as thin emaciated patients may not have sufficient muscle mass in certain areas.

Intramuscular injections should be delivered by inserting the needle with a dart-like action at 90 degrees to the skin, then withdrawing on the plunger and ensuring that the needle hasn't entered a blood vessel. The medication to be administered should then be injected and the needle removed. Apply gentle pressure with a gauze swab for ten seconds. Dispose of sharps safely, wash hands, check the condition of the patient and document on the prescription sheet.

There is evidence to recommend that the Z track technique be used as standard with the intramuscular injection technique as it is associated with less pain for the patient (Beyea and Nicholl, 1995). This was initially introduced for drugs that stained the skin such as iron for injection. Workman (2000) describes the technique (see Figure 7):

❑ Pull the skin downwards or to one side at the intended site.

❑ The needle is inserted and the injection given.

❑ Allow ten seconds before removing the needle to allow the medication to diffuse.

❑ On removal of the needle the retracted skin is released, causing the tissues to close over the deposit of medication and prevent it from leaking.

Figure 7
Z track technique

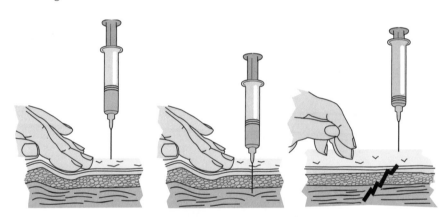

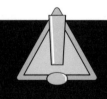
Note that the intramuscular route is not recommended in children, unless there is no other alternative, because of the potential for pain and trauma. Also, children have less muscle mass and perfusion, which will therefore affect drug absorption.

The main sites available for intramuscular injection include:

Deltoid muscle of the upper arm

This site is often used for vaccines such as hepatitis B and tetanus (see Figure 8). The injection should be given at a 90 degree angle to the skin. This area is only suitable for the injection of small volumes of fluids.

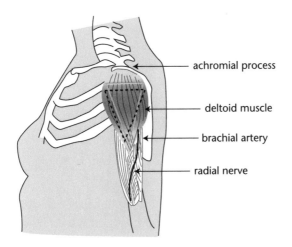

Figure 8
Deltoid
intramuscular
injection site

achromial process

deltoid muscle

brachial artery

radial nerve

Gluteus maximus muscle

See Figure 9: often referred to as the 'upper outer quadrant of the buttock', this site is commonly used although there have been reports of damage to the sciatic nerve. In the case of infants and children (prior to walking) it is not recommended as a suitable site (Trigg and Mohammed, 2006).

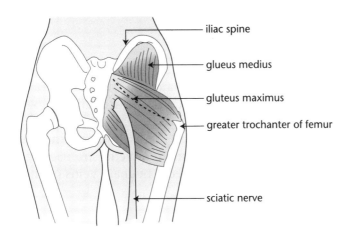

Figure 9
Gluteus maximus
intramuscular
injection site

iliac spine

glueus medius

gluteus maximus

greater trochanter of femur

sciatic nerve

Quadriceps muscle on outer aspect of femur

This is the traditional site commonly used for intramuscular injections and is a safe site for infants and young children (see Figure 10).

Figure 10
Quadriceps muscle
on outer aspect of
femur intramuscular
injection site

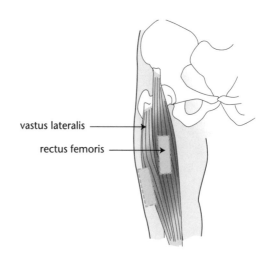

vastus lateralis ————

rectus femoris ————

Intravenous injection technique

See Chapter 5,
page 115.

Venepuncture, cannulation and fluid therapy will be explained briefly to help you to understand these procedures and so that you can assist medical staff and qualified practitioners effectively when they are preparing to administer medication via the intravenous route. For more information refer to Chapter 5.

The basic anatomy and physiology

The superficial veins of the upper limb of the arm are most commonly chosen for venepuncture. Veins situated in this area are numerous and more accessible, which ensures that the procedure can be performed efficiently with minimal discomfort to the patient. Superficial veins of the lower limb extremities can be used. However, there is a higher possibility of complications when these veins are used as the blood supply to this area can be diminished. The main veins of choice are (see Figure 11):

❑ median cubital veins;

❑ the cephalic vein;

❑ the basilic vein;

❑ the metacarpal veins.

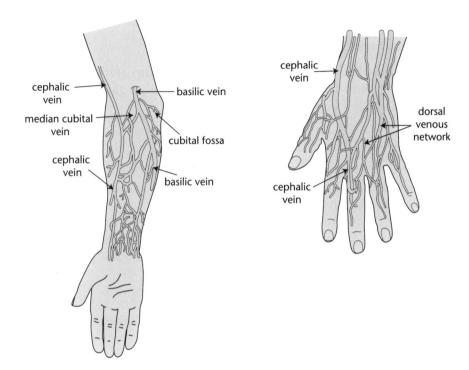

Figure 11
Common veins for venepuncture and cannulation

cephalic vein

median cubital vein

cephalic vein

basilic vein

cubital fossa

basilic vein

cephalic vein

dorsal venous network

cephalic vein

Skin preparation of the patient for venepuncture and cannulation

Asepsis is vital when performing venepuncture as the integrity of the skin is breached and an alien device is introduced into the circulatory system. The two major causes of microbial contamination are:

❑ cross-infection from practitioner to patient;

❑ the skin flora of the patient.

To minimise the risk posed by the patient's normal skin flora, firm and prolonged cleaning with an alcohol-based solution is advised. The cleaning should continue for 30 seconds in a circular action. The area then should be allowed to dry to:

❑ facilitate coagulation of organisms, thus ensuring disinfection;

❑ prevent a stinging pain on insertion of the needle due to the alcohol solution being present on the tip of the needle.

At this stage the skin of the selected venepuncture site must not be touched or repalpated before the procedure.

Equipment used for intravenous fluid therapy

Cannula (and needles)

These are sized by their diameter, which is called the gauge. The smaller the diameter, the larger the gauge. Therefore a 22-gauge cannula is smaller than a 14-gauge cannula.

Administration sets

These are commercially prepared in sterile packs. In the set you will find specialised sterile tubing with, at one end, a rigid trocar protected by a sterile sheath. At the other end is a protected Luer connector nozzle. At the trocar end the tubing widens into a drip chamber. An adjustable roller clamp surrounds the tubing below the drip chamber. This allows the flow of fluid to be regulated at the prescribed flow rate.

Burette sets

This is a specialised administration set for infusions when a volumetric infusion pump is not available and the patient needs a more accurate flow rate. The burette has a calibrated drip chamber with a roller clamp above and a roller clamp below the chamber. The chamber is filled with the amount of fluid prescribed in millilitres per hour and this fluid is infused over the hour. For the infusion to continue the drip chamber has to be refilled as prescribed when empty. Note that children should always have infused fluids via a volumetic infusion pump for a precise flow rate.

Intravenous infusions

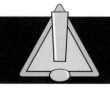

Be aware that as a student nurse you are not allowed to connect/reconnect or commence/recommence intravenous infusions of any kind nor set up or readjust any electronic pumps or syringe drivers.

For adults the prescriptions for intravenous fluids are usually written along the following lines: normal saline 0.9% 1 litre over 6 hours. In order to set up a manually controlled drip accurately by eye, you need to be able to count the number of drops per minute which will equate to the amount prescribed. The formula for this calculation is:

$$\text{Rate} = \frac{\text{Volume (in drops)}}{\text{Time (in minutes)}}$$

To calculate the volume in drops, you need to know how many drops of the fluid ordered are contained in 1 millilitre (ml). You should find this information on the packaging of the administration set. The volume in ml is then multiplied by the number of drops per ml to give the volume in drops. To find the rate in minutes, you need to change the hours into minutes by multiplying by 60. Some administration sets have no filter and are therefore unsuitable for giving blood. Since blood is thicker than clear fluid, fewer drops constitute a ml (usually 15 drops = blood, 20 drops = clear fluid).

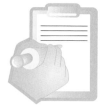

Example 1

You need to give 1 litre of normal saline in six hours. How many drops per minute?

Answer

$$\text{Rate} = \frac{1{,}000 \text{ ml} \times 20 \text{ drops}}{6 \times 60 \text{ minutes}} = 56 \text{ drops/minute}$$

Note that it is necessary to round to the nearest whole number.

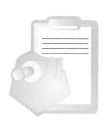

Example 2

A patient requires 500 ml over twelve hours. What is the flow rate?

Answer

500 divided by 12 is 41.66 ml/hr. If you do not have the facility to enter decimals then round to the nearest whole number. The answer would then be 42 ml/hr.

Figure 12
Example of a
volumetric infusion
pump

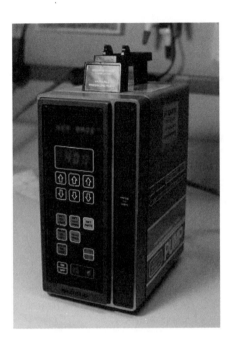

Intravenous pumps

There are many different types and makes of pump available (see Figure 12). You must be familiar with the type of pump used in your area of practice. There is evidence that many drug errors occur due to unfamiliarity with equipment. Intravenous pumps are always used to deliver infusions to children.

Syringe drivers

Small amounts of intravenous fluid, containing drugs, can be delivered using a syringe driver. Most of these drivers are designed for specific size of syringes (it is important to ensure you are using compatable equipment at all times), and can be adjusted to deliver a specific number of ml per hour.

Reconstituting drugs

Displacement values/volumes must be taken into account when reconstituting intravenous medication. Many drugs require reconstitution and most pharmacy departments offer a centralised intravenous additives service. Drugs are prepared under strict aseptic conditions using lamina flow chambers. However, there will still be times when drugs need to be reconstituted in the ward setting. This must be done in a clean environment, using aseptic technique and sterile equipment. This is a role that should be undertaken by a medical practitioner or a registered nurse who has undergone appropriate training.

Other ways of administering medication intravenously

Medication can be added to a volume of fluid for infusion via the bag or burette, or directly into the intravenous cannula through a bung near the entry site. Flush solutions, for example normal saline, should be used between bolus additions to ensure that incompatible drugs do not mix and, at the end of each administration, to ensure no drug remains in the line.

Safe practice

It was once considered an extended role for the qualified nurse but it has now become common practice for nurses to prepare and administer intravenous medication. In order to carry this out safely qualified nurses must demonstrate an in-depth knowledge of the potential risks and complications. Complications of intravenous therapy include the following:

❏ speed shock – an anaphylactic type reaction or circulatory overload resulting from insufficient control of administration;

❏ anaphylaxis – an extreme and generalised allergic reaction;

❏ extravasation/local infiltration – leakage and spread from vessels into the surrounding tissue, causing discomfort and **oedema** at the site;

❏ phlebitis – inflammation of the wall of a vein, a local response that manifests in inflammation;

❏ **bacteraemia** – a presence of bacteria in the blood, a sign of infection;

❏ **septicemia** – absorption of bacteria or their toxins from the bloodstream causing widespread destruction of tissue; sepsis can potentially be life-threatening (Fox, 2000).

The responsibilities of qualified nurses with regard to intravenous drug therapy and the detailed specifications of competencies for intravenous therapy have recently been published by the Royal College of Nursing (RCN), available at **www.rcn.org.uk**. There is no universal policy regarding the preparation and administration of intravenous drugs by student nurses. Individual hospital trusts will have their own set of protocols and guidelines.

Oxygen therapy

Oxygen is a colourless, odourless, tasteless gas which constitutes approximately 21 per cent of atmospheric air. Oxygen is essential for all tissues. However, some organs are more susceptible to the lack of oxygen (hypoxia) than others, for example, the brain, heart and kidneys. Adequate oxygenation is vital to prevent tissue damage. Hypoxia can occur for a number of reasons:

❏ failure of oxygen transport (oxygen is carried by the red blood cells), i.e. shock due to bleeding, cardiac problems, septic shock, and so on.

Basically shock, whatever the cause, relates to the inability to deliver oxygen to the tissues;

❑ cardiac diseases;

❑ pulmonary disease;

❑ poisoning, for example carbon monoxide;

❑ birth asphysia.

Oxygen is the first drug given in an emergency/resuscitation situation. The appropriate use of oxygen can be life-saving; however, at the same time, the appropriate use of oxygen is important. As with all drugs, oxygen can cause complications and involves risks. Oxygen must be administered with caution to patients whose respiratory drives are maintained by hypoxia, for example adults with chronic obstructive airways disease. These individuals retain carbon dioxide because of the reduced ventilation through their diseased lungs. For these patients the main respiratory stimulus is a falling PO_2 (pressure of oxygen) known as the hypoxic drive, thus if high levels of oxygen are given then their respiratory drive will diminish.

See Chapter 20, page 428.

Insufficient delivery of oxygen will lead to cell damage, hypoxia and, ultimately, cell death. Excessive oxygen use in some patients may lead to respiratory failure. As stated patients with chronic respiratory disease are particularly sensitive to the harmful effects of the incorrect delivery of oxygen, which is why it is important to provide the prescribed percentage of oxygen to the patient. For further information on oxygen therapy see Chapter 20, page 428.

Oxygen is a prescription drug

Oxygen is regarded as a drug and, therefore, should be prescribed by a doctor on the patient's prescription sheet. This should state the appropriate percentage and flow rate, which is litres per minute, to be given as well as the duration (Downie *et al.*, 1999).

Basically there are two options for oxygen therapy: firstly, to counteract hypoxia and to increase oxygen saturation levels, which would involve the use of medium to high concentrations of oxygen; secondly, to supplement oxygen levels without increasing carbon dioxide levels using low flow oxygen.

Oxygen delivery

Oxygen is provided in hospitals via a piped system with flow valves to connect onto the oxygen masks or in bottles (black body, white collar). Oxygen administration is a potentially dangerous procedure because oxygen supports combustion and can convert a spark into a flame. Therefore precautions to maintain safety must be taken in the immediate area of its use.

Oxygen devices

Nasal cannula

Oxygen can be delivered via a nasal cannula (see Figure 13). This is an effective method for delivering oxygen at low concentrations between 24 and 35 per cent. They have an advantage over face masks as they are less restrictive in terms of communication and feeding. They are commonly used in the child health setting because they are better tolerated than a mask. Nasal cannula and headboxes/hoods are an effective way of administering oxygen to children (Trigg and Mohammed, 2006). A headbox/hood should be used for infants to enable the oxygen percentage concentration to be measured more accurately.

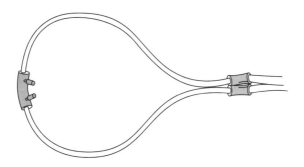

Figure 13
Nasal cannula

Face masks

These are the most common method for administering oxygen to adults (see Figure 14). A variety of masks are available. As a general rule care must always be taken to ensure that the mask fits snugly and in the correct position for efficient delivery of the drug. Fixed concentration venturi masks have the advantage of giving a known concentration of oxygen (in percentages). The oxygen masks are usually colour-coded and will indicate the percentage the patient will receive and the flow rate in litres per minute. They are available in 24/28/35/40/60 per cent concentrations. Medium concentration masks will deliver an oxygen concentration of between 40 and 60 per cent. These are commonly used in post operative recovery areas for short-term oxygen therapy following surgery. High concentration/non-rebreathing masks will deliver oxygen concentrations between 60 and 90 per cent. This method of oxygen therapy is used on trauma patients and post-cardiac arrest, and is generally for short-term use only.

Figure 14
A Venturi face mask

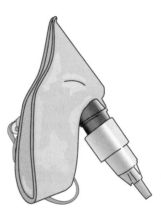

Observations and complications

Patients requiring long-term oxygen therapy will need humidified oxygen to prevent drying of the mucous membranes of the upper airway, as this can lead to chest secretions becoming sticky and difficult to expectorate.

Regular observations of the patient must be made while the patient is receiving oxygen therapy. If you are using a portable supply, check the cylinder regularly to ensure there is sufficient oxygen remaining in the cylinder. If humidification is being used the equipment must be changed as per the manufacturer's instructions to prevent infection. Humidifers are a common source of gram negative bacilli and viruses associated with the respiratory system (Pilkington, 2004).

Signs of inadequate oxygenation will present as:

❑ increased respiratory rate;

❑ increased pulse rate;

❑ confusion;

❑ agitation or reduction in conscious levels; and

❑ cyanosis.

Pulse oximetry (oxygen saturation monitor)

See also Chapter 20, page 432.

Pulse oximetry will detect hypoxia before clinical signs become apparent. The monitor is an electronic device which clips onto the patient's finger or ear lobe, or foot in the case of a small child, and gives a reading of the percentage of circulating haemoglobin that has oxygen molecules attached to it. So, a patient with 100 per cent saturation has oxygen molecules on all the haemoglobin. Normal saturation when breathing room air is between 96 and 100 per cent. Pulse oximeters have difficulty reading when the blood pressure is low, where there is excessive patient movement and when patients have false nails and/or nail polish. It will give an abnormally high reading in patients who have suffered carbon monoxide poisoning as it cannot differentiate between carbon monoxide and oxygen molecules attached to haemoglobin.

How saturation monitoring works:

❑ When haemoglobin is well saturated with oxygen it is red and has the capacity to absorb more light from the infrared probe on a saturation monitor.

❑ When haemoglobin has a lower oxygen concentration, the blood changes to a bluer colour and the amount of light absorbed from the red and infrared light that passes through the skin is reduced (Chandler, 2001).

❑ The photosensitivity of the haemoglobin enables the pulse oximeter to detect changes in blood and its oxygen concentration.

❑ The light-emitting part of the probe is placed on the top of one part of the body, for example the finger, and a photodetector is placed directly opposite the light source on the underside of the finger. The red and infrared light passes through the skin, enabling it to be picked up by the photodetector and interpreted.

It is important that the probe, and the area that it is going to be placed on, are clean. It is also vital to remove any nail varnish or, alternatively, to use a different site. A dirty probe, dirty skin or nails that have nail varnish on may give rise to inaccurate recordings. The probe must be fastened the right way up: the infrared light shines down through the skin, and on the opposite side the photodetector picks up a reading. It can be useful to turn the monitor on before starting to place the probe so that it can be determined from which side the probe is emitting the infrared light.

The probe and the lead can be secured by tape. The less the probe and lead move, the better the recording will be; motion artefact (irregular and scattered light paths), caused by movement of the probe, can lead to unreliable readings and can be a major problem in obtaining saturation readings. It is important to highlight that care must be taken when securing probes. The Medical Devices Agency (MDA) has had reports of skin being damaged from probes that have been fastened too tightly. Damage to the skin when using an oxygen saturation probe is a particular problem when they are used with children and neonates that have sensitive skin. The MDA recommends changing the probe site every two hours.

Professional responsibilities

Although the oxygen saturation monitor can detect hypoxaemia at a quicker rate than the nurse caring for the patient, it is crucial the nurse uses previous experience and powers of observation to detect a change in the patient's condition. Evidence suggests that the nurse and the patient can become dependent on the saturation monitor. This should not be allowed to happen. Saturation monitors should be used in conjunction with nursing skills and should not replace them.

All nurses who administer oxygen must have received training and supervised practice in the administration. It is the nurse's responsibility to ensure knowledge and skills are maintained from both the practical and theoretical perspective (Higgins, 2005). For further information read the articles by Casey (2001), Clark (2002) and Howell (2002).

Complementary medicine

Important nursing principles

The primary function of the Nursing and Midwifery Council (NMC) is to 'protect the public' by setting professional standards and giving advice and guidance to registered nurses, midwives and specialist community public health nurses. Registered nurses have a responsibility to deliver safe and effective care based on current evidence, best practice and, where applicable, validated research. (NMC, 2004)

Many members of the public seek treatment from a homeopath or buy 'over-the-counter' treatments, varying from basic vitamin supplements to plant remedies for eczema. Some members of the public take homeopathic and herbal medicines in conjunction with their traditional prescribed treatments. It is important to ensure that any homeopathic treatments or herbal remedies being taken are not contra-indicated with any prescribed medications the patient is taking and, if they are, to advise the patient accordingly. The patient and the multidisciplinary team should be involved in any discussion on what is acceptable and the alternative therapy should be prescribed accordingly. Any possible contra-indications should be explained to the patient so that they can make an informed choice. If there is conflict of interest and the patient insists on continuing, the conflict should be documented in the patient's care records. The Code states:

> You must ensure that the use of complementary or alternative therapies is safe and in the interests of patients and clients. This must be discussed with the team as part of the therapeutic process and the patient or client must consent to their use.

With regard to complementary and alternative therapies the NMC *Standards for medicines management* (2007) state that:

> Registrants must have successfully undertaken training and be competent to practise the administration of complementary and alternative therapies.

> Registrants are accountable for their practise and must be competent in this area (please refer to The NMC *Code of professional conduct: standards for conduct, performance and ethics*. You must have considered the appropriateness of the therapy to both the condition of the patient and any co-existing treatments. It is essential that the patient is aware of the therapy and gives informed consent.

> Complementary and alternative therapies may interact with other types of medicinal products and laboratory tests. All complementary and alternative medicines should be recorded alongside other medicinal products and prescribed on inpatient prescription charts.

Types of complementary medicine

Complementary medicine includes many different techniques and therapies for treating a patient and is an increasing feature of health care practice (see also Chapter 4, page 108). Traditional medicine (TM) is a term that is also used to cover a wide range of practices. Below are some of the common complementary therapies:

See Chapter 4, page 108.

- ❏ acupressure;
- ❏ acupuncture;
- ❏ Alexander technique;
- ❏ applied kinesiology;
- ❏ anthroposophic medicine;
- ❏ aromatherapy;
- ❏ Bach and flower remedies;
- ❏ chiropractic;
- ❏ cranial osteopathy;
- ❏ crystal therapy;
- ❏ healing;
- ❏ herbal medicine;
- ❏ homeopathy;
- ❏ hypnosis;
- ❏ iridology;
- ❏ kinesiology;
- ❏ massage;
- ❏ meditation;
- ❏ nutritional medicine;
- ❏ osteopathy;
- ❏ reflexology;
- ❏ reiki;
- ❏ relaxation and guided imagery;
- ❏ shiatsu;
- ❏ therapeutic touch;
- ❏ yoga, movement, dance, tai chi.

(Donnellan, 2001)

Despite growing public enthusiasm for such therapies, the medical profession on the whole regards any technique or substance that has not undergone extensive research and clinical trial with some scepticism. Much complementary medicine remains scientifically unproven. However, there is a growing body of evidence that certain complementary therapies are effective in given circumstances.

Many complementary therapies are based on the following principles:

❑ a focus on the patient not the disorder – find the cause not the symptom;

❑ the patient is a whole person who needs time, effort and understanding;

❑ mind, spirit and emotions have a huge impact upon the individual and their well-being;

❑ a gentle approach and a natural process, working with convention and not against it.

There are challenges ahead that relate to professional regulation and to a research-orientated culture. However, the boundaries between conventional and complementary medicine are shifting and complementary medicine is increasingly available on the NHS along with conventional treatments.

Summary

This chapter has identified some of the important aspects of the administration of medications, giving a broad introduction and incorporating the essential aspects of the Nursing and Midwifery Council Essential Skills Clusters (ESCs) in relation to medicines management. By applying the principles as described in the chapter, safety can be assured for both the patient and the practitioner.

Answers to activities:

Activity 1

1. Absorption

2. Distribution

3. Metabolism

4. Excretion

Activity 3

1. 2

2. 0.5 tablet

Activity 4

1. 210 mg

2. 100 mg

Activity 5

1. 1 ml

2. 10 ml

3. 30 mg

Suggested further reading

Dimond, B. (2003) 'Principles for the correct administration of medicines: 1'. *British Journal of Nursing.* 12(11): 682–5

Dimond, B. (2003) 'Principles for the correct administration of medicines: 2'. *British Journal of Nursing,* 12(12): 760–2

Gard, P.R. (2001) *Human pharmacology.* London: Routledge

Gatford, J.D. and Phillips, N. (2002) *Nursing calculations,* 6th edn. Edinburgh: Churchill Livingstone

Haigh, S. (2002) 'How to calculate drug dosage accurately: advice for nurses'. *Professional Nurse,* 18(1): 11–14

Kelly, J. (2001) 'Minimising potential side effects of medication at different ages'. *Professional Nurse,* 10(4): 259–62

References

Berman, A., Synder, S., Kozier, B. and Erb, G. (2007) *Kozier and Erb's fundamentals of nursing: concepts, process, and practice,* 8th edn. Pearson.

Beyea, S.C. and Nicholl, L.H. (1995) 'Administration of medications via the intramuscular group: an integrative review of the literature and research based protocol for the procedure'. *Applied Nursing Research,* 5(1): 22–3

Casey, G. (2001) 'Oxygen transport and the use of pulse oximetry'. *Nursing Standard,* 15(47): 46–53

Chandler, T. (2001) 'Oxygen administration'. *Paediatric Nursing,* 13(8): 37–42

Clark, A. (2002) 'Legal lessons: but his O_2 sat was normal!' *Clinical Nurse Specialist,* 16(3): 162–3

Department of Health (2004) *Building a safer NHS for patients – improving medication safety.* London: DoH

Donnellan, C. (ed.) (2001) *Complementary medicine.* Cambridge: Burlington Press

Downie, G., Mackenzie, J. and Williams, A. (1999) *Pharmacology and drug management for nurses,* 2nd edn. London: Churchill Livingstone

Downie, G., Mackenzie, J. and Williams, A. (2006) *Calculating drug doses safely.* London: Elsevier

Fox, N. (2000) 'Managing the risks posed by intravenous therapy'. *Nursing Times,* 96(30): 37–9

Higgins, D. (2005) 'Oxygen therapy'. *Nursing Times,* 101(4): 30–1

Howell, M. (2002) 'The correct use of pulse oximetry in measuring oxygen status'. *Professional Nurse*, 17(7): 416–18

Kanneh, A. (2002a) 'Paediatric pharmacological principles: an update. Part 1: drug development and pharmacodynamics'. *Paediatric Nursing*, 14(8): 36–42

Kanneh, A. (2002b) 'Paediatric pharmacological principles: an update. Part 2: pharmacokinetics: absorption and distribution'. *Paediatric Nursing*, 14(9): 39–43

Kanneh, A. (2002c) 'Paediatric pharmacological principles: an update. Part 3: pharmacokinetics: metabolism and excretion'. *Paediatric Nursing*, 14(10): 39–43

Little, K. (2000) Skin preparation for intramuscular injections'. *Nursing Times*, 96(46), NT Plus: 6–8

Mallet, J. and Dougherty, L. (2000) *The Royal Marsden Hospital – manual of clinical nursing procedures*. 5th edn. London: Blackwell Science

Medical Devices Agency (2001) *Tissue necrosis caused by pulse oximeter probes*. London: MDA

Nursing and Midwifery Council (2001) *UKCC position statement on the covert administration of medicines – disguising medicine in food and drink*. London: NMC

Nursing and Midwifery Council (2004) *Code of professional conduct: standards for conduct, performance and ethics*. London: NMC

Nursing and Midwifery Council (2007) *Standards for medicines management*. London: NMC

O'Connor, B. (2001) 'Inhaler devices: compliance with steroid therapy'. *Nursing Standard*, 15(48): 40–2

Pentin, J. and Smith, J. (2006) 'Drug calculations: are they safer with or without a calculator?' *British Journal of Nursing*, 15(14): 778–81

Peragallo-Dittko, V. (1997) 'Rethinking subcutaneous injection technique'. *American Journal of Nursing*, 97(5): 71–2

Pilkington, F. (2004) 'Humidification for oxygen therapy for non-ventilated patients'. *British Journal of Nursing*, 13(2): 111–15

Roberts, J. (2002) 'The management of poorly controlled asthma'. *Nursing Standard*, 16(21): 45–53

Trigg, E. and Mohammed, T.A. (eds) (2006) *Practices in children's nursing*, 2nd edn. London: Elsvier

Workman, B. (2000) 'Safe injection techniques'. *Primary Health Care*, 10: 43–9

Chapter 16

MEDICATION ERRORS, DRUG STORAGE AND CONTROLLED DRUGS

Paul Tipping

This chapter covers essential aspects of the Nursing and Midwifery Council (NMC) Essential Skills Clusters (ESCs) in relation to 'Medicines Management' (Sections 33–42). In particular, this chapter references the following sections.

Patients/clients can trust a newly registered nurse to:

Section 34 Work within the legal and ethical framework that underpins safe and effective medicines management.

Section 37 Order, receive, store and dispose of medicines safely in any setting (including controlled drugs).

Section 38 Administer medicines safely in a timely manner, including controlled drugs.

Section 39 Keep and maintain accurate records within a multidisciplinary framework and as part of a team.

Section 41 Use and evaluate up-to-date information on medicines management and work within national and local policies.

Introduction

In this chapter I intend to address three key elements in relation to medication management. The aim is to integrate these elements with the clinical scenario in this section in order to help you to think critically about some of the key issues. It will also allow you to reflect on issues that you may or may not have already seen in your clinical practice placements.

I will include current clinical guidelines and will reference the appropriate Nursing and Midwifery Council (NMC) Essential Skills Clusters (ESCs) for pre-registration nurses (NMC, 2007a). Note that there may be special procedures relevant to particular areas of practice that vary from those described here, especially with regard to the treatment of children. You should make yourselves familiar with your local documentation which will give you more detailed information specific to your local hospital Trust.

Medicines form a crucial part of the treatment of most, if not all, of our patients within the National Health Service (NHS). The Audit Commission

(2001) estimated that 40 per cent of nurses' time is spent dealing with medication so it is very important that you have a sound understanding of the key issues. The clinical and cost-effective use of medicines is important in meeting the needs of individual patients and the targets for the NHS. The National Patient Safety Agency (NPSA) supports this by reinforcing that safe medication is everybody's business in the NHS. They suggest that even small changes can make a difference in reducing harm to patients (Cousins, 2007).

Key documentation for nurses in relation to this chapter includes the NMC Guidelines for the Administration of Medicines. These guidelines have recently been updated (NMC, 2007). Other key documents are as follows.

Primary legislation

❏ The Medicines Act (1968) and supplementary amendments.

❏ The Misuse of Drugs Act (1971) and supplementary amendments.

❏ The Misuse of Drugs Regulations (1985) and supplementary amendments.

Also:

❏ Nursing and Midwifery Council (2004) *The code of professional conduct: standards for conduct, performance and ethics.*

❏ Department of Health (DoH) (2004) *Building a safer NHS for patients: improving medication safety.*

Medication errors

Medicine management is not just about the pharmacy service. It is about close multidisciplinary working between all health professionals dealing with medicines across the health economy, whether in or out of hospital. Errors can occur in any of the procedures relating to medicines including prescribing, dispensing, interpretation of the prescription and administration. With this in mind the National Patient Safety Agency (NPSA) was established in 2001. The aim of this organisation is to improve the safety and quality of patient care. Lord Warner has emphasised that both patient safety and improving the quality of care is at the heart of the current government's improvement strategy for the NHS (Department of Health, 2006).

There has been a lot of work carried out concerning the medication errors that occur in hospitals. Indeed, a recent study from Pirmohamed *et al.* (2004) indicates that up to 6.5 per cent of all patients admitted to hospital will experience medication-related harm. This is supported by the work of Davies *et al.* (2006) who suggest that up to 9 per cent of patients experience such harm.

What is a medication error?

The NPSA (2007a) has defined a medication error as:

> A preventable event that may cause or lead to inappropriate medication use or patient harm whilst the medication is in the control of health professional, patient or consumer.

A medication error may also be defined as:

> Any preventable event that may cause or lead to inappropriate medication use or patient harm, whilst the medication is in the control of the health care professional, patient or consumer. Such events may be related to professional practice, health care products, procedures, and systems including: prescribing, order communication; product labelling, packaging and nomenclature; compounding; dispensing; distribution; administration; education; monitoring; and use. (Audit Commission, 2001).

The most commonly occurring errors are omitted medicines, wrong medicines and wrong dose, strength or frequency of medicines. These make up in excess of 50 per cent of all medication incidents that are reported, with 28 per cent being wrong dose, strength or frequency (NPSA, 2007b).

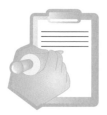

Activity 1.

Why do you think drug errors occur? List your reasons for drug errors.

Risk factors

There are many explanations for how and why medication errors might occur. There are, of course, always going to be risks associated with the administration of medication. It is therefore our responsibility as health care professionals, according to the NMC Code of Professional Conduct (2004) and the NMC ESCs (2007a), to make sure that we follow the general principles of medication administration across the health sector and age range. You also need to be aware of local policies and procedures. As a student, although you will be working under the supervision of your mentor, there is still an element of responsibility attached to your role. So take time while you are out on placement to understand relevant polices and procedures related to medication management, and ask your mentors to help you and support you with this process.

> *As a student nurse you should not be administering medication independently/autonomously.*

Some of the common risk factors involved in medicine administration include the following:

- ❏ staffing skill mix
- ❏ illegible prescription
- ❏ busy environment
- ❏ staffing shortage
- ❏ distraction
- ❏ communication (NPSA, 2007b)
- ❏ documentation (NPSA, 2007b)
- ❏ medical devices
- ❏ inaccurate prescription
- ❏ carelessness

- ❏ fatigue
- ❏ poor procedures
- ❏ poor reporting/auditing
- ❏ inadequate equipment
- ❏ complacency
- ❏ transfer of medication
- ❏ lack of knowledge around risk
- ❏ inexperience
- ❏ inaccurate application of the 5Rs
- ❏ poor drug calculations
- ❏ unsupervised practice.

Critical care and paediatric settings are particularly high-risk areas. These are where the prescribing and administration of many drugs with narrow safety margins occur, and these types of drugs are often associated in studies with high levels of errors. Extra precautions should be taken while working in these areas. Research suggests that over 50 per cent of drug errors are concerned with prescribing, and increased specialist pharmacist input would have a significant impact in reducing the number of adverse drug events. If a drug error has taken place then all relevant medicine containers, syringes, infusions and administration equipment involved in the error must be retained safely for examination.

Reporting

The reporting of medication errors is designed to protect patients and staff and to identify areas where improvements in practice need to be made. It is not designed to apportion blame or to be part of the disciplinary process. If we don't report all incidents of medication errors how can we improve the quality of care that we are delivering to our patients? It is difficult to obtain figures relating to medication errors as there is a low reporting rate. The figures that the NPSA often quote come from the reporting of incidents where harm has been caused. This is thought to be the tip of the iceberg (Department of Health, 2004). Figures released by the NPSA (2007b) suggest that the majority of medication incidents that have been reported resulted in no harm to the patients. The figure associated with this is 82.8 per cent of all incidents reported. The NPSA also estimates that medication errors could be costing the NHS more than £750 million each year in England. All elements of medication errors need to be reported as well as near misses such as, for example, a prescription error. The NPSA (2007b) reinforces this and states that there is rich learning to be gained from the data that is received. As a student working in your local hospital Trust you should make yourself familiar with the NPSA's Untoward Incident Reporting System, as well as reading the current NMC guidelines and seeking support from your mentor.

As medication errors are potentially very serious, if you have made a medication error, or have witnessed others making an error, you must report it. Remember it is our duty to protect patient safety. Be reassured that there are people to help and support you, whether in the Trust or at your education provider. Do not forget that the reporting of incidents or near misses is not about apportioning blame, but about looking at whether policy and procedures were followed and whether there could be anything to learn from the mistake.

Reporting adverse reactions

Your patients may experience reactions to the medications that they have been administered. This is not necessarily due to a medication error, but it is very important that these events are documented, the patient examined and the event reported to the Committee on Safety of Medicines (CSM). There is more information available about this in the Medicines and health care Products Regulatory Agency (MHRA) 'Yellow Card' scheme. The CSM particularly encourages the reporting of all suspected reactions in children. Make sure you report all adverse reactions, even if the reaction is well recognised like, for example, gastrointestinal bleeding with anti-inflammatory drugs. You do not have to be 100 per cent certain the drug caused the reaction, just be suspicious of a possible association and talk to your mentor about it.

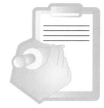

Activity 2.

While you are on placement in clinical practice take the opportunity to look up possible adverse reactions to drugs that have been prescribed to your patients in the British National Formulary (BNF).

Patient review

Remember, we have a duty of care (NMC, 2004), and the well-being of our patients is of prime importance following a medication error. Where the wrong drug, or the wrong dose of a drug, has been administered, or the drug has been administered incorrectly, the consultant responsible for the patient and the nurse in charge must be informed as soon as possible. The medical staff will decide whether any further action is needed in respect of patient management. As a student nurse, you must do the appropriate baseline observations and document them alongside the plan of care. Furthermore, remember that patients have the right to be informed of a medication error or near miss.

Medicine defect reporting

You also have a responsibility to the hospital Trust to follow their policy and procedures and alert staff to a defect where the product, as supplied by the manufacturer, is not of the expected standard. Defects may involve, for example, inadequate or incorrect labelling, ineffective packaging, contamination or discolouration of the medicine. If you have any suspicion that there is a defect do not use the drug and report it immediately to your mentor and the nurse in charge, who will inform the duty pharmacist.

Reducing the risks

The NPSA (2007a) has published recommendations to reduce the risk of medicines and medical device products by producing safer product designs like, for example, ready-to-administer medication or oral syringes for oral medication administration. They also advise safer storage of medications and separate cupboards for different products, and also recommend more involvement of patients. Some of these issues are addressed in the next section. One of the key elements for reducing risk remains the reporting of errors, no matter how small. Reporting a near miss or an error may prevent it from happening again. Remember that prevention is always better than cure.

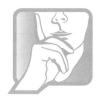

Reflection

How can you, as a student nurse, help to reduce medication errors?

How do we reduce medication errors?

See Chapter 15, page 284.

The answer is simple: follow the right protocols, policies and procedures, and do not allow yourself to get distracted (Department of Health, 2004). Remember the basic rules of drug administration, as addressed in Chapter 15. Think about yourself as a practitioner, know your limitations and seek help and support. Take some time to improve your knowledge about the medications that you are administering. Education and training are very important for all staff, and this should be a two-way process between your university and your clinical practice.

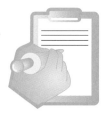

Activity 3.

While you are on placement in clinical practice make a list of common drugs that are used on the ward and find out as much as you can about them.

Where possible, try not to get distracted while carrying out a drug round. There have been a number of suggestions made about ways to achieve this, for example using a 'Do Not Disturb' sign on the drug trolley or wearing tabards which state 'Do Not Disturb Me!' Another idea is to let other staff know that you are undertaking the drug round so that they can listen for and respond to the nurse call bells.

The NPSA has set out seven priority areas for improving medication safety that support some of the issues we have looked at in this section. These priority areas are:

1. Increase reporting and learning from medication incidents.

2. Implement NPSA safe medication practice recommendations.

3. Improve staff skills and competences.

4. Minimise dosing errors.

5. Ensure medicines are not omitted.

6. Ensure the correct medicines are given to the correct patient.

7. Document patients' medicine allergy status (NPSA, 2007b).

The NPSA (2007a) states that there are more than 900 million prescriptions dispensed each year in the United Kingdom. On a positive note, remember that a majority of these will not involve errors as long as you follow local protocols and remain mindful of the issues discussed within this chapter.

Reflection

How would you feel if you were a patient and your nurse gave you the wrong medication? Reflect on this question and write a brief description of your feelings. Then consider how you might reassure a patient who has been given the wrong medication. What would you say to the patient and what information should you give them? Discuss your conclusions with your fellow students and with your mentor.

The storage of medication

We all have an important role to play when it comes to the storage of medications. There are many forms of medication storage. The NMC have created an ESC specifically in relation to the ordering, receiving and storing of drugs (Section 37) (2007a). The expectation in relation to this section is that you will be able to apply the knowledge of local trust policies to the safe storage of medications while in clinical practice. With this in mind, the aim of this chapter is to look at some of the key issues in relation to medication storage.

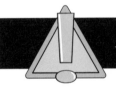

Remember that a hospital is a public place and, as such, the safe and secure storage of potentially dangerous substances, such as drugs, is paramount.

Once drugs arrive on the ward or in the department from the pharmacy it is important that the nurse in charge allocates an appropriately trained member of staff to check and put them away in the correct cupboards or trolleys. The only way you will learn to do this is to get involved while you are on placement.

Safety checks

Before any medication can be stored there are two safety checks that need to take place. The drugs will arrive in the clinical area in packaging and a visual check of these needs to take place. If the packaging has been tampered with or damaged, the medication should be returned to the pharmacy. The same applies to the drug label. There should be no alterations or changes to the labels. Additionally, all drugs are labelled with an expiry date and it is important to store the drugs in date order within the appropriate medication cupboard.

The storage of medication at an appropriate temperature

The MHRA (2001) sets out recommendations on how to store medications at appropriate temperatures. Local hospital Trusts will have their own variations on these recommendations, so you must familiarise yourself with your own local Trust policies.

Cold storage

There are a range of drugs that require cold storage. The information on temperature storage in relation to specific drugs can be found in the BNF and also in the manufacturer's guidelines. Any product requiring cold storage between 2°C and 8°C should be stored in a locked refrigerator designed for the storage of medication, and certainly not one that is used for the storage of food because of the risk of cross-contamination of the food stuff or the medication.

The minimum requirement for temperature monitoring is a thermometer that measures maximum and minimum temperatures, which can be put in with the drugs so that, as far as possible, it will not be affected by the opening and closing of the door. Good practice is to read and record the temperature daily and reset the thermometer, although it is advisable to check your local hospital policy. When storing medications in refrigerators avoid contact with the chiller plate or coil within the refrigerator as this may reduce the recommended temperature of the drug. This is particularly important in relation to high risk products such as, for example, vaccines. Think about how the drugs are placed in the fridge. The ideal position is with space around the drug to allow for the circulation of air. There are a very small number of specialist drugs that require freezer storage. However, the same principles apply to their management and storage. The temperature range recommended for these is below –5°C.

Room temperature storage

Most of the drugs that we see in clinical practice fall into this category. They are usually marked as 'Do not store above 25°C'. As long as the drug is stored at the recommended temperature, variation should not alter the stability or shelf life of the drug concerned. With this in mind, thought should go into where the drugs are stored. During periods of extreme heat or cold the drugs should be protected where possible. Therefore, where and how drugs are stored at room temperature is important. For example, they should not be stored in direct sunlight.

Caution – the clinical effectiveness of a drug may alter if it is stored at the wrong temperature.

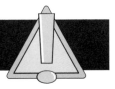

The location of medication cupboards and trolleys

An important aspect for the location of cupboards and trolleys is that medications should be stored in a convenient place for staff. This is to allow access and adequate space, but also so that the cupboard and/or trolley is in sight so they may be observed for security reasons. Cupboards and trolleys that are for medication storage should also be sited appropriately according to the nature and stability of the products they contain. Particular attention should be paid to the height of cupboards, to avoiding direct sunlight, to preventing contamination and to avoiding adverse temperatures, as these factors may pose a risk to staff, the drug itself or the patients.

Drug trolleys

These are lockable mobile storage units for medications and are used in a ward environment where mobile drug rounds may occur regularly. They should be stored as previously described but, when not in use, the trolley should be locked and secured to the wall as a safety measure. As we mentioned at the start of this chapter, hospitals are public places and medications are potentially dangerous if misused. During a drug round it is good essential practice not to leave the trolley open if it is unattended. If you do have to leave it then it should be locked. The keys for the drug trolley should be held by the person in charge of the ward.

Drug cupboards

A drug cupboard is a lockable but static unit which is wall mounted at a variety of heights, often in a clean utility room to which unauthorised personnel do not have access. There should be nominated cupboards for internally and externally-used medications. The keys should be held by the nurse in charge of the ward or clinical area, as they have overall responsibility for the activity on the ward or department. Regulations for the storage of substances hazardous to health are set out in the Control of Substances Hazardous to Health Regulations (COSHH) 1988. Common intravenous fluids and emergency drugs are the only medications that are not stored in a locked cupboard. However, emergency drugs do have to be in a sealed container.

Patients may have their own drug cupboards. This allows them to administer their own medication as prescribed. The use of this method is on the increase (possibly helping to reduce medication errors). Drugs are usually stored in a wall-mounted locked cabinet next to the patient's bed. The patient has the key and is responsible for it, but the policy on this may vary depending on local Trust procedures.

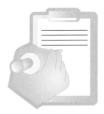

Activity 4.

Would it be a good idea to allow James Roper access to a drug cupboard? If not, why not?

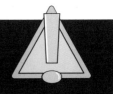

1. *Remember that ward or department medications are only for use with patients and are not for the use of members of staff or patients' relatives.*
2. *Do not forget that it is imperative that you follow the general principles of infection prevention and control when administrating medications.*

Controlled drugs

Controlled drugs today are an essential part of modern clinical practice. They are used for a wide variety of clinical conditions ranging from acute and chronic pain management to anaesthesia or palliative care. This section aims to give you an understanding of some of the key issues relating to controlled drug management and safety.

There has been a large amount of research work done on the safe management of controlled drugs following the Shipman enquiry (Department of Health, 2006). The key aspects following this investigation are:

❏ monitoring and inspection;

❏ prescribing of controlled drugs;

❏ the audit trail;

❏ information for patients;

❏ training and professional development.

(Department of Health, 2004)

The Department of Health has recently gone on to release guidance on the safer management of controlled drugs, which is intended to work alongside existing guidelines and legislation (Department of Health, 2007).

The definition of controlled drugs

Downie *et al.* (2003, p.12) offer this definition of controlled drugs: 'drugs of addiction which produce dependence such as diamorphine and pethidine'. The Misuse of Drugs Act 1971 and the Misuse of Drugs Regulations 1985 amended in 2006 regulate controlled drugs. They offer this definition: 'A "controlled drug" means a drug in Schedule 1, 2, 3, 4 or 5 of the Misuse of Drugs Regulations 1985 last updated 2006'. These regulations are quite detailed and, for many nurses, not relevant to clinical practice. Most drugs used in clinical practice are subject to Schedule 2 requirements. Should you wish to read more around the Schedule of Drugs look at the Misuse of Drugs Regulations 1985.

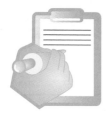

Activity 5.

Make a list of some of the common controlled drugs that you have seen being used in practice.

The prescription of controlled drugs

The prescription of controlled drugs should only be undertaken by an appropriately trained health care professional who is competent to do so, such as a doctor or nurse. Controlled drugs can also be administered under a Patient Group Directive (PGD) by appropriately trained members of staff such as, for example, some nurses or paramedics. In the past, the use of these drugs was restricted to hospitals, but they are now being used outside the hospital environment by district nurses and paramedics. Although their usage is now far wider, there are still strict requirements when it comes to controlled drugs. For example, doctors may not administer or authorise the supply of cocaine or diamorphine, or their salts, to an addicted person except for the purpose of treating organic disease or injury, unless they are licensed to do so by the Secretary of State. This illustrates the level of protection that exists around controlled drug management.

At times you may witness an instruction by telephone to a nurse to administer a controlled drug. This is generally not regarded as good practice so check your local Trust policy. There may be some instances where the medication has been previously prescribed and the prescriber is unable to issue a new prescription such as, for example, a community hospital that does not have a doctor on site, but where changes to the dose or route may be considered necessary. The use of information technology (either fax or e-mail) might be used. If this does happen then it should be followed up by a new prescription confirming the changes, ideally within 24 hours.

The storage of controlled drugs

There are detailed recommendations for how controlled drugs should be stored. Controlled drugs should not be stored anywhere unless there is an appropriately qualified member of staff on the ward or in the department where the drugs are to be kept. Whether the drugs are being used in hospital or out of hospital it is essential that they are stored according to national and local guidelines.

Controlled drugs should only be stored in a locked controlled drug cabinet reserved solely for this purpose. It is common practice for these cabinets to be inside an additional locked cabinet, although this is not required. There is often a red indicator light on these cabinets to inform staff that it is open. These cabinets should be secured to a wall, somewhere that is easily observed by staff. This sometimes causes much debate because if the cupboard is easily observed by staff then others can also see it. These cabinets also tend to be in areas that are busy, for example around the nurses' station or within patient areas, and this may lead to mistakes occurring. This is why it is important to follow the correct procedure and guidelines when dealing with medications to minimise risk.

The keys for the controlled drug cabinet should be held by the nurse in charge and kept separate from the main keys. Local arrangements will be made for the storage of spare keys or keys for areas which are not staffed 24 hours a day. Lost or stolen keys should be reported immediately to senior staff who will then follow local protocols.

If controlled drugs need to be refrigerated, they should be stored in a separate locked fridge solely for that purpose. If this is not possible then discussion will need to take place with the local pharmacy department. As with other drugs, controlled drugs should be kept in their original packaging and, where possible, should not be transferred to other storage containers.

The controlled drug register

Any area that stocks controlled drugs must hold a register of the drugs held. The purpose of the register is to monitor and record the usage and running balance of the drugs. The Royal Pharmaceutical Society of Great Britain (RPS, 2005) has produced guidance on the maintenance of a running balance. The Department of Health (2006) has published guidance that states that the 'nurse in charge' of the unit or department is responsible for ensuring regular stock checks take place and for maintaining accuracy of the running balance (see local policy), but daily checks are a minimum. These checks should be carried out by two members of staff, one a registered nurse and a second nurse or responsible person, for example a student nurse or senior health care worker (check local policy). Any movement of controlled drugs, whether for administration, disposal, or return to pharmacy, should be recorded. Any discrepancies should be brought to the immediate attention of the nurse in charge. An untoward incident form must be completed for actual and near miss controlled drug incidents.

Ordering and receiving controlled drugs

Any area with controlled drugs should also hold a drug ordering book. The nurse in charge of that area is responsible for maintaining a list of names, signatures and the grades of nurses who are authorised to order such drugs. There needs to be a balance of the level of stock that is held in the area, and overstocking or understocking should be avoided. Staff within the relevant areas will have an idea of the amount of controlled drugs that are used on a daily basis. Each item requested should be ordered on a separate page, including the date, signature and printed name of the person ordering the drugs. This request will then be forwarded to the pharmacy department where the order will be checked and the drugs prepared for collection or delivery (depending on local policy).

The delivery or collection of the drugs will be carried out by a member of the hospital staff with a valid identification badge. Upon arrival of the drugs to the area, a registered nurse must check the delivery, making reference to the original order. A signature will be required on the delivery record. These drugs should then be recorded in the area's controlled drug register, including the date received, quantity supplied and amended balance. This recording should be carried out by two members of registered staff. Senior staff and the pharmacy should be informed of any discrepancies. As a student nurse you will not be in a position to order controlled drugs, but check with your local hospital policy regarding students undertaking the checking procedure.

If there is a requirement for controlled drugs outside of pharmacy hours then your local hospital policy will inform you of the procedure to follow. There may be slight variations from Trust to Trust, so be sure to read up on this if you change Trusts.

The administration of controlled drugs

Controlled drugs have traditionally been checked by two registered nurses or midwives during the preparation and administration processes. This should always be the gold standard where two registered practitioners are available to undertake this process. However, at times, this might not be achievable, for example in community hospitals or during quieter night shifts. If it is detrimental to patient care not to give the drug, the registered nurse may use an appropriately trained health care worker as the second check. The person performing the check is verifying that the stock level of the particular drug corresponds to the drug register. If difficult drug calculations are required, then two registered members of staff must be involved in the preparation of the drug. Any mistakes in the register should be crossed out with a single line, then signed and dated.

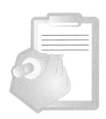

Activity 6.

Recap on the drug administration procedure in Chapter 15 and remind yourself of the 5Rs. How might you administer a controlled drug to James Roper?

There are some slight differences, specific to the administration of controlled drugs, in the administration procedure:

See Chapter 15, page 284.

❑ Check the stock level with the controlled drug register.

❑ Both staff members must sign the register and the patient's prescription chart.

❑ The nurse administering should perform an identity check at the patient's bedside.

❑ The dose administrated should be recorded.

❑ If any drug is left, it must be disposed of appropriately (see below).

❑ Amend the controlled drug register.

The disposal of controlled drugs

Controlled drugs must be destroyed in accordance with the laws specified in the Misuse of Drugs Regulations 1985. Your local pharmacy will have identified persons who are responsible for the disposal of these drugs. If controlled drugs are no longer required within your area then they must be sent back to the pharmacy department. The nurse in charge should inform the pharmacist of this. An entry must be made into the controlled drug register of the return of the drug involved and this should be signed by the appropriate members of staff.

Individual doses of controlled drugs which have been prepared but then not administered may be destroyed at ward or department level. A second qualified nurse should witness the destruction of the drug and a record should be kept in the controlled drug register, with both the nurses involved signing the register. Destruction should take place by rinsing the drug down the sink or sluice.

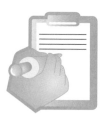

Activity 7.

While on placement and under the direct supervision of your mentor, get involved with the management of controlled drugs whenever possible. This will provide you with useful and safe practical experience.

Useful websites

Department of Health: **www.dh.gov.uk**

health care Commission: **www.healthcarecommission.org.uk**

National Institute for Health and Clinical Excellence: **www.nice.org.uk**

National Patient Safety Agency: **www.npsa.nhs.uk**

National Prescribing Centre: **www.npc.co.uk**

References

Audit Commission (2001) *A spoonful of sugar – medication management in NHS hospitals.* London: Audit Commission

Cousins, D. (2007) 'National Patient Safety Agency'. Online at: **www.npsa.nhs.uk/display? contentId=5807**

Davies, E.C., Green, C.F., Mottram, D.R. and Pirmohamed, M. (2006) 'Adverse drug reactions in hospital patients: a pilot study'. *Journal of Clinical Pharmacy and Therapeutics*, 31: 335–41

Department of Health (2004) *Building a safer NHS for patients: improving medication safety.* Online at: **www.dh.gov.uk**

Department of Health (2006) *Safer management of controlled drugs. changes to record keeping requirement.* Online at: **www.dh.gov.uk**

Department of Health (2007) *Safer management of controlled drugs: a guide to good practice in secondary care (England).* Online at: **www.dh.gov.uk**

Downie, G., Mackenzie, J. and Williams, A. (2003) *Pharmacology and medicines management for nurses*, 3rd edn. London: Elsevier Churchill Livingstone

Medicines and health care Products Regulatory Agency (2001) *Recommendations on the control and monitoring of storage and transportation temperatures of medicinal products.* Online at: **www.mhra.gov.uk**

Medicines and health care Products Regulatory Agency (n.d.) 'Pharmacovigilence "Yellow Card" scheme'. Online at: **www.yellowcard.gov.uk** (last accessed 20 July 2007)

Misuse of Drugs Act 1971. London: HMSO

Misuse of Drugs Regulations 1985, SI No. 2066, updated 2006. London: HMSO. Online at: **www.opsi.gov.uk**

National Institute for Health and Clinical Excellence (2007) Online at: **www.nice.org.uk**

National Patient Safety Agency (2007) *Safety in doses: improving the use of medications in the NHS.* Online at: **www.npsa.nhs.uk**

National Prescribing Centre (2007) *A guide to good practice in the management of controlled drugs in primary care (England)*, 2nd edn. Online at: **www.npc.co.uk**

Nursing and Midwifery Council (2004) *The code of professional conduct: standards for conduct, performance and ethics.* London: NMC

Nursing and Midwifery Council (2007a) *Essential Skills Clusters for pre-registration nursing programmes, Annexe 2.* Online at: **www.nmc-uk.org**

Nursing and Midwifery Council (2007b) *Guidelines for the administration of medicines.* London: NMC

Pirmohamed, M., James, S., Meakin, S., Green, C., Scott, A.K., Walley, T.J., Farrer, K., Park, B.K. and Brackenridge, A.M. (2004) 'Adverse rug reactions as cause of admission to hospital: prospective analysis of 18,820 patients'. *British Medical Journal*, 329: 15–19

Royal Pharmaceutical Society of Great Britain (2005) *Maintaining running balances of controlled drug stock.* Online at: **www.rpsgb.org.uk**

5 CARE MANAGEMENT

This part includes the following chapters:

Scenario: Teresa White

Teresa White is a 45-year-old female who enjoys a healthy active lifestyle. She has had no significant medical problems.

While driving to the local golf club Teresa is involved in a minor road traffic accident. She is admitted to the accident and emergency department of her local hospital. She is alert and orientated and can remember the details of the accident. She is aware that she hit her head on the windscreen, and reports no other injuries apart from a developing headache and a degree of blurred vision. Chapter 17 considers the assessment process and management and care for Teresa, including observations (temperature, pulse, respirations, blood pressure, neurological and blood glucose).

Teresa is admitted to the assessment unit for observation overnight. While she is there she starts to deteriorate (see Chapter 18 on early warning scores) and requires airway management. While Teresa does not require advanced life support, the requirements of the role of the advanced life support nurse are discussed in Chapter 19 to help develop your understanding of this aspect of nursing.

Surgery is performed on Teresa to relieve the intracranial pressure caused by a subdural haematoma. The requirements of pre- and post-operative care are covered in Chapter 20.

While she is recovering, Teresa develops a temperature. Specimen collection, in order to find out the cause of Teresa's temperature, is covered in Chapter 21.

Teresa makes an uneventful recovery and is discharged home after ten days.

Chapter 17

OBSERVATIONS

Sue Quayle

The Nursing and Midwifery Council has set standards to measure your performance in taking observations. The Essential Skills Clusters covered in this chapter are as follows:

Patients/clients can trust a newly registered nurse to:

Section 6 iii	Record information accurately and clearly on the basis of observation and communication.
Section 9 ix	Measure and document vital signs under supervision and respond appropriately to findings outside the normal range.
Section 10 v	Detect, record, report and respond appropriately to signs of deterioration and/or improvement.
Section 22 i-vii	Maintain effective standard infection control precautions.

Introduction

By the end of this chapter you will know how to accurately and efficiently record a patient's temperature, pulse respirations and blood pressure. Recording a patient's temperature, pulse and respiratory rate is vital for the early detection of any deterioration in the patient's condition (Kenward *et al.*, 2001). We will also cover neurological observations and blood glucose monitoring in this chapter.

Taking observations provides a good opportunity to get to know your patient. It is your chance to be able to put a name to a face and to determine the condition of your patient. While interpretation of the data is of vital importance it is also important to look at the patient holistically. Taking observations enables you to talk to the patient, to see whether they are in pain, if they are worried or if they are uncomfortable. Remember, verbal informed consent should always be obtained from the patient before starting observations procedures.

Observations

The interpretation of the data from the patient assessment is vital in determining the level of care a patient requires, providing an intervention or treatment and preventing a patient deteriorating from an otherwise preventable cause (Wheatley, 2005). The nursing assessment aims to provide an accurate picture of the current condition, whereas a medical diagnosis aims to provide a causal explanation for the patient's presenting signs and symptoms (Crow *et al.*, cited in Wheatley, 2005).

As Teresa has arrived in the accident and emergency department, a general set of observations will be taken. These include temperature, pulse and respirations (TPR) and blood pressure (BP). A set of neurological observations will also be performed along with an assessment of Teresa's blood glucose level.

Before you go to the patient's bedside, you must wash your hands (see Chapter 21, page 455). Knowing your patient's history and condition will enable you to decide if extra precautions are required. Multi-use equipment should also be thoroughly cleaned between each patient.

See Chapter 21, page 455.

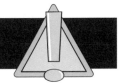

It is of vital importance that all observations are recorded accurately. Any observations outside the normal range should be acted upon appropriately.

Temperature, pulse, respirations and blood pressure (TPR, BP)

Temperature

Body temperature represents the balance between heat gain and heat loss and can be measured using various methods (Royal Marsden Hospital, 2005). Sites for temperature measurement are as follows:

❑ **Axilla** – under the arm. The thermometer must be well underneath the arm and underneath any clothing.

❑ **Oral** – under the tongue. If you are worried about a patient trying to bite the thermometer then use another method.

❑ **Tympanic membrane** – in the external auditory canal (outer ear).

❑ **Rectal** – in the rectum (rarely used these days).

❑ **Forehead** – some new thermometers have strips that are placed on the forehead. You may also encounter some modern electronic devices that measure body temperature on the skin surface.

There are many different types of thermometer available and they have different operating techniques (see Figure 1). It would be impossible to give a description of them here but you should become familiar with the

Figure 1
Thermometers

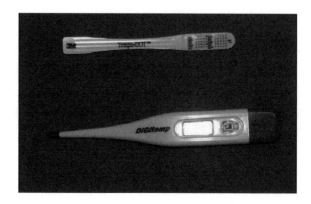

main types of thermometer used in your placement hospital. The traditional way of taking a temperature was by using a mercury thermometer, putting it under the tongue and leaving it in place for several minutes. The thermometer was read by recording the graduated scale that corresponded to the mercury level. Some of the new thermometers use a similar technique, but without the use of mercury.

The normal range of temperature is from 36.0 to 37.5°C (degrees Celsius). Values can vary with the site and with the technique. A low temperature is called **hypothermia**; a high temperature is called **hyperthermia** or **pyrexia**. Body temperature can alter due to illness, exposure of the body and drugs. Oral temperatures can be affected by any food or fluids the patient has taken recently. If a patient has recently taken hot or very cold food or fluids you should wait for 15 minutes before taking the temperature orally (Mueller Jarvis, 1976). Oxygen therapy can alter the patient's oral temperature, as can time of day, ovulation (in women), smoking and the temperature taker's technique. A temperature taken under the arm may produce a lower reading than that in the mouth. For this reason the site of taking the temperature should always be noted.

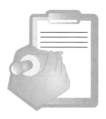

Activity 1.

Using a thermometer, record your own temperature and that of a friend. Assess the difference, after two minutes, between a temperature taken under the arm and a temperature taken orally.

Pulse

The pulse is an impulse transmitted by the contraction of the ventricles of the heart. It is commonly felt by **palpation** where an artery crosses a bony prominence (see Figure 2). Sites of possible pulse palpation include the following:

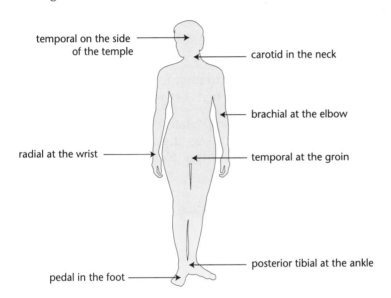

temporal on the side of the temple

carotid in the neck

brachial at the elbow

radial at the wrist

temporal at the groin

posterior tibial at the ankle

pedal in the foot

Figure 2
Sites of possible pulse palpation

- ❑ **Radial** – on the inside of the wrist above the thumb. This is the most common place to take the pulse for a routine reading as it is generally accessible.

- ❑ **Brachial** – on the inside of the elbow and on opposite side from the radial pulse (the inner aspect of the arm). This is where the pulse is felt prior to taking a blood pressure.

- ❑ **Carotid** – beside the trachea; an important site to remember as this is used to feel for a pulse during a cardiac arrest. Take unilaterally.

- ❑ **Temporal** – on the temple. A useful place to take the pulse in children.

- ❑ **Femoral** – in the groin. The pulse is often taken here if you are unable to obtain a pulse from the wrist. This site is often used in a patient deteriorating or during a cardiac arrest.

❏ **Popliteal** – just behind the knee. This is not often used as an area for taking the pulse but it is useful to know that it is there, especially if you are trying to assess the extent of the blood supply to the leg.

❏ **Posterior tibial** – just behind the ankle. This is often used in patients with breaks to bones or if there is poor circulation to the feet.

❏ **Dorsal pedis** – on the top of the foot. Often felt post-operatively, with injuries to the foot or when there is a problem with circulation.

❏ **An apex beat** can also be assessed by putting a stethoscope on the chest over the heart. When listening to the apex at the same time as feeling the radial pulse any deficits between the two can be obtained.

When assessing the pulse it is important not only to measure the beats per minute (bpm) but also to assess the rhythm, the quality and the elasticity (the springiness) of the artery. Normal and abnormal pulse rates are shown in Table 1.

Table 1
Normal and abnormal pulse rates (bpm)

Normal pulse	Slow pulse (bradycardia)	Fast pulse (tachycardia)
60 to 100	Less than 60	More than 100

A fast pulse can be an indication of low circulating blood volume as the heart beats faster to keep the blood pressure up, and this can be due to

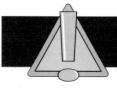

It is important to note that the pulse rates for children are different to adults and vary with age.

dehydration, stress, shock, pain and exercise. A low pulse can be caused by raised intracranial pressure, certain drugs and physical fitness. Irregular heart beats can be shown as an irregular pulse. The pulse may also change in pressure per beat. A weakness in the pulse may indicate decreased cardiac function (McCance and Huether, 2006).

To take a radial pulse, find the correct area as shown in Figure 3. Place the fingers over the site of the artery – you may need to move your fingers around until you find the pulse. Using a watch that shows seconds, count the number of beats felt within a one minute period. Document the rate.

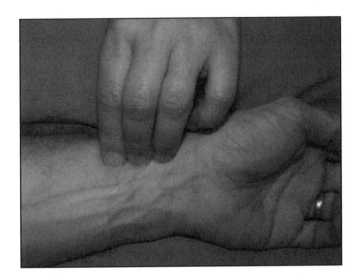

Figure 3
Taking a radial pulse

Activity 2.

With a friend, practise locating the different places used to take a pulse, particularly the brachial, radial and carotid (remembering to ask for permission before beginning). Count each other's pulse for a minute assessing rate, rhythm and strength.

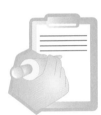

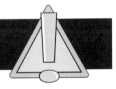

Do not use the thumb to take a pulse as you are more likely to record your own pulse than that of your patient!

Respirations

The function of the respiratory system is to supply the body with oxygen and to remove carbon dioxide. One respiration consists of an inspiration and an expiration. Assessment includes the rate, the rhythm and the quality. Observing respirations not only shows the rate and the rhythm, but also the effort that is taken. It is therefore important to assess how hard the patient is breathing, whether each side is moving equally or if the chest is moving in a see-saw action, what extra muscles are being used and any extra noises that might be heard such as wheezing, grunting, **stridor**, snoring, sighing and gasping. Other factors such as flaring of the nostrils should also be observed. All these can be signs of respiratory distress. Other signs, which may be less obvious, are signs that the patient is becoming anxious or tired. Respirations often show early signs of other problems. Over half the patients reviewed in a study by Kenward *et al.* (2001) had documented shortness of breath within 24 hours prior to a respiratory or cardiac arrest.

You take the respiration rate by observing the rising and falling of the patient's chest. When taking a respiratory rate you need to ensure the patient is not aware of what you are doing. It is easy to hold your own breath or to breathe really fast for a minute when you are aware someone is recording your breathing.

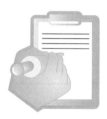

Activity 3.

Practise taking a patient's respirations while appearing to take the radial pulse. This apparent subterfuge will help you to gain an accurate respiratory rate.

Blood pressure

Blood pressure is the force of blood exerted on the wall of an artery. A normal blood pressure generally ranges from 100/60 to 140/90 mmHg. The upper figure represents the **systolic pressure**, while the lower figure represents the **diastolic pressure**. Both are measured in millimetres of mercury (mmHg).

❑ Systolic pressure is the maximum pressure of the blood exerted against the wall of the artery during ventricular contractions.

❑ Diastolic blood pressure is the minimum pressure of blood against the wall of the artery following closure of the aortic valve (Royal Marsden Hospital, 2004).

A low blood pressure is referred to as **hypotension**. A high blood pressure is known as **hypertension**. High blood pressure can be caused by:

❑ raised intracranial pressure;

❑ cardiovascular disease;

❑ stress;

❑ pain.

Low blood pressure can be caused by:

❑ low circulating blood volume (hypovalaemia);

❑ decreased cardiac output;

❑ dehydration;

❑ alcohol.

Shock is when the circulatory system is not able to work effectively to provide the required amount of circulation to the tissues (McCance and Huether, 2006, p.176). Types of shock include:

❑ cardiogenic shock (may be caused by a heart attack (myocardial infarction));

❑ hypovolaemic shock (due to massive blood loss or severe dehydration);

❑ septic shock (due to a severe systemic infection);

❑ anaphylactic shock (caused by a severe allergic reaction).

Shock induced hypotension is usually accompanied by a rapid pulse (tachycardia). Neurogenic shock, due possibly to meningitis, may also result in a lowered blood pressure but with a bradycardia rather than a tachycardia.

Blood pressure is taken manually by a device called a sphygmomanometer. Electronic devices are often used but will not be described in this book. If you come across these in your clinical placements, make sure you ask your mentor how they work. However, they should not be used at the expense of developing an expert manual technique.

Reflection

Review the cardiovascular system and think about some of the many diseases which could affect the patient's blood pressure.

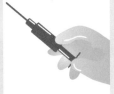

Taking a blood pressure

Before taking a blood pressure it is important to discover the approximate systolic pressure (see Figure 4). This can be obtained as follows:

1. Place the blood pressure cuff over the middle third of the arm.

2. While watching the sphygmomanometer dial, feel for the radial pulse.

3. Pump the cuff up slowly until the radial pulse disappears. The reading on which the radial pulse disappears is the systolic blood pressure.

4. It is important to estimate the systolic beat first so that the cuff is not over-inflated. This can cause a lot of unnecessary pain to the patient.

The technique for reading a patient's blood pressure is as follows.

1. Put the cuff attached to a sphygmomanometer around the middle third of the upper arm.

2. Ensure that the upper arm has no clothing on it or that any clothing underneath the cuff is a thin single layer and not creased. Jumpers or dressing gowns must be removed.

Figure 4
Measuring a
blood pressure

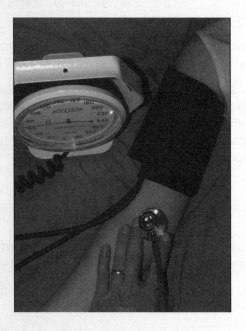

3. Close the valve on the pump. Trying to do this while keeping the stethoscope in place involves a lot of dexterity! One of the keys to taking a reliable reading is to learn to control the valve when pumping the cuff up and letting it down.

4. The stethoscope is placed in the ears (place the ear attachments facing slightly forwards as this follows the line of the ear canal). Use the flat side of the stethoscope to listen for the sounds.

5. The cuff is then pumped up 10 to 20 mmHg above the level of the systolic reading that you estimated earlier. Then let the air out of the cuff slowly, with the stethoscope over the brachial artery. If the cuff is let down too fast then you may not hear the sounds at the correct time resulting in an inaccurate reading. If it is let down too slowly then it can cause a lot of discomfort to the patient.

6. With the stethoscope on the brachial artery, you are listening for the **Korotkoff sounds**. When you hear the first clear pulse sound, the reading on the sphygmomanometer corresponds to the systolic pressure. As you continue to release air from the cuff, you will be able to hear the pulse. The level at which you can no longer hear the pulse through the stethoscope corresponds to the diastolic pressure.

Document accurately the readings when the sound appears (systolic) and then disappears (diastolic).

Hints for practice

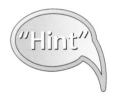

When taking a blood pressure the cuff must be over the middle third of the upper arm. If the cuff is too small or too large this is not possible. Most hospitals will keep a range of different size cuffs. Also, keep the stethoscope away from the tubes from the sphygmomanometer as this will create excessive noise. Finally, ensure that the head of the stethoscope is aligned in the correct way in order to hear properly.

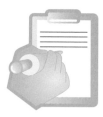

Activity 4.

Find a manual sphygmomanometer. Practise taking a manual blood pressure whenever possible to maintain your proficiency in this skill.

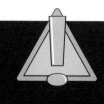

1. *The use of electronic devices is often a major part of patient assessment. The reliance on a machine for taking observations may be detrimental to patient care if other obvious cues to the patient's condition are not picked up, and may contribute to a superficial patient assessment (Wheatley, 2005).*
2. *Do not take a blood pressure on the arm of a patient who has an A-V shunt for kidney dialysis, or on the affected side of a patient who has had their lymph nodes removed for diseases such as breast cancer. Lymph oedema can affect readings after mastectomy.*

Oxygen saturation

The oxygen saturation is the percentage of oxygen circulating around the body. Normal values are 95 to 100 per cent. A saturation of below 70 per cent is life-threatening (Kozier *et al.*, 2002). Oxygen saturations fall when a patient has a reduced amount of oxygen circulating through the body.

See Chapter 15, page 317.

Oxygen saturations are obtained by taking a probe attached to an oxygen saturation monitor and placing it on the tip of the finger or toe over the nail. This obtains a reading by measuring the colour difference between oxygenated and deoxygenated blood (see also Chapter 15, page 317). Readings can be made more difficult if the patient has poor circulation to the fingers or toes or if there are fine movements such as tremors. Nail varnish and dirt can also act as a barrier to obtaining a good reading. It is possible to use some of the probes on the ear or the lip if necessary.

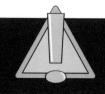

An oxygen saturation probe should never be used to take the pulse rate. It cannot assess the rhythm and quality. It also does not replace the respiratory rate observation as it measures blood oxygenation, not ventilatory function (Kenward et al., 2001).

Neurological observations

As Teresa has a head injury she needs a set of neurological observations and these are likely to be recorded on a chart similar to that shown in Figure 5. Note that it is recommended that in-hospital observations of a patient with a head injury should only be conducted by professionals competent in the assessment of head injury (NICE, 2003). However, as a student, you should take the opportunity to watch neurological observations being carried out while you are on placement and this section will help you to understand the procedure.

Head injury refers to any trauma to the head other than superficial injuries to the face (NICE, 2003). As the skull is a very hard structure there is little room to accommodate problems such as blood clots, tumours or oedema (Waterhouse, 2005). It is important to detect any problems early so that the appropriate treatment can be performed and possible brain damage prevented. Any patient who is at risk of deteriorating neurologically should have neurological observations carried out. This can include:

❑ patients who have had a head injury, especially if they have lost consciousness;

❑ patients who have had a stroke;

❑ those with brain tumours;

❑ those at risk of cerebral infection.

Neurological observations consist of the Glasgow Coma Scale (GCS), pupil size, pupil reactions, limb movements, temperature, pulse, blood pressure, respirations and blood oxygen saturation. The National Institute of Clinical Excellence (NICE, 2003) has published guidelines for head injuries. They state that neurological observations should be carried out:

❑ half hourly until the GCS is 15;

❑ half hourly for two hours;

❑ one hourly thereafter until condition improves;

❑ two hourly thereafter.

It should be noted that these are minimum requirements. If you are worried about your patient's condition, then you should increase the regularity of the observations.

Figure 5
An example of a
neurological
observation chart

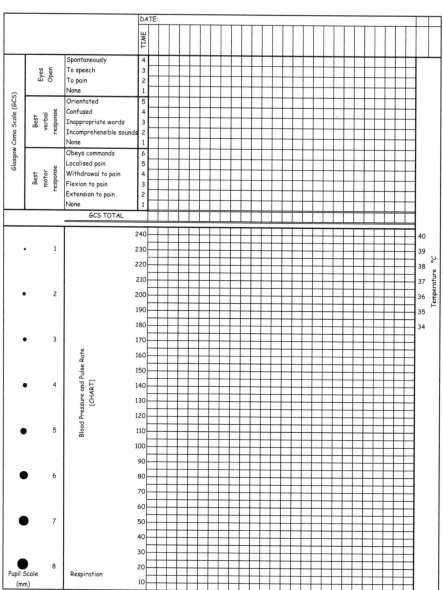

GCS evaluations

The GCS evaluates three categories that most closely reflect activity in the higher centres of the brain. These are:

❑ eye opening;

❑ verbal response;

❑ motor response.

A GCS of 15 indicates that the patient is functioning cerebrally. A deterioration of one point in the motor response or two points overall is clinically significant and must be reported to a senior member of staff. The GCS responses are as follows:

❑ Eye response:

- spontaneously – without the need for speech or touch;

- to speech – eyes open when spoken to;

- to pain – eyes open when pain evoked;

- none – no eye opening (unless closed due to injury).

❑ Verbal response:

- orientation – able to say the current year and month, where they are and why, and who they are;

- confusion – does not answer the above correctly;

- inappropriate words – random words;

- incomprehensible sounds – e.g. grunting, moaning or crying;

- none – not even following verbal or painful stimuli.

❑ Motor response:

- obeys commands – patient does what they are asked to do;

- localises - moves limb towards where pain is coming from;

- withdraws from pain – patient bends arm at the elbow but does not locate the pain;

- flexion to pain – the patient flexes the upper arm and rotates the wrist;

- extension – characterised by straightening of the elbow and internal rotation of the shoulder and wrist;

- none – no response to pain.

Pupil guide

Pupils are assessed to see if they are equal and reacting to light – this is sometimes abbreviated to 'PEARL' (pupils equal and reacting to light). Alterations in reaction, shape or size are a late sign of raised intracranial pressure. A pen torch is used and the pupil is assessed for size, shape and reaction. This is documented on the chart.

Limb movement

❑ Normal power – able to push the nurse away. Each limb must be tested separately.

❑ Mild weakness – able to push away but not with much power.

❑ Severe weakness.

❑ Flexion, extension, no response.

A doctor should urgently review a patient if any of the following occur:

❑ the development of agitation or abnormal behaviour;

❑ a drop in GCS of 1 point for over 30 minutes;

❑ any drop greater than 2 points;

❑ the development of severe or increasing headache or persistent vomiting;

❑ new or evolving neurological signs such as unequal pupils or asymmetry of limb or facial movements (NICE, 2003).

1. *Observations of infants and young children are very difficult and should only be performed by staff experienced in the observation of children with a head injury (NICE, 2003).*
2. *It should be noted that neurological bleeds are unlike other bleeds in the body. The bleeding does not cause a lowered blood volume and tachycardia but, instead, causes a raised blood pressure. Often the systolic blood pressure increases while diastolic stays the same and the heart rate will drop. The respiratory rate becomes irregular. The combination of these three factors is called Cushing's triad.*

Blood glucose monitoring

The body is monitored for blood glucose levels to discover the amount of sugar in the bloodstream. It is normal to maintain a blood sugar level of between 4 and 7 mmols per litre. When the body is unable to produce insulin, as with diabetes mellitus, the blood sugar levels rise. This is called hyperglycaemia. During illness, surgery, infection or stress, the blood sugar levels may rise in diabetic patients. Other patients may be diabetic and be unaware of it.

Hypoglycaemia is a low blood sugar level and can occur when the blood glucose level is unable to meet the metabolic demands of the body. A low blood sugar level can be caused by factors such as starvation, renal insufficiency which can cause infection, liver failure, insulin secreting tumours, salicylate (aspirin) poisoning and excess insulin in a diabetic, as well as resulting from some medications.

Taking a blood glucose level

On the ward a simple blood glucose level can be taken as follows.

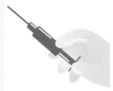

1. Wash hands and put on gloves.

2. Take a small prick of blood from the side of a clean finger of the patient, using a lancet.

3. Place the drop of blood onto a strip of blood glucose testing strips (read manufacturer's instructions first).

4. Insert this into the appropriate machine, which will then give a reading.

5. Ensure that the patient is not left bleeding afterwards.

6. Dispose of sharps correctly.

7. Dispose of gloves and wash hands.

As with thermometers, there are so many different machines on the market that it would be impossible to describe each one here. Familiarise yourself with the type of blood glucose monitor that is used in your hospital/clinical area.

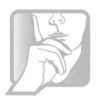

Reflection

Look at the blood pressure, pulse, respirations and temperature of a patient. See how the observations relate to each other and to the patient's medical history.

Summary

By now you should have a better theoretical and practical knowledge of how to measure:

❑ temperature;

❑ pulse;

❑ respirations;

❑ blood pressure;

❑ oxygen saturation;

❑ neurological observations;

❑ blood glucose.

As you take your observations you will also have learnt that you must gain consent from your patient. Infection control procedures must be adhered to throughout and, importantly, always document what you have measured and talk to your supervisor if you have a concern about a patient's condition.

Acknowledgements

Thanks are due to Dr Jenny Wilson, MBChB, MRCGP, GP Bedford.

Further reading

McCance, K. and Huether, S. (2006) *Pathophysiology: the biological basis for disease in adults and children*, 5th edn. St Louis, MO: Mosby

References

Andrews, T. and Waterman, H. (2005) 'Packaging: a grounded theory of how to report physiological deterioration effectively'. *Journal of Advanced Nursing*, 52(5): 473–81

Kenward, G., Hodgetts, T. and Castle, N. (2001) 'Time to put the R back in TPR'. *Nursing Times*, 97(40): 32–3

Kozier, B., Erb, G., Berman, A. and Snyder, S. (2002) *Kozier and Erb's techniques in clinical nursing: basic to intermediate skills*, 5th edn. Englewood Cliffs, NJ: Pearson Prentice Hall

McCance, K. and Huether, S. (2006) *Pathophysiology: the biological basis for disease in adults and children*, 5th edn. St Louis, MO: Mosby

Mueller Jarvis, C. (1976) 'Vital signs – how to take them more accurately and understand them more fully'. *Nursing*, 6(4): 31–7

National Institute for Clinical Excellence (2003) *Head injury: triage, assessment, investigation and early management of head injury in infants, children and adults*. London: HMSO

Royal Marsden Hospital (2004) *Manual of clinical nursing procedures*, 6th edn. Oxford: Blackwell

Waterhouse, C. (2005) 'The Glasgow Coma Scale and other neurological observations'. *Nursing Standard*, 19(33): 56–64

Wheatley, I. (2005) 'The nursing practice of taking level 1 patient observations'. *Intensive and Critical Care Nursing*, 22: 115–21

Website

www.rcn.org.uk/resources/mrsa

Chapter 18

EARLY WARNING SCORES – THE DETECTION OF DETERIORATION

Sue Quayle

The Nursing and Midwifery Council has set standards to measure your performance in taking observations. The Essential Skills Clusters covered in this chapter are as follows.

Patients/clients can trust a newly registered nurse to:

Section 6 iii	Record information accurately and clearly on the basis of observation and communication.
Section 9 ix	Measure and document vital signs under supervision and respond appropriately to findings outside the normal range.
Section 10 v	Detect, record, report and respond appropriately to signs of deterioration and or improvement.
Section 22 i–vii	Maintain effective standard infection control precautions.

What is the Early Warning Score?

Early detection of the deterioration of a patient's condition is essential in order to be able to respond appropriately. This chapter introduces you to the importance of understanding what can happen to your patient's condition. You will be introduced to the concept of the Early Warning Score (EWS). The EWS consists of a simple calculation made when the patient's temperature, pulse, respirations, blood pressure and conscious level are recorded. This calculation results in a score that will indicate if the patient requires urgent treatment, is an imminent emergency or an emergency. It is vital that you are able to detect the deterioration or potential deterioration in a patient's condition early and that you are able to respond appropriately. In the previous chapter you learnt how to take a temperature, pulse, respiration rate and blood pressure, and you were introduced to the Glasgow Coma Scale and blood glucose monitoring. This chapter will help you to learn how to use the EWS to identify the deteriorating patient and plan the appropriate care.

The NICE guidelines state that a physiological track and trigger system should be used to monitor all adult patients in an acute hospital setting. All patients in the acute ward environment should have at least one set of vital sign observations and an Early Warning Score recorded every

12 hours. The frequency of these observations should increase when abnormal physiology is detected (NICE, 2007). The Early Warning Score (EWS) or Physiological Observation Track and Trigger System (POTTS) has been developed to assist the identification of critically ill ward patients and those at risk of deterioration (Wheatley, 2005). The EWS provides nurses and doctors with a concise and unambiguous way of communicating deterioration, while giving them confidence in using medical language. It also provides them with commonly agreed criteria against which deterioration can be measured (Andrews and Waterman, 2005). Simple physiological observations identify high-risk in hospital patients. Those who die are often inpatients for days or weeks before death allowing doctors to be able to intervene and, hopefully, change the outcome (Goldhill and McNarry, 2004).

The need for the EWS is highlighted by examples of sub-optimal care such as those reported by McQuillan *et al.* (1998). They showed that life-threatening problems with the airway, breathing and circulation were being missed, misinterpreted and mismanaged. In two studies, up to 84 per cent of patients demonstrated warning signs in the hours before cardio-respiratory arrest (Schien *et al.* and Smith and Wood, cited in Kenward *et al.*, 2001). Over half the patients reviewed in a study by Kenward *et al.* had documented shortness of breath within 24 hours prior to a respiratory or cardiac arrest.

Calculating the EWS

The monitoring of vital signs involves not just taking a measurement but also the interpretation of the measurement you have recorded. It is also important to be able to monitor and interpret the changing trends of vital signs over time. At this point it's probably a good time to review your basic knowledge of the different types of shock (see Table 1). This will help you predict what could happen to the patient so you will be able to respond proactively with the appropriate treatment.

The clinical signs of shock are similar to many other conditions, which may make diagnosis difficult. The body's compensatory mechanisms can also mask many of the signs of shock for a while (McCance and Huether, 2002).

Table 1
Different types
of shock

Hypovolaemic shock	Due to a lack of circulating blood volume. Commonly caused by bleeding or dehydration.
Cardiogenic shock	Caused by reduction of the heart's ability to function properly.
Neurogenic shock	Disruption of sympathetic tone causing a widespread vasodilation.
Septic shock	Due to overwhelming infection that causes systemic vasodilation. Eventually the cardiac output is not enough to compensate for the vasodilation.
Anaphylactic shock	Sensitivity to an antigen or allergen causing vasodilation.

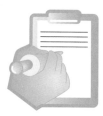

Activity 1.

Look up the different types of shock outlined in Table 1. What do you think might happen to the temperature, pulse, respirations and blood pressure when these types of shock occur?

The EWS is a simple system calculated using five main parameters. These are pulse, blood pressure, respiratory rate, temperature and the level of consciousness (called AVPU and described in more detail below). The sum of these parameters creates the EWS and is used in the hospital observation chart for the patient. Some parameters which are also used are urine output and oxygen saturation and are also listed below.

❏ Temperature – hypothermia or hyperthermia may be an indication of an infection and sepsis.

❏ Pulse – in shock the pulse rate may rise rapidly. The patient's sympathetic nervous system compensates and may increase the heart rate and the respiratory rate long before the blood pressure starts to fall (Ahern and Philpot, 2002). In neurogenic shock bradycardia may be present.

❏ Respiratory rate – it is well documented as being one of the best indicators of high-risk patients (Subbe *et al.*, 2003).

❏ Blood pressure – blood pressure may only lower later on in shock. Ahern and Philpot (2002) state that hypotension occurs after tachycardia and should be treated urgently.

❑ AVPU – is a simple, decreasing assessment of the level of consciousness of the patient. The letters stand for:

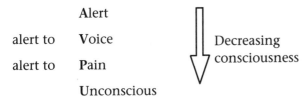

	Alert	
alert to	Voice	Decreasing
alert to	Pain	consciousness
	Unconscious	

A score of a P or U will also be backed up with a low Glasgow Coma Scale reading. There are many reasons for a decreased level of consciousness. It may be a result of direct intercranial pressure or arise from other causes such as altered blood chemistry levels.

❑ Urine – to function correctly the kidneys need to receive an adequate blood supply. Normal urine output should be 1.5–2.0 litres every 24 hours (Ahern and Philpot, 2002). To measure urine output accurately the patient may be catheterised and the urine measured hourly. If a patient triggers the EWS a fluid balance chart should be commenced immediately.

❑ Oxygen saturation – the NICE guidelines state that this should also be measured (NICE, 2007).

The idea is that small changes in each of the seven parameters described above, when looked at together, will show signs of deterioration earlier than a change in a single parameter (Rees, 2003). Any overall changes in the patient's condition can then be detected earlier and the patient can be treated sooner to prevent any further deterioration, and hopefully before they need emergency action. Remember that the higher the EWS score, the sicker the patient and the more urgent the situation.

It should be noted at this point that the pain scale is a different scoring system. 'Alert to pain' in the AVPU assessment is not the pain score. Different hospitals will have a pain scale which may be calculated separately from the EWS. However, pain is an important indicator that there is a problem, and any patient complaining of severe or worsening pain should be assessed and reported even if the EWS is not triggering a response. Patients may also be on a nausea or sedation score. Again these must also be assessed and reported on if necessary.

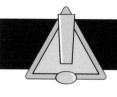

It is important to note that paediatric and midwifery EWS scores may be calculated in a completely different way.

See Chapter 19, page 382.

It is important to perform an ABCDE assessment on any patient who is triggering on the EWS. This assessment is described in Table 2. See also Chapter 19, page 382, on basic and advanced life support for more detail on airway management.

Table 2
The ABCDE assessment

Airway	If the patient can talk clearly and can cough or swallow then the airway is clear. If not call for help.
Breathing	Assess the patient's breathing. If the patient is not breathing adequately, then call for help.
Circulation	Take the pulse and blood pressure. Assess the colour of the patient, capillary refill and urine output. Call for help if abnormal.
Disability	Assess the level of consciousness. Either use AVPU or the Glasgow Coma Scale. A blood glucose level may also be taken.
Exposure	Taking a history, reviewing charts, results and investigations.

Some Trusts may require a calculation of the EWS. This may be documented on the observation chart. Other hospitals may have an observation chart with areas coloured in such a way that as you record your measurements in the coloured area you know that that parameter is triggering action. It is important to find out what your Trust uses.

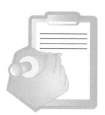

Activity 2.

Have a look at the example of an Early Warning Score chart (shown in Figure 1.). Can you relate the chart to what you have learnt so far in this chapter? How does it compare to the EWS charts used in your own clinical area?

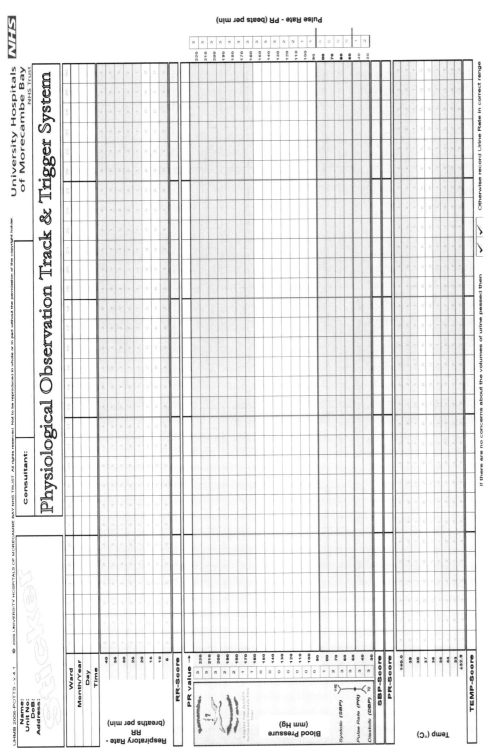

Figure 1 Early Warning Score chart (reproduced with kind permission from Morecambe Bay NHS Trust)

Figure 1
continued

Urine Rate (mls per hr) ↑301	3	3	3	3	3	3	3	3	3	3	3	3	3	3	3	3	3	3	3	3	3	3	3	3	3	3	3	3	3	3
201 - 300	2	2	2	2	2	2	2	2	2	2	2	2	2	2	2	2	2	2	2	2	2	2	2	2	2	2	2	2	2	2
30 - 200	0	0	0	0	0	0	0	0	0	0	0	0	0	0	0	0	0	0	0	0	0	0	0	0	0	0	0	0	0	0
10 - 29	1	1	1	1	1	1	1	1	1	1	1	1	1	1	1	1	1	1	1	1	1	1	1	1	1	1	1	1	1	1
↓9	3	3	3	3	3	3	3	3	3	3	3	3	3	3	3	3	3	3	3	3	3	3	3	3	3	3	3	3	3	3
Catheter Y/N																														
Urine-Score																														
Responsiveness-Score																														
TOTAL EWS																														
INITIALS	1	2	3	4	5	6	7	8	9	10	11	12	13	14	15	16	17	18	19	20	21	22	23	24	25	26	27	28	29	30

Responsiveness-Score	Agitated &/or Confused	Awake	Verbal	Pain	Unresponsive
	1	0	1	2	3

There are other important primary observations on the reverse side. Turn over

UHMB 2006-POTTS - v.4.1

SaO_2 Sats. (%)	1	2	3	4	5	6	7	8	9	10	11	12	13	14	15	16	17	18	19	20	21	22	23	24	25	26	27	28	29	30

Oxygen Therapy

Route: Trachy Mask (**TM**) or Nasal Cannulae (**NC**) or Face Mask (**FM**)

O_2 Route																														
O_2 Volume																														

Pain:		0		1		2		3	
	at rest...		no pain		slight pain		intermittent pain		continuous pain
	with movement...						moderate pain		severe pain

Pain Score																														
PCA Total (4-hourly)																														
Delivered/Demanded	/	/	/	/	/	/	/	/	/	/	/	/	/	/	/	/	/	/	/	/	/	/	/	/	/	/	/	/	/	/
Epidural ✓																														
Local Anaesthetic Infusion ✓																														

Nausea & Vomiting (N&V):	0	no N&V	1	mild to moderate N&V	2	severe N&V

N&V Score																														
Anti-emetic given ✓																														
Blood Glucose																														
Actioned ✓																														

DAILY WEIGH / FLUID BALANCE

If patient's weight increases day on day, they may be in fluid retention.
Check patient's weight every 24 hours and tally fluid balance.

Weight (Kg)																														
Fluid Balance (ml)																														
GCS																														
INITIALS	1	2	3	4	5	6	7	8	9	10	11	12	13	14	15	16	17	18	19	20	21	22	23	24	25	26	27	28	29	30

The *ghosted* column numbers above match *ghosted* column numbers on chart over page. If replicating chart, ensure both sides are copied on A3 paper.

University Hospitals NHS
of Morecambe Bay
NHS Trust

Patient Observation Protocol

Figure 1
Early Warning Score Chart (reproduced with kind permission from Morecombe Bay NHS Trust)

A full set of patient EWS observations must be recorded every four hours unless other instructions have been issued. Other important observations, on the reverse of the chart, must also be recorded at the same time.

h   Plot observations in chart area as normal and record their values (see sketch showing respiratory rate (RR) data).   *Charting in this way ensures observations can be tracked over time but also ensures that records can be easily and accurately recovered at a later date.*

h   Blood pressure and pulse rate (PR) occupy the same chart area - therefore record systolic and diastolic BP (SBP and DBP) as described on left axis. Plot PR as usual and record reading in the spare box at the top of the chart area.

h   Note that the urine record is not a linear scale but five ranges. Record the urine rate (mls per hour) in the correct range.

h   For PR observations - values falling above the   red line   and below the   blue line   require scoring.

h   All other observations require scoring if falling on a shaded (blue   area of chart.

h   Score values are   *ghosted*   behind the relevant box in the chart, except   SBP and PR. The SBP-score instruction is located to the left of the chart area. The PR-score instruction is located to the right of the chart area.

h   Enter a score for each observation (including zeros) in the relevant yellow box, sum the values in each yellow box and enter result in bright yellow 'TOTAL EWS' box at the bottom of chart.

h   Sign the "INITIALS" box and ensure date and time are clearly written on chart.   A qualified nurses must counter-initial the observation when it triggers the protocol below, thus indicating that the appropriate action has taken place.

Note: Patient ID and consultant name occur on one side of chart only, therefore photocopy both sides of the chart.

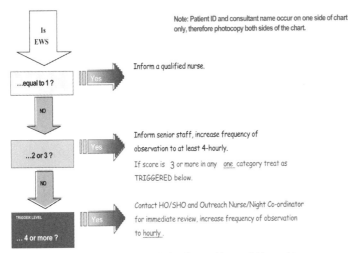

Is
EWS

...equal to 1 ?   Yes   Inform a qualified nurse.

NO

...2 or 3 ?   Yes   Inform senior staff, increase frequency of observation to at least 4-hourly.
If score is 3 or more in any   one category treat as TRIGGERED below.

NO

TRIGGER LEVEL

... 4 or more ?   Yes   Contact HO/SHO and Outreach Nurse/Night Co-ordinator for immediate review, increase frequency of observation to hourly .

Doctor should seek senior advice as needed from registrar and/or consultant.

Some patients will regularly have observation measurements that may be normal for them but may trigger a score on the set parameters. Patients in this situation may be placed on a Modified Early Warning Score (MEWS). If parameters are to be changed it is important that this decision is made with a doctor and the new values documented in the appropriate places.

EWS – taking action

It is important that you are not only able to recognise the need for early detection of a critical illness but also able to ensure that the correct intervention is made in a timely manner. The NICE guidelines have set specific levels at which they feel a patient should receive intervention. These are graded on three levels, using a score between 1 and 3:

❑ Low – where the observations are increased and the nurse in charge is alerted.

❑ Medium – where the team who has primary responsibility for the patient is alerted urgently and, at the same time, a team is alerted that is competent in acute illness.

❑ High – emergency call to a team with critical care competencies and diagnostic skills (NICE, 2007).

Studies have shown that a score of 3 often requires urgent attention. In most hospitals a score of 3 or more requires a response from the doctor. This should then result in the patient's management being changed to prevent further deterioration (Rees, 2003). A score of less than 3 does not necessarily mean that no action needs to be taken. However, a score of 3 or more generally means that action should be taken. If a score of 3 or more is recorded in a single parameter then most hospitals require that urgent action should be taken. Some hospitals use different parameters and it is important that you find out your Trust's protocol for patient observations. An example of the Lancashire Teaching Hospitals NHS Trust's calculation protocol is described in Figure 2.

	3	2	1	0	1	2	3
RR		<8		9–14	15–20	21–29	>30
HR		<40	41–50	51–100	101–110	111–130	>131
RESPONSE			Confused/ agitated	Alert	Voice	responds to pain	Unresponsive
Sys BP	<70	71–80	81–100	101–199		>200	
TEMP		<35		35.0–38.4		>38.5	
URINE				>500 ml/24 hr	250–500/24 hr	<250/24 hr	
			>150 ml/hr		<30 ml/hr	<15 ml/hr	

Where RR = Respirations, HR = Heart Rate

Figure 2
Lancashire Teaching
Hospitals NHS
Trust's calculation
protocol

If a total EWS score is 6 or more then urgent action should be taken. A score of 9 usually requires the calling of the cardiac arrest team. Many hospitals provide an action plan. This is used to provide a logical sequence of events that are to be carried out to ensure that the correct treatment is given. An example of an action plan is shown in Figure 3.

Activity 3.

Practise taking a set of observations on a friend and calculate the Early Warning Score using the calculation protocol in Figure 2.

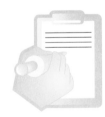

Reflection

Review the different signs of shock again. Reflect on the way in which these signs may appear on the Early Warning Score chart in Figure 1.

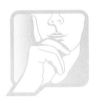

Figure 3
An action plan

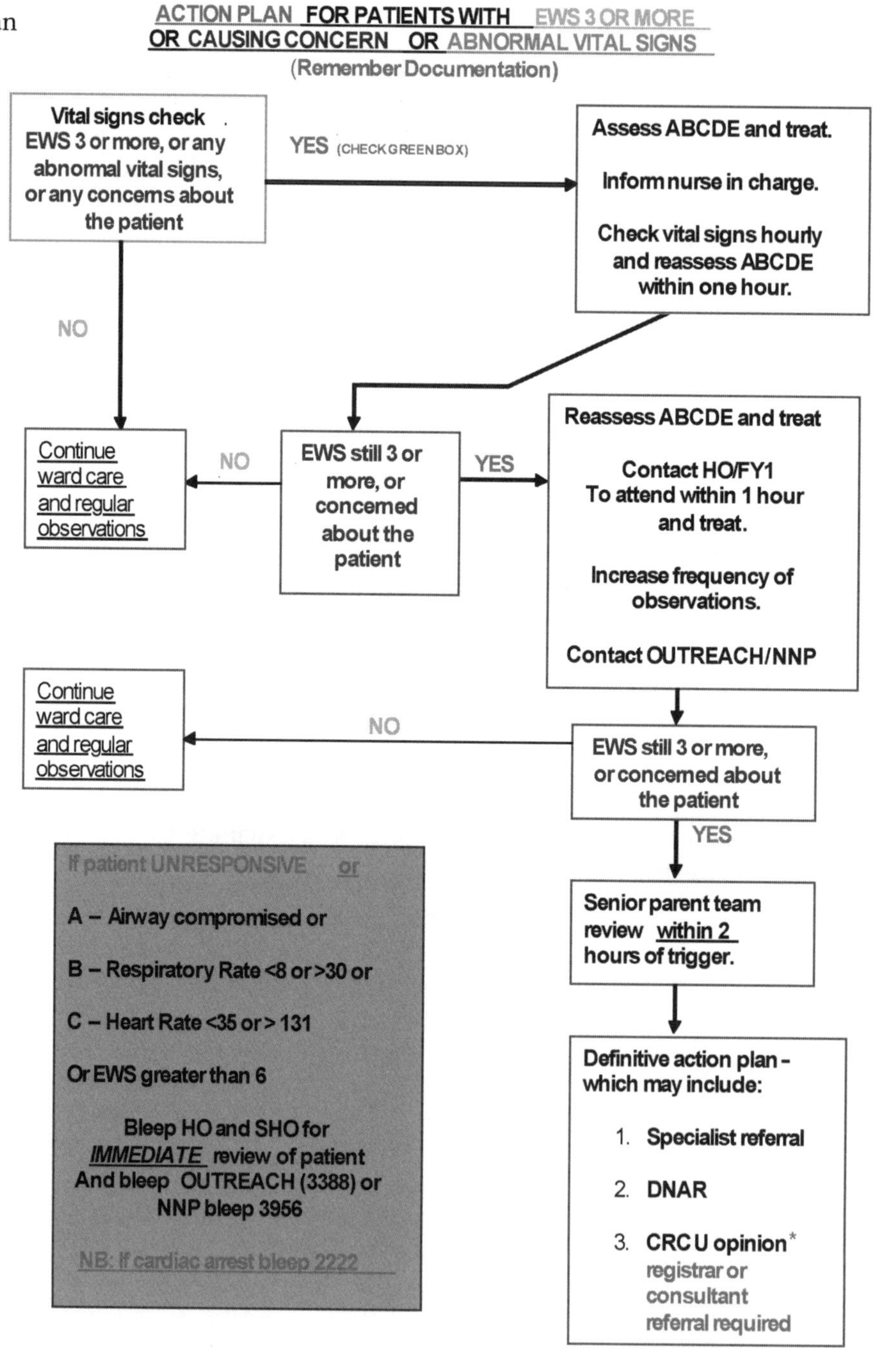

ACTION PLAN **FOR PATIENTS WITH** EWS 3 OR MORE
OR CAUSING CONCERN   OR ABNORMAL VITAL SIGNS
(Remember Documentation)

Vital signs check .
EWS 3 or more, or any
abnormal vital signs,
or any concerns about
the patient

YES (CHECK GREEN BOX)

Assess ABCDE and treat.

Inform nurse in charge.

Check vital signs hourly
and reassess ABCDE
within one hour.

NO

Continue
ward care
and regular
observations

NO

EWS still 3 or
more, or
concerned
about the
patient

YES

Reassess ABCDE and treat

Contact HO/FY1
To attend within 1 hour
and treat.

Increase frequency of
observations.

Contact OUTREACH/NNP

Continue
ward care
and regular
observations

NO

EWS still 3 or more,
or concerned about
the patient

YES

If patient UNRESPONSIVE   or

A – Airway compromised or

B – Respiratory Rate <8 or >30 or

C – Heart Rate <35 or > 131

Or EWS greater than 6

Bleep HO and SHO for
IMMEDIATE review of patient
And bleep OUTREACH (3388) or
NNP bleep 3956

NB: If cardiac arrest bleep 2222

Senior parent team
review within 2
hours of trigger.

Definitive action plan –
which may include:

1. **Specialist referral**

2. **DNAR**

3. **CRC U opinion**[*]
   registrar or
   consultant
   referral required

The outreach team

Outreach teams have been established in many hospitals to provide support for the care of patients on general wards. Usually, they are called to see a patient you are worried about. They will then help with the care of your patient. You will need to find out if there is an outreach team in your hospital or, if not, you need to know who to call and at which trigger stage. The outreach team has been developed to:

❏ avert admissions by identifying patients who are deteriorating and either helping to prevent admission to ICU or ensuring that admission to a critical care bed happens in a timely manner to ensure the best outcome;

❏ enable discharges, by supporting the continued recovery of discharged patients on wards and, post-discharge from hospital, with their relatives and friends;

❏ share critical care skills with staff on the wards and in the community, ensuring the enhancement of training opportunities and skills practice and to use information gathered from the ward and community to improve critical care services for patients and relatives (Department of Health, 2000).

Documentation

Documentation of the recording of observations is of vital importance. Without this there is no patient record to refer to and no opportunity to review the patient's history. The person who could remember every set of a patient's observations on a shift would be exceptional! If a patient's vital signs have not been documented then it is difficult to prove that they have been measured at all. Wood and Smith (1998) (cited in Kenward *et al.*, 2001) found that, having identified some of the most sick patients in the hospital, the documentation of many of their vital signs was absent.

When documenting the EWS it is important to document and report your concerns as well as recording the numbers themselves. Any findings should be reported along with any action taken. The patient's response to treatment should also be documented along with any further action to be taken. If no change has occurred then this should also be documented.

A hospital ward is often a busy place so documentation should be clear and concise so that it efficiently communicates the patient's condition to the reader. Observation charts are designed so that a clear trend can be seen visually. A graph which is clear and concise makes it easier to detect a deteriorating patient.

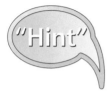

Hint for practice

Figure 4 shows what I think is the easiest, most effective method of recording a patient's blood pressure. Connecting the diastolic and systolic pressures with an arrow gives a quick indication of an improving, stable or deteriorating trend.

I have also found it useful if the pulse is recorded in red. (First check with your Trust to make sure this is acceptable.)

Figure 4
Documenting pulse and blood pressure

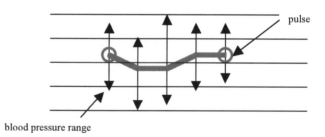

pulse

blood pressure range

It is important that you are aware of the basic pathophysiology of what the patient could be experiencing. This knowledge means that you can try and prevent the next stage in the deterioration process.

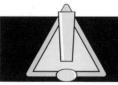

It has been well documented that the respiratory rate is often not recorded (Wood and Smith, 1998, cited in Kenward et al., 2001). This is extremely poor practice.

Observations in today's working environment

In reality, in the working environment today, many of the observations are obtained by the health care assistant. In fact, many staff nurses may not spend time with the patient. This increases the nurse's responsibility through the added dimension of personnel management (Boucher,

1998). Despite this, the responsibility for detecting patients who are deteriorating lies with the qualified staff (Wheatley, 2005). It is therefore very important that, as a student, you report any change in condition immediately. Many patients present with multiple diagnoses and their responses to medical treatment are often multifaceted and often unpredictable (Boucher, 1998). It is, therefore, necessary to report not only what is written on the observation chart but any other signs and symptoms which may be seen.

An Australian study found that nurses who were worried about the condition of their patients often based their criteria not on the observations themselves but on things such as patient's colour, coldness or clamminess as well. The importance of past experiences must be recognised (Cioffi, 2000). It is therefore important that nurses report not only on the physiological parameters recorded, but also on changes in rhythm, changes in breathing patterns, use of accessory muscles and changes in colour when taking the respirations. When taking a pulse it must be noted if it is weak or thready, as this may be an early indication of shock. There may also be occasions where a nurse may feel the patient's condition has changed, but they cannot express exactly how. Such worries should be listened to and the patient's condition assessed.

Reflection

Think of the times when you have used the Early Warning Score when it has triggered action. Did you follow an approved action plan?

Summary

By now you should have a better theoretical and practical knowledge of how to:

❏ accurately document patient observations;

❏ calculate an Early Warning Score;

❏ respond appropriately to a triggering EWS.

Remember the following:

❏ Always ask the patient's consent before you begin your observations;

❏ Always adhere to the infection control procedures (they are for your protection as well as for your patient's protection);

❏ Always document what you have measured and talk to your mentor if you have a concern about a patient's condition.

Acknowledgements

The author would like to thank Katie Swarbrick, Consultant Nurse Critical Care (Outreach) Lancashire Teaching Hospitals NHS Foundation Trust; Dr Jenny Wilson, MBChB, MRCGP, GP Bedford; and University Hospitals of Morecambe Bay NHS Trust.

Further reading

McCance, K. and Huether, S. (2002) *Pathophysiology: the biological basis for disease in adults and children*, 4th edn. St Louis, MO: Mosby

References

Ahern, J. and Philpot, P. (2002) 'Assessing acutely ill patients on general wards'. *Nursing Standard*, 16(47): 47–54

Andrews, T. and Waterman, H. (2005) 'Packaging: a grounded theory of how to report physiological deterioration effectively'. *Journal of Advanced Nursing*, 52(5): 473–81

Boucher, M.A. (1998) 'Delegation alert'. *American Journal of Nursing*, 98(2): 26–32

Cioffi, J. (2000) 'Recognition of patients who require emergency assistance: a descriptive study'. *Heart and Lung: Journal of Acute and Critical Care*, 29(4): 262–8

Department of Health (2000) *Comprehensive critical care: a review of adult critical care services*. London: HMSO

Goldhill, D.R. and McNarry, A.F. (2004) 'Physiological abnormalities in early warning scores are related to mortality in adult patients'. *British Journal of Anaesthesia*, 92(6): 882–4

Kenward, G., Hodgetts, T. and Castle, N. (2001) 'Time to put the R back in TPR'. *Nursing Times*, 97(40): 32–3

McCance, K. and Huether, S. (2006) *Pathophysiology: the biological basis for disease in adults and children*, 5th edn. St Louis, MO: Mosby

McQuillan, P., Pilkington, S., Allan, A., Taylor, B., Short, A., Morgan, G., Nielson, M., Barrett, D. and Smith, G. (1998) 'Confidential enquiry into quality of care before admission to intensive care'. *British Medical Journal*, 316: 1853–8

National Institute of Clinical Excellence (2007) *Acutely ill patients in hospital: recognition and response to acute illness to adults in hospital*. London: HMSO

Rees, J.E. (2003) 'Early Warning Scores'. *World Anaesthesia*, 17(10): 1–5

Subbe, C.P., Davies, R.G., Williams, E., Rutherford, P. and Gemmell, L. (2003) 'Effect of introducing the Modified Early Warning Score on clinical outcomes, cardiopulmonary arrest and intensive care utilisation in acute medical admissions'. *Anaesthesia*, 58(8): 797–802

Swarbrick, K. (2007) *Draft Trust policy for reducing risk of deterioration and prevention of cardiac arrest*. Lancashire Teaching Hospitals NHS Foundation Trust

Wheatley, I. (2005) 'The nursing practice of taking level 1 patient observations'. *Intensive and Critical Care Nursing*, 22: 115–21

Chapter 19

AIRWAY MANAGEMENT AND LIFE SUPPORT

Simon Dykes

The aim of this chapter is to develop the skills and knowledge required to safely manage the airway of a deteriorating patient and carry out life support procedures. In this chapter, in addition to other general ESC requirements, you will cover the following skill requirements.

Patients/clients can trust a newly registered nurse to:

Section 9   Respond appropriately by seeking assistance from a senior colleague when faced with sudden deterioration in patients'/clients' physical or psychological condition or emergency situations (e.g. abnormal vital signs, patient/client collapse, cardiac arrest, self-harm, extremely challenging behaviour, attempted suicide).

Airway management

Introduction

Our scenario concerns a 45-year-old woman named Teresa who originally attended the accident and emergency department with an isolated head injury and who subsequently suffered an acute severe headache with blurred vision. As a result of these symptoms the patient was admitted to the surgical assessment unit and is now under your care. A health care assistant who has been attending to Teresa has called for your assistance as she appears to be unwell and has a reduced respiratory rate. After ensuring it is safe to approach the patient, the first thing you do is to check for responsiveness by simply speaking loudly and clearly, saying 'are you all right?' while shaking Teresa gently by the shoulders. As the scenario develops we will explore the necessary skills and knowledge required to support your patient's condition.

Recognition of airway obstruction

Airway obstruction in patients can be very subtle and can be easily missed by health care professionals (Nolan *et al.*, 2005). What is important is that when we are assessing any patient's airway we also use our hearing as well as our sight. If we were to miss a fully or partially occluded airway, assisting the patient's ventilations by whatever means will be ineffective and, of course, detrimental to our patient's condition as their hypoxia will worsen.

In a patient who has had an acute collapse it is essential that we look for respiratory effort by looking at chest movement, listen for respiratory effort and noises, and feel for respiratory effort by placing one hand on the patient's chest. Adopting this technique will allow us to easily identify if there is a partially occluded airway for us to deal with.

Types of partially occluded airway noises

With a partially occluded airway, air entry to the lungs is reduced and is usually noisy.

❏ Inspiratory stridor once heard is seldom ever forgotten. This is a noise that is created by an obstruction somewhere within the larynx and above it. The obstruction can be caused by either a foreign body or a narrowing within the upper airway, and it will result in a harsh inspiratory noise.

❏ Snoring is caused by an occlusion of the posterior portion of the pharynx; usually this is caused by the tongue. Poor airway management, which is incorrect airway manipulation in the form of head tilt, chin lift and jaw thrust, can also result in obstruction. Correct airway management techniques will rectify this.

❏ Gurgling is highly suggestive of fluid within the upper airways. This should be rectified as quickly as possible to prevent the fluid not only blocking the airway but also from entering the lungs. This can be rectified by postural drainage (turning the patient on their side to drain the fluid) or by using the appropriate suction equipment. It is essential that you have had the appropriate training before using suction apparatus as incorrect techniques can be detrimental to the patient.

Check for obstructions

Prior to opening the airway with the appropriate method, you will need to examine the airway to ensure there are no foreign bodies or obstructions visible. This can simply be achieved by opening the mouth and making a visible inspection.

Finger sweeps

If you can clearly see a foreign body within the airway it may be of benefit to perform a finger sweep to remove the object. To do this you should be wearing disposable gloves. Placing your index finger into the airway, attempt to hook out the obstruction (see Figure 1). Never perform 'blind' finger sweeps as this can move the object further down the airway worsening the obstruction. The obstruction must be clearly visible and easily reached. People who perform this manoeuvre must also be very aware that, should the patient start fitting, the clenching of the patient's teeth could cause severe injury to the rescuer.

Figure 1 Finger sweeps

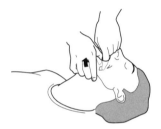

Opening the airway

Patients requiring resuscitation often have an obstructed airway, which is frequently caused by the loss of protective reflexes. Basic airway opening procedures should be employed, i.e. the head tilt/chin lift or the jaw thrust. Whichever airway opening technique you use, the underlying principle remains the same – you are removing the tongue from the posterior portion of the pharynx, thus enabling a free passage of ventilation, be that the patient's own breathing or ventilation by mechanical means. The head tilt/chin lift (see Figure 2) and the jaw thrust (see Figure 3) are the two basic airway opening techniques for us to use to ensure our patient is ventilating adequately. Both are simple yet very effective and can mean the difference between a pink and oxygenated patient and a blue hypoxic patient.

Figure 2
Head tilt chin lift

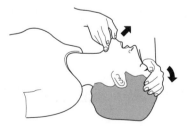

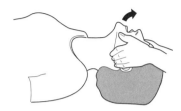

Figure 3
Jaw thrust

To perform a head tilt/chin lift manoeuvre, place one hand on the forehead of the patient. Place the fingers of your other hand on the bony prominence of the patient's jaw, moving the chin upward and tilting the head backwards. This should be achieved with gentle pressure and done so with care.

In the case of suspected spinal injury, a jaw thrust should be performed. This particular method is ideal for opening the airway in a patient with suspected cervical spine injury, as it involves no backward displacement of the spine. The head remains in the neutral position, pressure is applied at the angle of the jaw and the jaw is lifted forward, which will pull the tongue forwards. It is an extremely useful method of opening the airway, but obviously requires a two-handed action and will be difficult to maintain over time.

Using suction

Suction should always be readily available in hospitals. Use a rigid wide bore suction catheter (Yankeur) to remove large volumes of liquid, such as blood, saliva and vomit, from the upper airway. To remove smaller volumes of fluid, such as airway secretions, it may be more appropriate to use a soft suction catheter. When suctioning a patient with a rigid catheter insert the suction tube into the mouth as far as you can see, and suction as you withdraw it from the mouth.

You must have formal training before using suction equipment. Never perform 'blind' suctioning when clearing your patient's airway. Always ensure that you can see where you are aspirating, so that you can ensure you avoid direct trauma to the patient's airway. Suctioning a patient's airway with a rigid suction catheter can easily cause trauma to the delicate membrane linings so suctioning should be done with care. It also important to remember that while you are using suction equipment to clear your patient's airway, the patient is not receiving supplemental oxygen and, as a result, may start to become hypoxic.

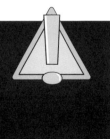

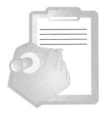

Activity 1.

How would you know that a patient is hypoventilating?

Securing and maintaining the airway

As previously mentioned, our patient Teresa has suddenly deteriorated and now has a reduced respiratory rate and is obviously hypoventilating. Once we have established a patent and clear airway, our next step is to aid the patient by securing and maintaining the clear airway with the use of an appropriately sized oropharyngeal airway (see Figure 4), sometimes referred to as a guedel.

Figure 4
Oropharyngeal airways

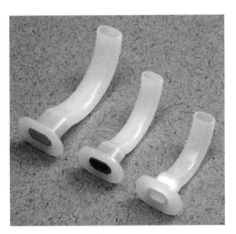

The oropharyngeal airway is a curved plastic tube that consists of a flange, a lumen and an outer reinforced section. There are many sizes available for use with patients of all ages. The airway is designed to fit neatly between the tongue and the hard palate of the mouth. A correctly sized airway should be one that sits neatly with the flange section resting just above the patient's front incisors.

The correct method for sizing an oropharyngeal airway is to measure from the angle of the jaw to the front incisor, as shown in Figure 5. If the airway rests at the teeth then it is the correct size. If it slips back into the airway it is too small and if it protrudes from the mouth it is too big.

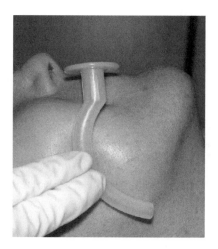

Figure 5 The correct method for pre-sizing an oropharyngeal airway

During insertion of the airway if the patient becomes intolerant or shows visible signs of rejecting the airway, then they do not need one. Indeed there is a strong possibility that your patient will vomit, causing further resuscitation and airway problems.

(a)   (b)

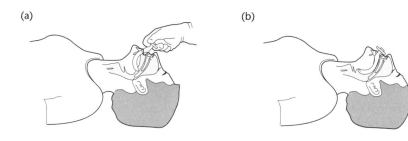

Figure 6 a and b Inserting an oropharyngeal airway

To insert the airway (see Figure 6 (a) and (b)) it is put into the mouth upside down as shown in (a) and then rotated through 180° as it passes beyond the hard palate (b). As our patient's condition has suddenly deteriorated and we have rectified the occluded airway, it is necessary for us to ensure that we offer further protection and prevent the tongue from falling backward and causing a further airway obstruction.

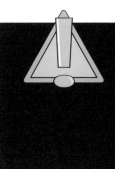

Never guess the size of an oropharyngeal airway for your patient. It is good practice to always use the measuring technique prior to insertion as all of our patients have different anatomical proportions. Once the oropharyngeal airway is in place, this does not mean that the airway is now totally protected. The airway is still in danger from occlusions such as vomit and blood. If our patient vomits with the airway in place, then this fluid will not only block the airway, it will also cause long-term pulmonary complications. Always keep rechecking the patient's airway.

Breathing

Once we have corrected and supported our patient's airway, it is now necessary for us to assess the respiratory status and effort being made by the patient. Teresa is clearly not breathing as she should be as her respiratory rate is now less than ten respirations per minute. As Teresa's ventilations are inadequate to perfuse her tissues with the necessary oxygen, it will now be necessary for us to support and aid her breathing with the use of mechanical means and with supplemental oxygen.

Mouth-to-mouth rescue breaths

A rescuer's expired oxygen content is only 16–17 per cent. Therefore rescue breaths must be replaced as soon as possible by ventilation with oxygen-enriched air (Resuscitation Council, 2005a). Mouth-to-mouth ventilation (Figure 7) is the most basic method of delivering rescue breaths. While pinching the nose closed and offering a degree of head tilt/chin lift, the rescuer seals their mouth around the patient's mouth and delivers a breath over one second. The rescuer must then remove their mouth from the patient's mouth to allow for expiration. However, if other means of ventilating our patient are available, then these should be used first as there is obviously a risk of cross-infection with unprotected mouth-to-mouth ventilation and it is not recommended.

Pocket mask ventilations

The pocket mask (Figure 8) is widely used and available within the hospital setting. They are very similar in construction to a face mask used during anaesthesia, and have a one-direction valve to allow the patient's expired air to be taken away from the rescuer. Typically, these face masks are transparent to allow for blood or vomit to be seen within the airway.

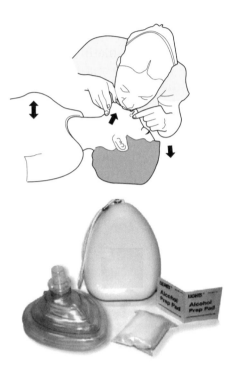

Figure 7
Mouth-to-mouth
ventilations

Figure 8
An example of a
pocket mask

Supplemental oxygen can also be added to the mask by attaching the appropriate tubing to the oxygen port. To use the pocket mask, breathe into the mask for one second through the one-way valve, ensuring there is adequate chest rise (Figure 9). When ventilating any patient by any method it is essential to give each rescue breath over one second and to give a ventilatory volume that corresponds to visible chest movement of the patient.

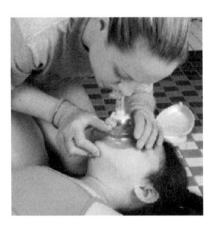

Figure 9
Use of a pocket
mask

Bag, valve and mask device (BVM)

The BVM (Figure 10) is used for ventilating patients making little or no respiratory effort. When using the mask you use a C-grip method (sometimes referred to as the 'anaesthetist's grip'), with the thumb and forefinger around the mask and the remaining fingers around the angle of the jaw, pulling the jaw up to meet the mask (Figure 11). To provide ventilation in this manner it is necessary to extend the neck and perform a head tilt/chin lift manoeuvre. The alternative jaw thrust manoeuvre is required in suspected cases of cervical spine injury. The bag is then squeezed to provide ventilations to the patient.

Figure 10 Bag, valve and mask

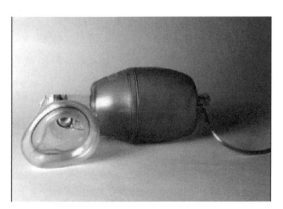

Figure 11
Ventilation with bag, valve and mask

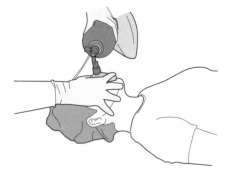

Always check that, whatever method of ventilation you use, you allow the casualty to breathe out between ventilations and that you can see the chest rise and fall with ventilation. With the oxygen reservoir in place and oxygen attached, you can deliver high concentrations of oxygen, which is obviously of critical importance. When connecting oxygen to the device ensure it is set to 15 litres per minute on the flow meter. Each breath needs to be delivered over approximately one second and with a volume which corresponds to normal chest movement.

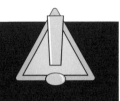

When using the BVM it is important not to 'snatch' the bag as, in doing so, you will ventilate the patient too aggressively. This may force some of the ventilation into the patient's stomach, possibly inducing aspiration of the stomach contents.

When using a bag, valve and mask it is usually necessary to use an oropharyngeal airway (guedel) to keep the airway open. This also makes it easier for you to ventilate the patient. An oropharyngeal airway helps to prevent backward displacement of the tongue. It is also useful to give some form to the mouths of patients who have no teeth. However, if the patient has good close-fitting dentures, then these should be left in place.

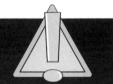

Poor technique when ventilating a patient using any of the devices mentioned is obviously potentially catastrophic, as we may be starving the patient of an adequate oxygen supply.

The Resuscitation Council UK (2006) advises us that using a bag, valve and mask with an appropriate airway opening manoeuvre requires skill, experience and practice. Therefore, as a model of good practice, bag and mask ventilation is better with two people (Figure 12), with one person squeezing the bag and the second person applying an effective seal with the face mask.

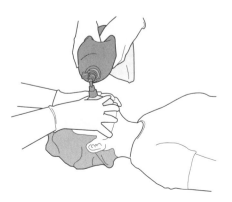

Figure 12
Two-person technique for bag, valve and mask ventilation

Airway management summary

❑ Initially you were called to assist with a 45-year-old woman who was making some abnormal respiratory sounds. The situation was approached with safety as the first priority.

❑ The next step saw us checking for a response from the patient using a verbal command and a shake at the shoulders.

❑ Recognising that there was food debris inside the airway, this was removed with finger sweeps and suctioning.

❑ Realising that there was in fact an airway problem, we adopted the head tilt/chin lift method to open up the airway.

❑ An oropharyngeal airway was used to aid our airway management.

❑ Teresa, our patient, was discovered to be hypoventilating and, as a result, was ventilated with a pocket mask and a bag, valve and mask with supplemental oxygen.

Table 1 provides an overview.

Table 1
Airway management summary

Airway support	Ventilatory support
❑ Head tilt/chin lift	❑ Mouth to mouth
❑ Jaw thrust	❑ Pocket mask
❑ Finger sweeps	❑ Bag, valve and mask
❑ Suction	❑ Supplemental oxygen
❑ Oropharyngeal airway	

Basic life support

The aim of the second section of this chapter is to introduce and develop the skills and knowledge required for effective basic life support.

Background

Cardiac arrest affects about 700,000 people per year across Europe (Resuscitation Council, 2005a). Basic life support is the foundation for any attempt at subsequent advanced life support and, should the basic techniques be inadequately performed, then this will not only reduce the prognosis for the patient but will also reduce the effectiveness of any further advanced interventions. Indeed, the latest evidence from the Resuscitation Council suggests that the focus of any resuscitation attempt should be efficient basic life support with additional early and safe defibrillation.

The purpose of basic life support is to maintain adequate ventilation and circulation until means can be obtained to reverse the underlying cause of the cardiac arrest. In order to maintain life and function effectively a constant supply of oxygen is required to all parts of the body. The brain in particular will become severely damaged if deprived of oxygen for just a few minutes. To ensure that there is enough oxygen supplied to the brain there are three elements which must be maintained and supported:

❑ Airway – this must be clear to enable oxygen to pass to the lungs;

❑ Breathing – to deliver the oxygen to the lungs;

❑ Circulation – to pump the oxygen from the lungs to the rest of the body.

If any of these physiological responses are absent then the necessary support and assistance will be required. Basic life support consists of the following elements:

❑ initial assessment;

❑ airway maintenance;

❑ expired air ventilation (rescue breathing);

❑ chest compression.

Basic life support implies that no equipment is employed other than a protective device (Resuscitation Council, 2005a). In hospital a pocket mask is used. For information about the use of the pocket mask during life support attempts please see page 388 in this chapter, regarding airway management and ventilatory support.

See page 388, this chapter.

Adult basic life support

The following algorithms are taken from the Resuscitation Council (2005a) guidelines. The first algorithm shows the sequence of basic life support for an out-of-hospital arrest for the lay person (see Figure 13), which will allow you to compare and contrast the two approaches to dealing with a cardiac arrest. However, no matter where you are, whether in hospital or out of

Figure 13
Out-of-hospital basic
life support
sequence

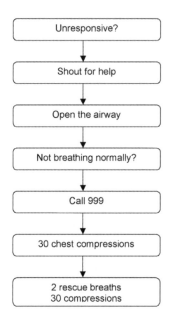

hospital, the philosophy of basic life support remains unchanged. It is of vital importance that, as health care professionals, we are comfortable with the basics before we move to the more advanced aspects of life support. After all, there may be times when you are called to assist with a collapsed member of the public while away from the hospital. This possibility emphasises the need for all health care professionals to be totally familiar with the basic sequence of life support.

As you can see, this is a very simplistic approach to basic life support, but it is one which must be understood among the general public and all UK health care professionals.

Adult basic life support algorithm (in-hospital resuscitation)

The second algorithm (Figure 14) is a continuation of the out-of-hospital life support sequence. Here there is an expectation that the health care professionals attending to the patient are adept at recognising a collapsed patient with no breathing or pulse. The focus is on the early identification of the cardiac arrest and calling for the necessary support, which in this case is the resuscitation team. Looking at the sequence of

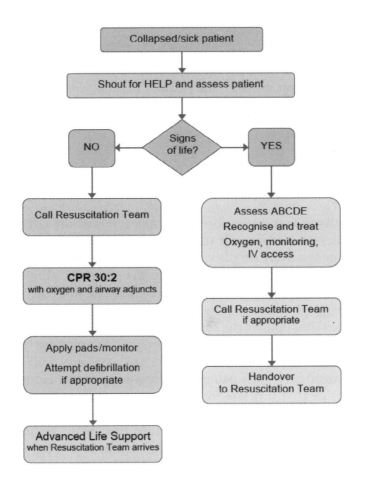

Figure 14
Adult basic life support algorithm (in-hospital resuscitation) reproduced with the kind permission of the Resuscitation Council UK

events we can clearly see the inclusion of advanced interventions; these will be carried out and performed by the appropriately trained personnel within the resuscitation team. The priority here is for you to ensure that effective basic life support is being performed. Advanced life support practicalities will be addressed in the next section of this chapter.

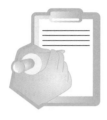

Activity 2.

To ensure that we deliver sufficient amounts of oxygen to the brain during life support, which three aspects must be supported effectively?

Hint: See page 393 in this section.

Basic life support sequence

Ensuring personal safety

Before anyone commences basic life support it is essential that they make sure it is safe to approach the patient. This could mean considering something relatively simple such as, for example, that you are attending to a collapsed patient on the floor and the patient is lying on a slippery surface. Here it would be very easy to rush to attend to the casualty and, in doing so, become injured yourself. Or you might be in a more dangerous situation where, for example, a patient has sustained a shock from an electrical power source. Before you do anything else you must ask yourself whether the power source has been turned off and it is safe for you to attend to the patient. Before we can render aid to anyone we must ensure that it is safe for us and our colleagues. In addition, note that the wearing of disposable gloves is strongly advocated, if these are available, to prevent cross-infection. In our particular scenario your patient Teresa is lying in bed in a semi-recumbent position and has been found in a collapsed condition by a health care assistant.

Check the patient for responsiveness

If you discover a collapsed patient it is essential that you call for help before attempting life support. Once the call for help has been made, then you must check for responsiveness by simply speaking loudly and clearly, saying 'are you all right?' while shaking the patient gently by the shoulders. Should assistance arrive at this point, then these actions may be performed together.

If the patient does respond

If the patient does respond to your voice (and/or shaking of the shoulders), urgent assistance is still required as the patient is obviously in a collapsed condition. Unless the airway is obviously obstructed then the patient should be left where you found her. If the patient has a blocked airway then it will be necessary for you to ensure the patient has a clear airway. The procedure for this is described in the first section of this chapter.

See page 383, this chapter.

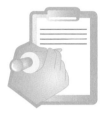

Activity 3.

How would you know that the patient had an occluded airway?

Hint: See the section on airway management on page 382.

If the patient does not respond to a verbal command

Ensure that the patient has been turned onto their back and in a supine position. Now, it is vital that you stick to a structured approach and follow the **A**irway, **B**reathing and **C**irculation check (ABC). Look in the mouth and ensure it is free from debris and foreign bodies. Now apply the correct airway-opening technique to the patient as above – either a head tilt/chin lift or, if you suspect a cervical spine injury, a jaw thrust.

Keeping the airway patent and open, look, listen and feel for signs of breathing for no longer than ten seconds. Those health care professionals who are more experienced may do a check of the carotid pulse at the same time as assessing the breathing status. The pulse check, like the breathing check, should take no longer than ten seconds. Figure 15 shows how the rescuer looks, listens and feels for breathing, while Figure 16 shows the carotid pulse check.

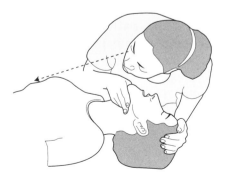

Figure 15
Breathing check

Figure 16
Carotid pulse check

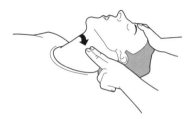

You gently shake Teresa by the shoulders and speak to check for responsiveness but there is no response to your initial interventions.

If the patient is breathing normally

Place the patient into the recovery position (shown in Figure 17), ensure help is on the way and keep reassessing the patient's airway and breathing.

Figure 17
The recovery
position

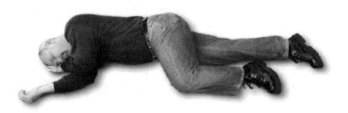

If the patient has a pulse but is not breathing

See page 408, this
chapter

In this case urgent assistance and support will be required. Ensure the patient has a clear airway and commence supportive respiratory ventilation, with supplemental oxygen. Be prepared to carry out cardio-pulmonary resuscitation (CPR) as the patient may suffer a cardiac arrest at any moment. As the patient is not breathing it may be necessary for the patient to be ventilated more appropriately with the use of a mechanical ventilator once the patient has been intubated (for intubation see the final section of this chapter on advanced life support). The patient would need to be transferred as soon as practically possible to an appropriate high tech area, such as an intensive care unit. In our identified scenario, however, Teresa has a pulse although she is not breathing adequately.

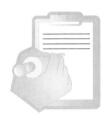

Activity 4.

1.   We have identified that Teresa is not breathing properly and has a pulse. What do we need to do to support Teresa's respirations?

Hint: see the paragraph above and the section on airway management.

2.   Who would you call to give you assistance?

Hint: See the in-hospital resuscitation algorithm on page 395.

Now that we are successfully supporting Teresa's ventilatory status and the appropriate personnel are on the way, it is necessary for us to discuss other practicalities of basic life support.

If there is no pulse or no signs of life

Once you have identified that the patient has no signs of life, it will be necessary to commence CPR. This should follow the sequences identified within the previous algorithms. See Figures 18 and 19.

(a)

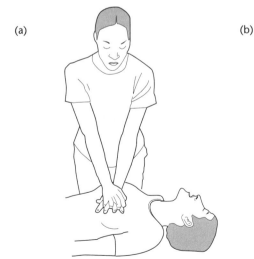

(b)

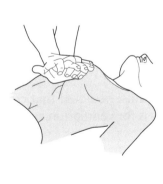

Figure 18
Cardiac compressions

Figure 19
Compression and
release

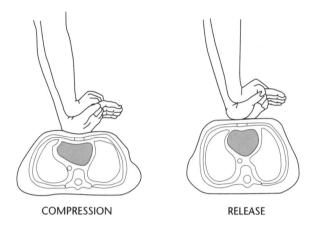

COMPRESSION   RELEASE

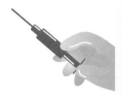

1. Place the heel of one hand in the centre of the chest with the heel of the other hand on top.

2. Interlock your fingers, keeping away from pressing on the patient's abdomen or the lower bony portion of the sternum.

3. Position yourself vertically above the patient's chest and, with your arms straight, press down on the sternum at a depth of 4–5 cm. After each compression, release the pressure on the chest but do not lose contact between your hand and the patient's chest. The chest should be compressed 30 times. Repeat at a rate of 100 compressions per minute.

4. After the first 30 compressions, ventilate the patient twice, then resume compressions. This 30:2 ratio should be performed for two minutes (five cycles).

5. It must be noted that compressions should not be interrupted, unless it is for ventilation and or defibrillation.

The diagrams in Figure 19 highlight the importance of ensuring that, once the chest has been compressed, we release the pressure to allow the heart to refill ready for the next compression.

Post-resuscitation care

The goal for any life support attempt is to regain a circulation; however, this is only the start of post-resuscitation care (Resuscitation Council,

2005a). You may regain a circulation with your attempts at life support yet the patient may still not be breathing spontaneously. If this is the case then it will be necessary for you to support the patient's airway and ventilations. The post-resuscitation care phase begins as soon as you have established a return of spontaneous circulation. At this stage the patient will require urgent transfer to a high tech area to allow for further care and support once they are stable enough to do so.

Summary

❏ Our patient Teresa was discovered in a collapsed condition so you first called for further assistance from the appropriately trained personnel.

❏ On initial assessment you identified that there was inadequate respiration, although Teresa had a pulse.

❏ To support Teresa's respirations, you placed the airway into the correct position (head tilt/chin lift) and assisted her ventilations. Basic life support attempts must follow the structured approach identified in the algorithms in Figures 13 and 14.

❏ As health care professionals, we must be adept at the basic skills as this is ultimately what makes resuscitation endeavours truly effective.

❏ You will need to study and practise the basic life support techniques discussed within this section to be truly efficient and competent.

Advanced life support

Introduction to advanced life support

The aim of this next section is to introduce you to the concept of advanced life support. Previously in this section we have looked at basic airway management and basic life support. It is vital that as health care professionals we are able to demonstrate effective basic practices before we can develop our advanced skills. Also, advanced life support has no place without effective basic life support. If you carry out advanced life support without the necessary basic skills this would be to the detriment of patient care. Therefore this section will seek to develop the knowledge and understanding of advanced life support, using our scenario as an example.

Let us recap on the current scenario. Your patient has been admitted from the accident and emergency department to the surgical assessment unit after suffering an isolated head injury, followed by a period of headaches and blurred vision. Our patient, Teresa, is normally fit and well and enjoys an active lifestyle. You have been called to her bed by a health care assistant who has alerted you to the fact that the patient is in a collapsed condition. Your initial assessment discovered that the patient did not respond to your voice or shaking of the shoulders, had a poor respiratory effort and had a carotid pulse. As a result, and after following the structured approach of airway, breathing and circulation, you commenced ventilatory support using a pocket mask. You have also managed to raise the alarm and have contacted the crash team to assist and attend the patient. Although Teresa has not suffered a cardiac arrest while in your care, it is of vital importance that you understand the role of the nurse when supporting the process of advanced life support. To fulfil this, it is necessary for us to now explore and broaden our knowledge and understanding of advanced life support practicalities.

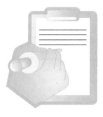

Activity 5.

Basic life support recap (hint: see the sections on airway management and basic life support).

1.   Name two ways of opening a patient's airway.

2.   Name four causes of airway obstruction.

3.   How do you measure an oropharyngeal airway prior to insertion?

4.   What is the ratio of compressions to ventilations?

5.   What is the recommended number of chest compressions per minute?

What is advanced life support?

Advanced life support complements basic life support. It is a sequential chain of actions that includes invasive techniques and therapies that not only support the patient but also seek to reverse the possible causes of the cardiac arrest. Such advanced interventions include:

❑ defibrillation;

❑ intravenous cannulation;

❑ advanced airway management;

❑ specific drug usage.

I will now describe each of these interventions in more detail. It can be helpful if the interventions of advanced cardiac life support (ACLS) are seen together as a chain of survival. Figure 20 shows how the sequence of events occurs in a logical and timely manner, from the recognition of a problem with our patient, through to the advanced life support interventions.

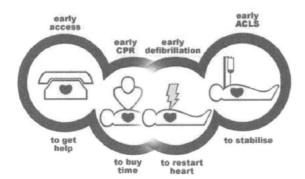

Figure 20
The chain of survival

Defibrillation

There are many makes of external defibrillator on the market these days but there are only two main types – the manual defibrillator and the automatic defibrillator. The automated variety is commonly called an automated external defibrillator or AED (see Figure 21). Defibrillation is the use of a carefully controlled electric shock, administered through a device on the exterior of the chest wall, to restart or normalise heart rhythms. Manual defibrillators (see Figure 22) monitor and record the cardiac rhythm and can also produce a printed copy of the rhythm. It must be noted here that this printed copy is not the same as the more detailed rhythm analysis generated by a 12-lead electrocardiogram.

Figure 21
Automated
defibrillator

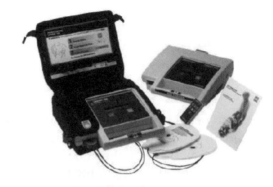

Figure 22
Manual defibrillator

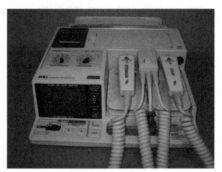

The term 'fibrillation' pertains to the action of the heart muscle when it 'quivers' in an uncoordinated fashion producing no cardiac output and, therefore, the patient is said to be in **cardiac arrest**. This term also relates to a particular cardiac rhythm known as **ventricular fibrillation** (VF). To 'defibrillate' means to use a controlled electrical shock, in the form of a dual current, to stop the 'quivering' of the heart muscle.

When do you defibrillate a patient?

It is important to know when and when not to defibrillate a patient. When the resuscitation team arrive to give you assistance, the first thing to do is to monitor the patient's cardiac rhythm. This must be done as a priority as certain rhythms respond well to defibrillation. We have already identified that VF (see Figure 23) is an indication for defibrillation. Another rhythm that can respond to defibrillation is **ventricular tachycardia** (VT) (see Figure 24). Here it is important to note that VT can be either pulseless or pulsed. It is, of course, VT with no pulse that should receive an electrical shock. It must be noted that the other two rhythms identified within the cardiac arrest scenario are known as

pulseless electrical activity (PEA) (see Figure 25) and **asystole** (see Figure 26). Pulseless electrical activity can be any rhythm that has the ability to generate a pulse, but a pulse will be absent from the patient. There is co-ordinated electrical activity within the heart, but mechanically the heart has failed. PEA can take many forms and is not always represented by the rhythm shown in Figure 25. Asystole is an absence of all electrical and mechanical activity within the heart. These two rhythms should be treated with ventilation and chest compression, not defibrillation.

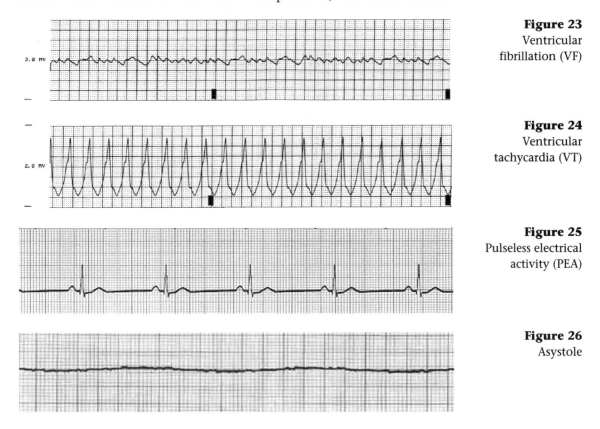

Figure 23
Ventricular
fibrillation (VF)

Figure 24
Ventricular
tachycardia (VT)

Figure 25
Pulseless electrical
activity (PEA)

Figure 26
Asystole

Defibrillation and safety

Of all the advanced clinical interventions, the technique of defibrillation carries a great risk to the user if performed inappropriately. Defibrillation can seriously injure or even result in death if health and safety aspects are ignored. As a result, and because during defibrillation we are using electricity to stun the heart muscle, specific safety factors must be employed and followed.

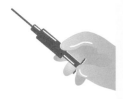

For safe defibrillation

1. The paddles (from which the electrical charge is delivered) should be in one of two places at all times: either securely clipped into the defibrillator or on the patient's chest. The paddles should never be waved around in the air or left next to the patient on the bed or floor, etc.

2. Before the electrical charge is delivered, the operator must ensure that everyone is clear from the patient and that no one is touching any part of the patient. This is also true for the operator: they must ensure that they too are not in contact with the patient during electrical discharge. All this should be accomplished with a clear, loud command of 'Stand clear' and this should be accompanied with a visual check to ensure it is safe to proceed and defibrillate the patient. It should be noted that if an AED is being used, this will give verbal commands to the user.

3. Before defibrillation takes place, it is essential that the 'paddle field' is clear. The 'paddle field' simply means the area of the patient's chest where the paddles will lie. Typically (and it is good practice) we define the area of defibrillation as the patient's entire chest. To ensure this area is clear it will be necessary to remove anything that will conduct electricity, such as jewellery, either around the neck or at the nipple. GTN (glyceryl trinitrate) patches, used to treat angina, must also be removed as these too may conduct electricity.

4. Perspiration must be removed prior to defibrillation as electricity and water do not mix. It is also essential that patients who are obviously wet (due to urinary incontinence for example), and who are lying in a wet environment, are dried prior to defibrillation. Patients who are lying on a metal surface must be moved onto a non-metallic surface prior to defibrillation. For example, if you were called to a patient who had collapsed on a fire-exit stairwell, which is typically made from metal, you must move the patient first. Although all hospital beds and trolleys typically have metal bases, this does not put the operator or resuscitation team at risk as the patient will invariably be lying on a mattress of some description.

5. During resuscitation attempts, any supplemental oxygen that is being used may inadvertently enrich the atmosphere close to the

defibrillation field. Therefore the oxygen should be either turned off or removed prior to defibrillation as a spark caused during the electrical discharge (although rare) may cause combustion.

6. Gel pads should be applied to the chest prior to defibrillation. These focus the charge and prevent electrical burns to the patient's chest.

Paddle placement

Figures 27 and 28 show where defibrillation paddles should be placed on a patient's chest wall when using the automatic or the manual variety of defibrillator. One paddle is placed under the patient's right clavicle (known as the sternum position) and the other placed on the left side of the chest so that it is just above the rib margin (known as the cardiac apex position). These positions are the same which ever defibrillator is used.

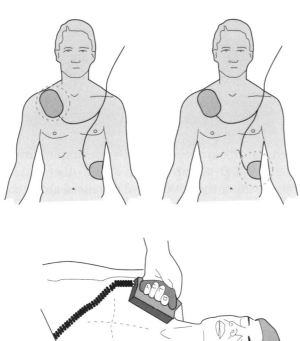

Figure 27
Paddle placement during automatic defibrillation

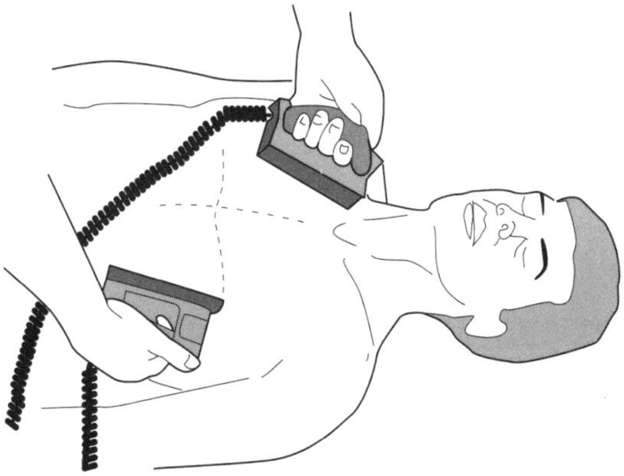

Figure 28
Paddle placement during manual defibrillation

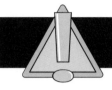

Never attempt defibrillation if you have not completed the appropriate training programme endorsed by your employing Trust.

Advanced airway management

Before we continue looking at the advanced ways to protect our patient's airway, let's recap on the basics.

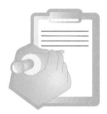

Activity 6.

List four basic methods of maintaining a clear airway.

Hint: See the section on airway management in this chapter (page 382).

Advanced airway management interventions are supplemental to basic airway management. The following is an introduction to the various techniques.

Nasopharyngeal airways

The nasopharyngeal airway (see Figure 29) is a simple curved tube with a flange at one end and an atraumatic tip at the other end. This device is placed into the nostril of the patient and advanced along the floor of the nose. This device is useful when the oral airway is totally occluded and unable to be opened.

Figure 29
The nasopharyngeal airway

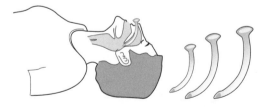

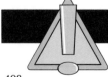

Formal training is required prior to using a nasopharyngeal airway.

Laryngeal mask airway

Laryngeal mask airways (LMA) (see Figure 30) are widely used by anaesthetists. They are also used for the unconscious patient with absent airway reflexes and are used to provide effective ventilations. This particular device consists of a wide-bore tube with an inflatable cuff at the distal end which, when inflated, forms a seal around the laryngeal opening. The use of the LMA provides a clear and relatively protected airway that can be inserted without the need for intubation skills (which will be discussed later). It has a standard connection allowing the use of other resuscitation equipment such as a bag, valve and mask.

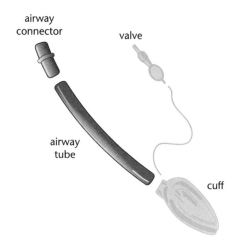

airway
connector

valve

airway
tube

cuff

Figure 30
A laryngeal mask
airway

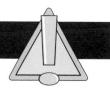

Formal training is required prior to the use of a laryngeal mask airway.

Endotracheal intubation

This technique is said to be the 'gold standard' of airway management. Other airway maintenance techniques, ranging from the basic through to the more advanced, are unable to protect the airway as effectively as endotracheal intubation. Although nurses are not expected to perform intubation, you may be required to assist and support the actual process. The process of intubation involves the passing of a special tube through the patient's larynx, where it is temporarily fixed in place (see Figure 31 (a) and (b)). This intervention, typically performed by doctors, anaesthetists and paramedics, carries with it certain risks. The largest risk of all is the incorrect placement of the tube into the patient's oesophagus. If this is not identified quickly it will cause severe hypoxia and, ultimately, death.

Figure 31
Endotracheal
intubation

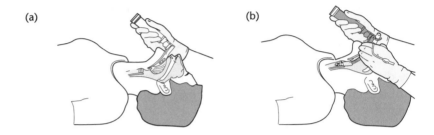

(a)   (b)

Figure 32 explains the different parts and mechanics of an endotracheal tube. Endotracheal tubes are supplied in various sizes and should be appropriately sized for different patients.

Figure 32
An endotracheal
tube

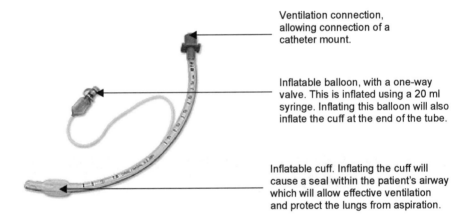

Ventilation connection, allowing connection of a catheter mount.

Inflatable balloon, with a one-way valve. This is inflated using a 20 ml syringe. Inflating this balloon will also inflate the cuff at the end of the tube.

Inflatable cuff. Inflating the cuff will cause a seal within the patient's airway which will allow effective ventilation and protect the lungs from aspiration.

Figure 33 shows the equipment required for endotracheal intubation. It is essential to pre-check this equipment as it will be required in an emergency situation and must be ready. Supplemental oxygen, suction equipment and a correctly-sized airway adjunct in the form of an oropharyngeal airway should accompany any attempts at intubation.

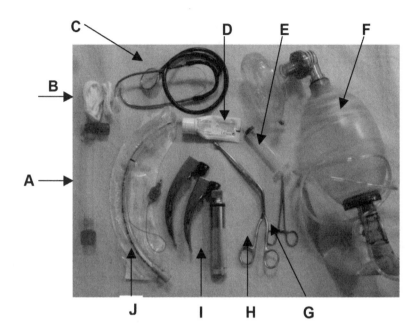

Figure 33
The equipment
required for
endotracheal
intubation

A Catheter mount – once the tube has been successfully placed past the vocal cords, the catheter mount is then connected to the endotracheal tube which will allow connection of the bag, valve and mask.

B Ribbon/gauze tie off – once the patient has been successfully intubated, the endotracheal tube is secured into place by tying the gauze around the tube and then securing it to the patient.

C Stethoscope – this is used to confirm correct placement of the tube, ensuring that lung sounds can be heard on both sides of the chest. This is also used to help avoid oesophageal intubation.

D Lubricating jelly – this is applied to the distal end of the tube and will help the tube pass without causing trauma to the airway.

E 20 ml syringe – the syringe is used to inflate the balloon and cuff using approximately 10 ml of air.

F Bag, valve and mask – this is used to ventilate the patient once intubated.

G Spencer Wells clamps – should the one-way valve fail at the inflatable balloon, these clamps can be applied to prevent further air loss.

H Magill forceps – these can be used to retrieve foreign objects located deep within a patient's airway, under direct vision in unison with the laryngoscope handle and blade.

I Laryngoscope with blades – once the patient's airway has been opened, the laryngoscope blade is used to visualise (i.e. allow the doctor to see) the vocal cords. Once visualised the tube is passed through the cords.

J Endotracheal tube – when correctly placed this is used to ventilate the patient. A cuff at the end of the tube causes a sealing effect, protecting the airway further and allowing effective ventilations to take place.

Figure 31 (a) and (b) shows the operator holding a laryngoscope in the left hand and lifting the tongue away, allowing visualisation of the vocal cords. Once the cords have been identified the operator can then proceed to pass the tube through the cords. Once the tube is past the cords, a balloon at the end of the tube is inflated giving an effective seal and preventing the risk of aspiration. The patient may now be effectively ventilated with a bag, valve and mask.

The latest evidence suggests that the airway should be secured early during advanced life support. This means that the patient can be connected to an appropriate ventilator immediately, allowing the performance of continuous cardiac compressions with minimal interruptions. Once the patient has been successfully intubated, the patient can be ventilated with a bag, valve and mask or an automatic ventilator.

It must be stressed that formal training is required to perform intubation skills. However, as a nurse, you may be required to assist with this procedure. Therefore it is essential that you know what equipment is required and what it is used for.

Peripheral intravenous access

See Chapter 5, page 123.

Peripheral intravenous access during life support will allow us to administer specific cardiac arrest drug therapies and fluids that support and compliment effective basic life support and defibrillation. The technique of intravenous access is also referred to as cannulation (see also Chapter 5). It is typically achieved using an appropriately sized cannula or Venflon™ (these two names are used interchangeably) as shown in Figures 34 and 35. The Venflons™ that are used to gain intravenous access come in different sizes with varying colours. Once the

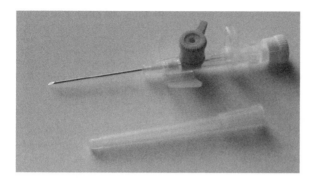

Figure 34
Cannula or
Venflon™

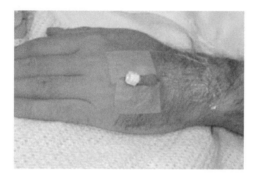

Figure 35
I/V cannula in situ

patient has been successfully cannulated, this entry into the patient's venous system can be repeatedly used for drugs or fluids. Intravenous access is typically achieved in one of the patient's arms, although the external jugular vein may be used during cardiac arrest as it is more efficient and effective for drug therapy because it lies in closer proximity to the heart.

It must be noted that during cannulation the sharp stylet is removed from the cannula leaving a plastic tube inside the patient's vein. Cannulation is therefore hazardous as there is a potential for a needle stick injury.

Formal training is required prior to performing cannulation and intravenous access skills.

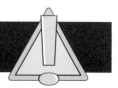

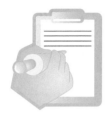

Activity 7.

Using the website address below, research and describe the following drugs used during advanced life support;

❑ adrenaline (epinepherine)

❑ atropine

❑ amiodarone

❑ magnesium.

Website: **www.resus.org.uk/pages/als.pdf**

The process of advanced life support

Now that we have looked at the individual skills associated with advanced life support, you need to have an appreciation of how they are all put together. The following algorithm in Figure 36 is taken from the Resuscitation Council's Advanced Life Support guidelines (2005b). As you look at the algorithm you can see that pivotal to the process is basic life support and defibrillation.

References and further reading

Nolan, J.P., Deakin, C.D., Soar, J., Bottiger, B.W. and Smith, G. (2005) *European Resuscitation Council guidelines for resuscitation 2005*. Elsevier – see Section 4: Adult advanced life support; Section 2: Adult basic life support and automated external defibrillation, Resuscitation 2005; 67S1, S39-S86, Elsevier. Online at: **www.erc.edu/index.php/guidelines_download_2005/en/**

Resuscitation Council (UK) (2005a) *Adult basic life support*. London: Resuscitation Council. Online at: **www.resus.org.uk/pages/bls.pdf**

Resuscitation Council (UK) (2005b) *Adult advanced life support*. London: Resuscitation Council. Online at: **www.resus.org.uk/pages/als.pdf**

Resuscitation Council (UK) (2006) *Immediate life support*, 2nd edn. London: Resuscitation Council

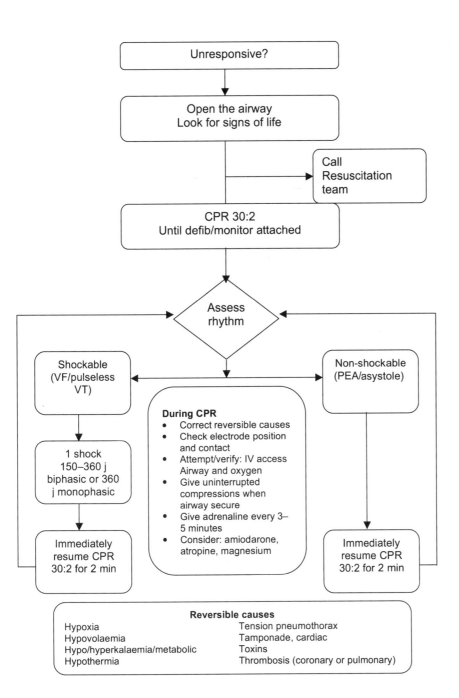

Figure 36
Advanced life
support algorithm
adapted from the
Resuscitation
Council (2005b)

Chapter 20

PRE- AND POST-OPERATIVE CARE

Alison Eddleston

This chapter relates to the following Nursing and Midwifery Council (NMC) Essential Skills Clusters (ESCs) for pre-registration nursing programmes.

Sections 1–8 of Care Compassion and Communication
Sections 9–18 and 20 of Organisational Aspects of Care
Sections 22–26 of Infection Prevention and Control
Sections 27–32 of Nutrition and Fluid Management
Sections 34–36 and 38–42 of Medicines Management.

Introduction

This chapter aims to provide a comprehensive review of the assessment, monitoring and support needed to safely manage the patient from pre-operative assessment to post-operative care. It will do this by:

❑ developing the necessary knowledge and skills required to manage the care and support of the patient in the pre-operative period, including:

– patient assessment;

– screening and investigation;

– patient consent and information;

– documentation;

– premedication and fasting.

❑ developing the necessary knowledge and skills required to manage the care and support of the patient in the post-operative period:

– patient assessment;

– monitoring strategies;

– nursing management.

In the UK there are approximately 5,000,000 anaesthetics given annually, with the majority of patients recovering from anaesthesia without any problems (Sewell and Young, 2004). Patients who are in the initial stages of recovery from anaesthesia and surgery are highly dependent and require a significant amount of nursing care and interventions to support them through the post-operative period (Young and Purdy, 2006). Therefore, an important part of a nurse's role is to prepare patients pre-operatively by planning the appropriate care and identifying the support required to manage these patients post-operatively.

Within this chapter the following key issues will be explored: patient assessment, monitoring and support, and the role of the nurse. The chapter will also include a selection of reflective exercises for you to undertake and will draw on the patient scenario used elsewhere in Part 5. These tools are designed to help you expand your knowledge and support clinical learning.

Scenario review

Throughout Part 5 you have been reviewing the care and management of Teresa after her road traffic accident. This has involved following Teresa's journey from assessment in the accident and emergency department to her deterioration in the ward environment and her medical emergency. In Chapter 19, Teresa was resuscitated whilst on the ward. What happened next is that, following implementation of resuscitation guidelines and intubation, a decision was made to transfer Teresa for further radiological investigation in the form of a computerised tomography (CT) scan and additional monitoring and support. A provisional diagnosis of an intracerebral bleed was considered due to Teresa's head injury. The CT scan confirmed the provisional diagnosis that a subdural haematoma is the cause of Teresa's deterioration. In view of the above findings Teresa is now to be transferred to the operating department for stabilisation and surgery.

Pre-operative care

Pre-operative assessment is an important part of patient care. It establishes that the patient is as fit as possible for both surgery and anaesthesia and has consented to undergo the procedure (Royal College of Anaesthetists, 2004a).

The aim of pre-operative assessment is to reduce peri-operative morbidity and mortality by identifying patients who require additional assessment and investigations prior to surgery. It also provides the patient with an opportunity to discuss their fears and anxieties by providing supportive information (Janke *et al.*, 2002). Pre-operative assessment should take place early in the patient's journey, in order that all the requirements for essential resources and possible obstacles can be anticipated before the day of the operation. However, this may be difficult in the case of emergency surgery (Royal College of Anaesthetists, 2004a). A patient's journey from pre-operative assessment to post-operative care involves a variety of different professionals and departments. All these personnel contribute to the care given to the patient and this process requires both communication and teamwork skills.

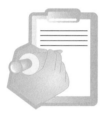

Activity 1.

Write a list of all the professionals and departments you think would be involved in the patient's journey from pre-operative care to post-operative management. Once you have written your list, review the essential personnel and departments that would be needed if your patient was either an emergency admission or a planned admission.

The pre-operative assessment process

Pre-operative consultation by an anaesthetist is essential for the medical assessment of a patient before anaesthesia for surgery or any other procedure (Royal College of Anaesthetists, 2004a). This involves undertaking an acute patient assessment through physical history taking and a clinical examination. The aim of this process is to obtain a complete picture of the patient, by not only reviewing the presenting problems but also reviewing the patient's fitness for surgery. It is also an opportunity to take into consideration any additional information that may affect the patient's journey such as, for example, chronic illness and social and family well-being.

The main focus of the physical examination is to review the patient's fitness for anaesthesia. One of the most important aspects of the physical examination is to assess whether the cardiovascular system (see Figure 1) will be able to cope with the trauma and stress of surgery. Also, it is important to ensure that there is adequate respiratory function and the patient's airway is able to maintain oxygenation.

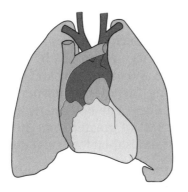

Figure 1
The respiratory and cardiovascular system

The American Society of Anaesthesiologists has developed a classification system known as the Patient Physical Status Classification System. It is commonly used to assess a patient's overall risk of anaesthesia. Patients who are above category two are identified as at risk of requiring additional support either intra-operatively or post-operatively.

Activity 2.

1. Review both the respiratory and cardiovascular systems and think about the diseases and illnesses that could affect a patient's anaesthesia.

2. Visit the web address **www.frca.co.uk** and search for the American Society of Anaesthesiologists' Physical Status Classification System. Using this information, review the patient information in Table 1 and attach a category of risk (ASA Grade) in each case.

3. Now review the above information and highlight the key issues that you think are important in the pre-operative assessment of our patient Teresa.

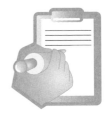

Table 1
Patient information

ASA Grade	Definition
	15-year-old boy who is undergoing surgery following a severe laceration to his right knee.
	65-year-old lady with significant respiratory problems due to chronic pulmonary obstructive disease, who is undergoing a total hip replacement.
	70-year-old man who is having emergency surgery for a leaking aortic aneurysm operation.

Undertaking pre-assessment screening

Non-medically trained staff such as nurses and other multiprofessionals play a crucial role in the screening process by providing the anaesthetist with relevant information and identifying and instigating investigations. Pre-anaesthesia screening includes reviewing a patient's height and weight and body mass index. The body mass index is used to identify risks due to obesity. A BMI of greater than 30 may lead to increased mortality and morbidity and is therefore a risk during an operation.

The National Institute for Clinical Excellence (NICE) (2003) identified that around five million elective surgical procedures are performed by the NHS in England and it has been routine practice to test patients pre-operatively for unsuspected conditions. This routine testing has resulted in unnecessary delays, inconvenience and cancellations. In view of this, NICE (2003) produced a clinical guideline to support pre-operative testing that improves patient care. The guideline recommends the investigations listed in Table 2 are undertaken subject to the patient's circumstances. This is endorsed by the Royal College of Anaesthetists (2004) who state that each Trust should have in place agreed policies, protocols or guidelines that support the investigations in Table 2.

Table 2
Recommended pre-operative investigations (NICE, 2003)

❏ Plain chest X-ray	❏ Random blood glucose
❏ Resting electrocardiogram	❏ Urine analysis
❏ Full blood count	❏ Blood gases
❏ Renal function	❏ Lung function
❏ Haemostasis (clotting)	❏ Pregnancy
	❏ Sickle cell anaemia

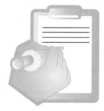

Activity 3.

1. Review the above investigations and document the following information for your future learning:

    – how these tests are undertaken including the type of specimen required;

  - precautions needed when carrying out these investigations (for patients and staff);

  - infection control issues related to these investigations;

  - the appropriate accompanying documentation;

  - the personnel to contact;

  - normal values for blood analysis.

See Chapter 21, pages 463–6.

2. Read the section on urinalysis in Chapter 21 of this book.

3. Identify the key investigations that Teresa will require prior to her emergency surgery.

See Chapter 21, pages 463–6.

Vital signs

A patient's vital signs will also provide the assessment team with key information regarding a patient's fitness for surgery and anaesthesia. Careful assessment of temperature, pulse, blood pressure and oxygen saturations will provide a baseline recording that will enable signs of deterioration to become evident.

Activity 4.

Refresh your knowledge and review Chapter 17 on observations.

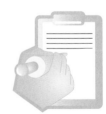

Patient information

All patients have the right to give or withhold consent to medical treatment (James, 2004). Patients also have an interest in what is going to happen to them and what to expect during a medical encounter (Association of Anaesthetists of Great Britain and Ireland, 2006). The process of obtaining consent is a crucial part of pre-operative care and management and requires specialist knowledge and skills in order to provide the patient or their representative with the appropriate information. Patients also have the right to withdraw consent as long as they have been supplied with adequate information and have the capacity to understand and make a balanced decision (Association of Anaesthetists of Great Britain and Ireland, 2006). No other person can consent to treatment on behalf of any other adult.

The treating doctor is responsible for ensuring that a patient has consented to treatment. Patients who do not have the ability to make decisions may be treated without consent if it is in their best interests (Association of Anaesthetists of Great Britain and Ireland, 2006). Examples of such patients include the critically ill and those with mental health problems. Children under the age of 16 are not deemed competent to consent to treatment, unless the doctor decides that the child has sufficient intelligence and understanding. This is known as the Gillick competence (Association of Anaesthetists of Great Britain and Ireland, 2006). For further information on consent see Chapter 14, page 276–9.

See Chapter 14, pages 276–9.

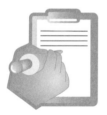

Activity 5.

1.   The Department of Health (DoH) has issued a model consent policy, the documentation for which can be obtained from **www.dh.gov.uk**. Visit the website, search for 'consent' and check your knowledge and understanding by becoming familiar with the consent form. You will also be able to review all the issues listed by viewing the Department of Health (2001) document *Consent – what you have a right to expect: a guide for adults.*

2.   After reviewing the information about patient consent, identify the key issues that are pertinent to Teresa's pre-operative assessment and future management.

Psychological preparation

The psychological preparation of a patient in the pre-operative period plays a key role in reducing anxiety, which in turn leads to decreased dependence and a smooth transition into the post-operative period.

Providing patients with both verbal and written communication regarding peri-operative practice and answering questions will help to allay any fears and anxieties (Janke *et al.*, 2002).

Reflection

Imagine you are about to visit the operating department for the first time.

1.   What would be your concerns, fears or anxieties?

2.   What type of information would you like to receive?

3.   What type of information is there available for patients?

Documentation and record-keeping

Good record-keeping is a mark of the skilled and safe practitioner and supports the communication and dissemination of information between members of the interprofessional health care team (Nursing and Midwifery Council, 2005). As discussed previously, good communication skills are an essential component of pre-operative care. Good verbal and written communication skills will mean that not only are the patient and their family kept informed but also that you will provide valuable information that will help to facilitate any intra-operative nursing needs (Hurley and McAleavy, 2006).

A systematic written record needs to be undertaken by all members of the multiprofessional team involved in the pre-operative assessment process. Outlined within this documentation will be the patient's clinical history, examination and the screening and investigations undertaken. Additional supporting evidence will be provided by the informed consent obtained from the patient and a record of the written and verbal information given to the patient. All this information will formulate a pre-operative checklist to ensure a patient's safety and smooth transition from pre-operative to post-operative care.

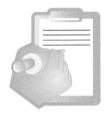

Activity 6.

Review a pre-operative checklist used on your surgical placement and compare it with the information provided in this chapter. This will enable you to become familiar with the information needed for your future learning and development.

Additional considerations

Premedication

Premedication is the administration of medication, usually an analgesic or antiolyix, prior to anaesthesia. This is an important component of anaesthetic practice as it can help to relieve anxiety, alleviate post-operative pain and facilitate a smooth transition to anaesthesia. In order to have maximum benefit best practice standards recommend premedication be given correctly two hours prior to induction to block a pre-operative stress response (Garrioch, 2004).

Pre-operative fasting

Patients have traditionally been denied food and drink for six hours before the induction of general anaesthesia as it was thought to reduce the incidence of pulmonary aspiration of gastric contents (Smith, 2004). Bothamley and Mardell (2005) state that fasting patients prior to surgical procedures is an accepted part of normal peri-operative practice. However, the length of fasting appears to vary considerably. In a major review of pre-operative fasting Brady *et al.* (2003) highlighted that there was no difference in the volume or pH of gastric contents whether the patient was fasted for a short or long period. Therefore, based on the evidence above, it appears safe for most patients to drink clear fluids two to three hours before a general anaesthesia.

The role of the nurse

Within the pre-operative period the nurse has a supporting role to play during the assessment process. This includes communicating and liaising with the multiprofessional team, patients and their families to provide written and verbal information to support the patient's journey. The nurse's role also involves the planning and preparation of patients for the intra-operative period. This is achieved through the assessment of patient care, documentation of screening and investigations as well as reviewing premedication and fasting protocols.

Summary – pre-operative care

The section above explored the key issues required to manage the care and support of the patient in the pre-operative period. Issues highlighted include patient assessment, screening and investigation, patient consent and information, documentation, premedication and fasting.

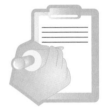

Activity 7.

Review the issues discussed and plan the pre-operative care and management of Teresa with respect to the following issues: patient assessment, screening and investigation, patient consent and information, documentation, premedication and fasting.

Post-operative care

Post-anaesthesia recovery is a continuous process that cannot be considered complete until the patient returns to their pre-operative physiological state (Sewell and Young, 2003). This recovery period may take a number of days or weeks as both anaesthesia and surgery produce a series of hormonal and stress responses that affects the homeostasis of the body.

Scenario review

Initially, Teresa is admitted to the intensive care unit for further neurological support following a craniotomy to remove the subdural haematoma and the insertion of an intracranial pressure monitor. As Teresa continues to make good progress the decision is made to transfer her to the surgical/neurological ward for further post-operative management.

Postoperative assessment

All patients who have undergone an operation, under either general or regional anaesthesia, are at risk of compromise to their airway, breathing and circulation. Until they have regained control of their airway, demonstrated cardiovascular stability and are able to communicate, patients must be cared for in the recovery area by appropriate trained staff, on a one-to-one basis (Royal College of Anaesthetists, 2004b).

Post-operative assessment involves both monitoring and supporting the patients through this crucial period of recovery. Close monitoring of both respiratory and cardiovascular observations enables any signs of deterioration to be acted on promptly. This requires you to develop skills of observation, inspection and auscultation (listening to, for example, heart and lung sounds). Directly observing your patient and their activity requires you to look for key information. This information can also be obtained by listening to sounds produced by the body and touching your patients. By getting to know your patients through observation, touch and listening, you will be able to assess changes in a patient's airway and breathing (respiratory), circulation (cardiovascular) and disability status (neurological) (Resuscitation Council, 2005).

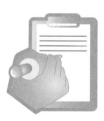

Activity 8.

1. What kind of information can be obtained through direct observation to help you assess a patient's recovery from anaesthesia and surgery?

2. Review and refresh your knowledge and skills on the key observations required to support a patient's cardiovascular system (see Chapter 17).

Scenario review

On admission to the surgical/neurological ward Teresa is alert and orientated and, apart from a slight headache, has no complaints. She is to be monitored from a cardiovascular and respiratory perspective for a further 24 hours, utilising both cardiac monitoring and pulse oximetry. Teresa's observations reveal a body temperature of 37°C, a heart rate of 90 bpm and a blood pressure of 150/90 mmHg. Supplementary oxygen at a concentration of 40 per cent is being administered via a simple face mask.

Monitoring and support

Post-operative monitoring and patient support is an essential element of a nurse's role following surgery and anaesthesia as this is the time period when a patient is considered most vulnerable and has the potential to develop complications of both the respiratory and cardiovascular system. Close monitoring of both these systems will enable the nurse to identify and provide the appropriate care and management to help resolve the types of complications discussed in the following sections.

Respiratory support and monitoring

Following surgery and anaesthesia, respiratory and airway problems can account for up to 30 per cent of all complications (Sewell and Young, 2003). Respiratory complications usually occur as a result of the following processes: obstruction to the airway, hypoxaemia (low levels of oxygen within the bloodstream) and hypoventilation (inadequate respiration). The monitoring and support required depends on the severity of the problem but may include initiation of oxygen therapy, airway management and ventilatory support. Patients with significant respiratory complications need to be managed within the critical care setting where more detailed observations and ventilatory support can be provided.

Airway management

Observation and maintenance of a patient's airway is of vital importance in the immediate post-operative period (Young and Purdy, 2006). There are two potential complications that require close observation – airway obstruction and laryngospasm. Airway obstruction can occur as a result of the loss of the normal protective reflexes due to anaesthesia. The use of artificial airway management tools used to maintain anaesthesia may cause irritation of the larynx and result in laryngospasm. Both these complications require immediate treatment and interventions to maintain airway patency.

See Chapter 19,
page 382.

Considerations for practice

(See also Chapter 19, page 382.)

❑ Airway assessment – look, listen, feel.

❑ Patient positioning.

❑ Respiratory observations.

❑ Airway management techniques.

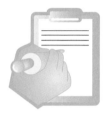

Activity 9.

Review and refresh your knowledge by referring to Chapters 17 and 19.

Oxygen therapy

Oxygen is transported around the body by two methods – 3 per cent is dissolved in the blood plasma and 97 per cent is bound to the haemoglobin molecule. It is administered in the post-operative period to help support the reversal of anaesthesia through the transport of anaesthetic gases across the alveolar/capillary membrane so that they can be excreted from the body (Hughes, 2004). It is also administered to correct and treat hypoxaemia (insufficient levels of oxygen in the blood), which is a potentially life-threatening complication. Close monitoring and titration of oxygen therapy is an essential part of a nurse's role to ensure patients' safety and effective treatment.

Dosage and prescription

Oxygen therapy should be prescribed and titrated according to patient need and monitored for effectiveness via pulse oximetry and arterial blood gas analysis. As oxygen therapy is a prescribed treatment, the following parameters should be documented on the patient's prescription chart: percentage, flow rate, duration of therapy, device to be used and monitoring of treatment (Bateman and Leach, 1998). When managing an acutely ill patient in either the emergency situation or the deteriorating situation the following oxygen guideline is advocated: high flow 15 l/min through either a partial rebreathing system or non-rebreathing system (Smith, 2000). You may also see oxygen prescribed as a percentage, e.g. 40 per cent, or written as the following symbol F_IO_2 (fraction of inspired oxygen), e.g. F_IO_2 0.4.

Low flow devices

Low flow devices such as nasal cannula and simple face masks draw in supplementary oxygen with room air to deliver a percentage range of oxygen. A nasal cannula (see Figure 2) delivers an F_IO_2 from 0.24 to 0.40 and requires a flow rate for an adult of 0.5–6 l/min. They are inexpensive and well-tolerated. Simple face mask devices (see Figure 3) deliver F_IO_2 from 0.24 to 0.60, which requires a flow rate 5–10 l/min. It is important to note that a minimum flow rate of 5 l/min is required to prevent re-breathing of exhaled gas with these devices.

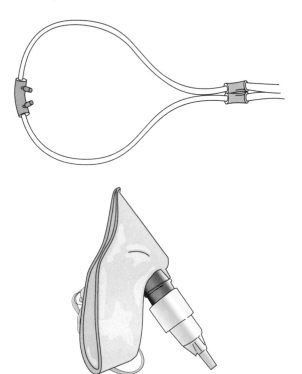

Figure 2
Nasal cannula

Figure 3
Simple face mask

High flow devices

High flow devices deliver oxygen at rates above normal inspiratory flow and therefore, in contrast to low flow devices, supply a fixed percentage or F_IO_2.

Examples of high flow devices include a partial rebreathing system (Figure 4) or a non-rebreathing system (Figure 5).

Figure 4
A partial rebreathing system

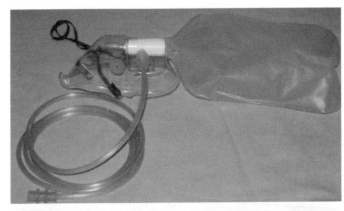

Figure 5
A non-rebreathing system

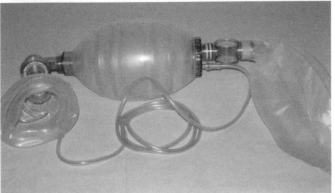

Complications

Oxygen is a dry gas that can dehydrate exposed mucous membranes (Gallacher, 2004). Particular areas vulnerable to drying are the mucous membranes in the patient's nose and mouth. Care and support to maintain adequate humidification are essential in order that patients are happy to comply with treatment. Additional support may be given by moistening the mucous membranes with humidification therapy and regular oral hygiene.

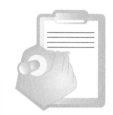

Activity 10.

1. Review the information about oxygen therapy devices given here and in Chapter 15. This will help you to understand the different types of masks available and to support the correct device for the patient's condition.

2. On reviewing the above information with respect to oxygen therapy identify the key issues that are pertinent to Teresa's post-operative management and assessment.

Applying the patient's oxygen device requires care and attention, as incorrectly securing the oxygen therapy can lead to either pressure damage to the ears and nose or ulceration of the patient's mucous membranes due to the device being fitted too securely. Also, a tightly fitting device could cause the patient to feel claustrophobic and result in increased anxiety levels and non-compliance with treatment. Alternately, if a device is secured too slackly, then it could be that the patient requires an additional increase in therapy because inadequate therapy is being delivered due to a loose device.

Once the device is in place and treatment has commenced, the prescribed therapy requires monitoring to ensure effective treatment is delivered. Two areas of concern are oxygen toxicity and the loss of respiratory drive in chronic respiratory patients due to high levels of circulating carbon dioxide, which could affect a patient's breathing pattern.

Patient and operator safety is crucial to effective delivery and treatment of oxygen therapy. Oxygen, as previously discussed, is a dry gas that is highly combustible and, as such, requires special precautions to be taken. Patients and staff should note the dangers to themselves and special precautions should be taken to avoid flammable substances and smoking in the vicinity. Considerations for practice include:

❏ patient comfort and safety;

❏ application of the mask;

❏ choosing the correct delivery device for the patient's clinical condition;

❏ prescribed treatment – flow, duration, device;

❏ monitoring of the therapy;

❏ patient safety – identification of the appropriate cylinder, fire hazards, etc.

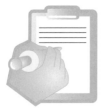

Activity 11.

Review the above considerations in the light of your own knowledge and experience of managing patients receiving oxygen therapy while on placement.

Monitoring oxygen therapy

The pulse oximeter is a useful device for evaluating the oxygen status of patients in a variety of clinical settings (Casey, 2001), as it measures and reports oxygen saturation (SpO_2). It provides non-invasive, continuous information that shows the availability of oxygen haemoglobin in the blood. The pulse oximeter utilises light emissions from the tissues to monitor arterial and venous blood flow and so measure the percentage of haemoglobin that is saturated with oxygen. This information is relayed to the pulse oximeter and displayed as a waveform or numerical percentage. The information is relayed to the oximeter using a probe which contains two light-emitting diodes, one emitting red light and the other emitting infrared light, and a photodetector (see Figure 6).

Figure 6
Pulse oximetry
sensor and probe

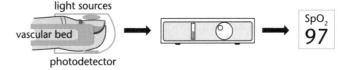

The normal percentage range considered when titrating a patient's oxygen parameters is 95–100 per cent. However, it is important to note that all patients are individuals and, as such, may have their own therapeutic range against which oxygen is titrated.

Complications

When monitoring and recording a patient's pulse oximetry reading, the following information needs to be considered in order to maintain patient safety and provide effective and accurate titration of treatment. If you consider that the pulse oximeter detects oxygen saturation via a light sensor, then either too much or too little light will affect the reading. This is because the sensor is not able to detect true arterial and venous blood flow. Two other factors that may distort a patient's reading due to disruption in the light source are motion (movement) and equipment failure. Misinterpretation of readings due to too much light may be caused by the environment being too bright or be the result of a spotlight being placed directly over the patient. If the sensor receives too little light it will not be able to detect the patient's blood flow. This may occur because the probe is not in the correct position or because the probe is the wrong size for the patient. This is known as optical shunting.

Another possible complication is motion artefact. This occurs when blood flow to the finger (or other part of the body) to which the oximeter probe is attached is affected by movement. For example, if a patient is moving their hand around, the pulse oximeter may detect a reading but, due to increased blood flow to the hand, the reading may be inaccurate. You will need to determine if the reading is accurate before recording its value.

Considerations for practice, especially after surgery, are either a low haemoglobin level or the presence of anaemia. As the pulse oximeter measures oxygen saturation levels it reflects the ability of the haemoglobin molecule to transport oxygen around the body. However, additional investigations may also be required to determine a patient's overall oxygenation status. This will include a blood gas analysis, which will be able to assess for hypoxaemia by sampling arterial blood. For example, a patient with a haemoglobin level of 8 g/dl could display a reading of 95–100 per cent SpO_2 reading via the pulse oximeter but, as there is a reduction in the amount of circulating haemoglobin, this could result in the amount of oxygen available for distribution to the tissues being reduced. This may mean that the patient has not enough circulating oxygen for their needs and additional therapy may be required to prevent hypoxaemia.

Patients post-anaesthesia and surgery often experience central nervous system complications such as shivering and induced hypothermia. This can result in the patient being cold to the touch. Also, post-operative patients are vulnerable to changes in their cardiovascular circulating volume due to loss of body fluid through trauma, the disease process and treatment regimes. For example, they may lose body fluid due to vomiting, diarrhoea or diuretic therapy. As a result, the patient may have low blood pressure and reduced perfusion to the tissues. Therefore it may be difficult to obtain an accurate pulse oximetry reading and a variety of sites, such as the ear, finger, nose and toe may need to be accessed to achieve an accurate reading. Alteration in cardiovascular volume can be restored through intravenous fluid replacement. Temperature regulation can be supported by using the appropriate warming strategies to meet the patient's needs such as, for example, additional blankets, warming devices and heated fluids.

Additional considerations

As previously discussed, pulse oximetry assesses oxygen saturation readings by detecting arterial and venous blood flow to monitor oxygen haemoglobin levels. So, any factor that either affects or alters the detection of a blood flow may lead to inaccurate readings. Therefore, when monitoring a patient pre- and post-operatively, the following issues may affect a patient's reading:

❑ the presence of oedema;

❑ venous pulsation;

❑ intravascular dyes;

❑ nail polish.

The presence of limb oedema in a patient can influence a pulse oximetry reading by causing venous pulsation. Venous pulsation can occur as a result of the excessive fluid in the tissues being compressed by the sensor, which may lead to an increase in venous blood flow. Causes of venous pulsation to be aware of are a tightly fitting sensor or the use of a non-invasive blood pressure monitoring device on the same limb as the sensor. The use of intravenous dyes for patient investigations may also influence pulse oximetry readings. This results in the sensor not being able to detect a reading due to alterations in the light absorbency of the blood. Examples of intravenous dyes include methylene blue, isosulfan blue and indiocyanine green. Finally, when monitoring a patient's SpO_2 reading, the presence of nail polish can hinder the sensor's ability to detect an arterial and venous blood flow. Chan *et al.* (2003) undertook a small-scale study that reviewed the effect of fingernail polish on pulse oximetry. Readings were taken from polished and unpolished hands using one of ten colours. Results revealed slightly lower pulse oximetry readings with black or brown polished nails compared with readings with unpolished nails. However, when the probe was orientated so that the light was parallel to light nail polish, the reading was not affected.

Considerations for practice

❑ Review oxygen transport and the application of pulse oximetry.

❑ Monitoring and patient safety:

– sensor application;

– complications;

– additional factors such as intravenous dyes.

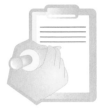

Activity 12.

1. Review the above considerations to develop your own knowledge and experience of managing patients receiving oxygen therapy.

2. Monitor your own saturation reading and see what effect the following complications have on your reading: light, motion and venous pulsation. Compare and contrast the readings displayed.

3. Review the information on pulse oximetry monitoring and identify the key issues that could affect Teresa's care and management.

Cardiovascular support and monitoring

Following surgery and anaesthesia close physiological monitoring is crucial if you are to detect early signs of cardiovascular compromise (Ang *et al.*, 2002). Common cardiovascular complications often experienced in the post-operative period include hypotension, hypertension, myocardial ischaemia and cardiac dysrhythmias.

Hypotension and hypertension

A change in a patient's blood pressure post-operatively is a common occurrence and can often result in both hypotension and hypertension. These changes usually occur as a result of the body trying to compensate for the patient's general ill health, loss of fluid or inadequate fluid replacement, pre-operative starvation and pain (Behar *et al.* 2007). Post-operative hypotension is often related to anaesthesia and, as such, usually ceases to be a problem following post-anaesthetic recovery. Hypertension is commonly associated with pre-existing peripheral vascular disease and pain (Young and Purdy, 2006).

One of the major causes of hypotension in the post-operative patient is loss of fluid from the intravascular space (bleeding) and/or the extravascular space (vomiting, diarrhoea and sweating leading to generalised dehydration), which can contribute to hypovolaemia (Behar *et al.*, 2007). Therefore, accurate monitoring and assessment of a patient's cardiovascular status is crucial to ensure adequate fluid replacement and to prevent the life-threatening complications of shock. The aim of fluid management in surgical patients is to support the maintenance of fluid levels in both the intracellular and extracellular spaces to maintain homeostasis (Hughes, 2004).

Considerations for practice

❏ Cardiovascular assessment – look, listen, feel.

❏ Cardiovascular observations.

❏ Fluid balance.

❏ Additional considerations:

- cardiac monitoring;

- central venous monitoring;

- pain assessment (see Chapter 4).

Cardiovascular assessment

Assessment of the cardiovascular system utilises the following skills: direct observation, palpation and auscultation. These skills are needed when assessing a patient's vital signs such as, for example, pulse and blood pressure. Direct observation allows you to assess a patient's general condition with regard to their cardiovascular status. This can be achieved by undertaking a general assessment of the patient's overall condition and includes the following assessment data: height and weight, BMI and health history.

Clinical assessment of the patient through looking at their colour and touching them provides vital information about a patient's peripheral circulation and fluid status. Alteration in a patient's colouring, for example signs of blueness (cyanosis), pallor and greyness, requires a more detailed examination and could indicate poor oxygen delivery to the tissues. The presence of warmth and a good blood supply to the peripheral areas, especially to the hands and feet, demonstrates a good circulatory status.

By using direct observation skills you can also assess a patient's fluid status. Signs of dryness when examining the patient's tongue and skin (**turgor**) could indicate the presence of dehydration, whereas a patient who is sweating and has a raised temperature may require additional fluid to compensate for any additional losses.

Initially patients are often cold and peripherally shut down post-operatively, needing close observation until their body temperature returns within normal limits. (A patient's peripheral circulation can be assessed by their colour, touch and warmth.) (see Chapter 10, page 227).

See Chapter 10, page 227.

Cardiovascular observations

The frequency of the clinical cardiovascular observations depends on the stage of recovery, nature of the surgery and the clinical condition of the patient (Sewell and Young, 2003). The following cardiovascular observations should be recorded as a minimum: blood pressure, pulse, heart rate and rhythm. Additional information that can support a patient's cardiovascular assessment includes: monitoring a patient's level of consciousness; oxygen saturations, body temperature, pain assessment and fluid status. For example, following surgery and anaesthesia, patients often experience extraordinary fluid losses. There are a number of bodily systems that can be affected by fluid losses; these are:

❑ cardiovascular (blood volume);

❑ gastrointestinal (nausea and vomiting);

❑ renal (urine output);

❑ respiratory (work of breathing);

❑ skin (sweating).

Additional intravenous fluids may need to be given during the post-operative period to correct any deficiencies noted. This may take the form of a fluid challenge which is where a bolus of intravenous fluid, usually between 250 ml and 1 litre, is given over a short time span (usually 30 minutes) to compensate for volume reduction. However, it is important to be aware that excessive fluid replacement can lead to significant complications in cardiac vulnerable patients. Therefore, detailed monitoring and support with regard to replacement, resuscitation and maintenance of fluid balance is an essential component of post-operative care (Behar *et al.*, 2007).

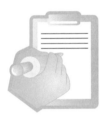

Activity 13.

Review and refresh your knowledge of these observations by referring to Chapters 10 and 17.

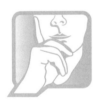

Reflection

Think about somebody that you know – a patient, relative or friend – who has recently undergone surgery and anaesthesia and review the following points.

❑ What type of surgery/operation did they have (e.g. gastrectomy)?

❑ Which bodily systems did this effect (e.g. gastrointestinal tract, kidneys, etc.)?

❑ How would their fluid balance be affected (e.g. nil by mouth, vomiting, diarrhoea or bleeding, poor urine output leading to dehydration)?

Cardiac monitoring

Another potential cardiovascular complication that may occur within the post-operative period is an alteration of the cardiac rhythm. Disturbances of cardiac rhythm are also known as **arrhythmias** and **dysrhythmias**. Some arrhythmias have the potential to adversely alter a patient's cardiovascular status and are life-threatening, for example ventricular fibrillation or asystole. However, within the post-operative period, arrhythmias or dysrhythmias often occur as a result of either pre-existing cardiac disease or electrolyte and acid base balance disturbances (see Table 3). Therefore treatment should be directed at managing the underlying cause (Sewell and Young, 2003).

		Table 3
❑ Sinus bradycardia	❑ Ventricular ectopic heart beats	Common
❑ Sinus tachycardia	❑ Ventricular tachycardia	arrhythmias seen in
❑ Atrial fibrillation	❑ Elevated T waves	the post-operative
		period

It is important that you are able to recognise disorders of the cardiac rhythm so that you can support a patient's cardiovascular monitoring throughout the post-operative period. This can be achieved by becoming familiar with the anatomy and physiology of the conduction system and reviewing the PQRST complex (see Figure 8).

Another consideration is the placement of ECG electrodes and the attachment of leads. This is an area that you may be asked to become familiar with in order to support the monitoring process.

Cardiac monitoring (Olive, 2005)

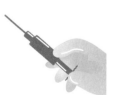

1. Explain the procedure to the patient and obtain consent.

2. Prepare the skin according to the electrode manufacturer's instructions.

3. Place the electrodes and attach the leads (see Figure 7):

   – red – right midclavicular line just below clavicle;

   – yellow – left midclavicular line just below clavicle;

   – green – left midclavicular line at the 6th–7th intercostal space.

4. Switch on the monitor.

5. Set alarm limits according to patient's normal/abnormal parameters.

Figure 7
Lead placement

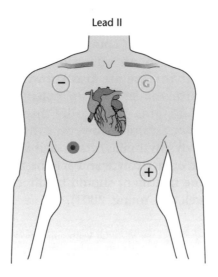

Lead II

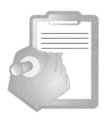

Activity 14.

Refresh your knowledge of the anatomy and physiology of the conduction system:

1. Review in detail the cardiac cycle and the waveforms produced (see Figure 8).

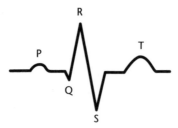

Figure 8 PQRST complex

2. Identify and become familiar with the following cardiac rhythms:

- sinus rhythm;

- sinus bradycardia;

- sinus tachycardia;

- atrial fibrillation.

3. Review the above information and highlight the cardiovascular support and management that Teresa will require for the next 24 hours.

Central venous access devices

The use of central venous access devices has become common practice within the acute care setting. These devices (see Figures 9 and 10) are often referred to by the following names: long lines, central catheters, Hickman or Broviac catheters (Hamilton, 2006). It has been estimated that approximately 200,000 central venous catheters are inserted annually in a wide range of clinical settings (NICE, 2002).

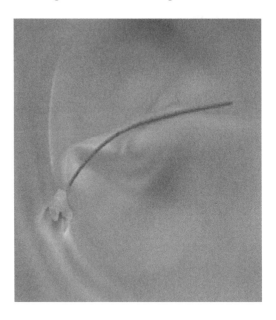

Figure 9
Single lumen central
venous access line

Figure 10
Multiple lumen
central venous
access line

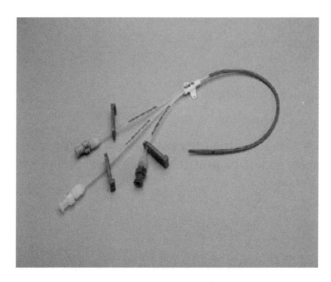

The main use of a central venous access device within the post-operative period is for monitoring central venous pressure (CVP). Central venous pressure is measured by the insertion of a catheter into a large vein. The catheter is advanced along the vein until the tip is at the entrance to the right atrium of the heart. The normal CVP range is 3–10 mmHg (5–12 cmH$_2$0) (Laight *et al.*, 2006).

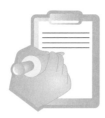

Activity 15.

1.   Review Figure 11, which provides you with a visual guide to support your developing knowledge and understanding about measuring a patient's CVP. This will enable you to become familiar with the information needed for your future learning and development.

2.   Document the following information for your future learning:

   – the procedure for undertaking a CVP recording;

   – complications of a central venous access device;

   – documentation needed.

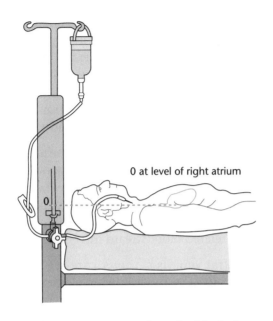

Figure 11
Central venous
monitoring

0 at level of right atrium

Measuring a patient's CVP can provide valuable information about the following cardiovascular parameters:

❑ cardiac function;

❑ venous return;

❑ venous tone;

❑ pulmonary vascular resistance.

Reviewing the above parameters will provide a helpful guide for supporting a patient's cardiovascular system and monitoring fluid replacement requirements (Bahar *et al.*, 2007). Additional indications for using a central venous access device include large venous access for intravenous drug administration and nutritional support.

The Health Act 2006 *Code of Practice for the Prevention and Control of health care Associated Infections* states that effective prevention and control of health care associated infections have to be embedded into everyday practice and applied consistently by everyone (Department of Health, 2007). Bloodstream infections associated with central venous catheter insertion are among the most dangerous of complications, worsening the severity of the patient's underlying ill health, prolonging the period of hospitalisation and increasing the cost of care (Pratt *et al.*, 2007).

All health care professionals involved in the management of a central venous access device have a vital role to play in maintaining patient safety and providing safe delivery of intravenous therapy (Hamilton, 2006). One initiative that has been developed to reduce the risk of health care associated infection is the high-impact intervention which uses a care bundle approach to reduce the risk of infection related to clinical procedures which produce a risk of infection (Department of Health, 2007).

The Department of Health (2007) recommends the use of the *High impact intervention no.2: central venous catheter care* as good practice. This care intervention is based on national evidence-based guidelines for preventing health care associated infections and expert advice to provide a central venous catheter care review tool that aims to reduce the incidence of catheter-related bloodstream infections.

The elements of central venous catheter care are designed to support clinical practice and consist of the following elements, namely insertion and continuing care, details of which are outlined in Table 4.

Table 4
High impact intervention no 2: central venous catheter care bundle

Insertion element reviews	Continuing care reviews
❑ Catheter type	❑ Regular observation of site
❑ Insertion site	❑ Catheter site care
❑ Alcoholic Chlorexidine Gluconate skin preparation	❑ Catheter access
❑ Prevent microbial contamination	❑ No routine catheter replacement

Source: Department of Health (2007).

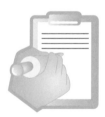

Activity 16.

Visit the Department of Heath website **www.dh.gov.uk** and check your knowledge and understanding by becoming familiar with the elements of *High impact intervention no. 2: central venous catheter care*. You will also be able to review all the issues listed by reading the other high-impact interventions designed to reduce health care-associated infections such as MRSA. Read, for example, about the Department of Health (2005) *Saving lives campaign – the delivery programme to reduce health care associated infections (HCAI).*

Neurological assessment

During anaesthesia there is a marked change in a patient's neurological status. The patient moves from a continuum of unconsciousness to a conscious state following reversal of anaesthetic agents (Young and Purdy, 2006). The majority of patients move along the continuum with no ill effect. However, a small percentage may require further respiratory, cardiovascular and neurological monitoring and support because of complications that are due to delayed emergence from anaesthesia, pain, temperature regulation and post-operative nausea and vomiting.

Considerations for practice

Neurological assessment:

❑ delayed emergence from anaesthesia;

❑ level of consciousness;

❑ blood glucose monitoring;

❑ neurological observations.

Additional considerations:

❑ pain assessment;

❑ temperature regulation;

❑ post-operative nausea and vomiting.

Neurological observations

Delayed emergence from anaesthesia may result from a number of causes, such as the residual effects of anaesthesia drugs and metabolic disturbances due to fluctuating blood glucose and electrolyte levels, for example hypo- or hyperglycaemia and hypo/hypernatrimia (low/high blood sodium levels). However, prolonged unconsciousness may signify that a more sinister event has occurred such as a cerebral vascular event or a cardiac event such as stroke or myocardial infarction (Sewell and Young, 2003). These problems are often observed during the initial period of recovery from anaesthesia in the post-anaesthetic care environment. Formal assessment of a patient's neurological function is only necessary if normal recovery becomes prolonged (Young and Purdy, 2006).

Neurological assessment provides both the basic tool for diagnosis of neurological deficit and the means of measuring progress. This assessment should be completed on admission and should be undertaken at regular intervals in order to determine the patient's progress (Dawson and Shah, 2006). The additional use of advanced neurological observations and assessment tools, such as, for example, the Glasgow Coma Scale, may be required.

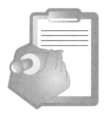

Activity 17.

Review the information in Chapter 17 on neurological observations and blood glucose monitoring, and review Chapter 19 on life support.

Pain management

Pain following surgery is inevitable for many patients and certain issues such as a patient's age, gender and culture play a key role in their ability to cope with this (Kitcatt, 2003). Basic post-operative analgesia includes opioids, non-steroidal anti-inflammatory drugs and paracetamol. Opioid analgesics work by depressing the appreciation of pain and their effects may reduce anxiety. Paracetamol and anti-flammatory drugs can provide a baseline for pain relief (Baxter and Chinn, 2006). Supplementary analgesia can be given using patient-controlled analgesia, epidural and regional blocks (Behar *et al.*, 2007).

Epidural analgesia

Epidural analgesia is highly effective at controlling acute pain after surgery as it combines excellent pain relief with minimal side effects to provide high patient satisfaction (Weetman and Allison, 2006). Opioids and local anaesthetics are the most common analgesics and can be delivered either by direct single injection or by a catheter that has been inserted through a needle into the epidural space (Pasero, 2003) (see Figure 12). Once the epidural space has been located, there are three potential drug administration methods available: bolus (single injection), continuous infusion and patient-controlled analgesia. However, while this is an effective pain-relieving strategy it is not without its complications. Complications are usually associated with the drugs used and the risks associated with the epidural catheter. Epidural management requires knowledge, skill and competence in order to support patient safety and minimise any potential for harm.

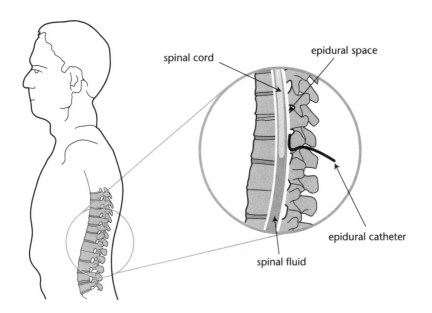

Figure 12
Epidural placement and catheter

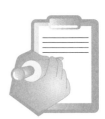

Activity 18.

Review the different types of post-operative analgesia outlined in Table 5 and identify the specific side effects for each type of drug so that you are familiar with the different types available.

Table 5
Types of post-operative analgesia

Type of drug	Example	Side effects
Opioid	Morphine, pethadine, fentanyl	?
Non-steroidal anti-inflammatory	Diclofenac	?
Patient-controlled analgesia	Morphine, diamorphine	?
Epidural	Bupivaciane 0.0625 to 0.125%	?

Patient-controlled analgesia

See Chapter 4, page 104.

Patient-controlled analgesia (PCA) is a safe and effective tool for managing moderate to severe pain (Macintyre, 2001). (See also Chapter 4, page 104.) Drug delivery is a continuous infusion method of, usually, a low-dose opioid and anti-emetic, which allows for additional bolus doses to deal with any patient breakthrough pain experience (Baxter and Chinn, 2006). As discussed above, epidural analgesia can also be administered using this method. Complications are usually associated with the drugs used and the risks associated with patient competence.

The drug administration equipment consists of a continuous delivery infusion pump that enables additional bolus drug administration via a designated handheld device (see Figure 13). It is suitable for any adult who is cognitively and physically able to use the equipment and can understand that pressing the button will result in pain relief (Pagero and McCaffery, 2005). A key safety feature of this type of delivery method is the lock-out period. This is the period of time during which another dose of the patient-controlled analgesia cannot be delivered, no matter how many times the patient presses the button.

Figure 13
Patient-controlled analgesia device

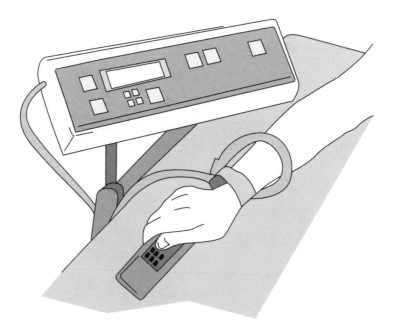

Pain assessment

Pain assessment is a complex skill (Briggs, 2001) that requires good communication and teamwork skills to ensure that the patient receives the appropriate pain management for their need. There is a variety of pain assessment tools available to support the needs of the post-operative patient. It is important to develop an awareness of the different types available, and also to review the policies and protocols that govern pain management in your Trust as these will vary depending on individual Trust requirements.

Considerations for practice

❑ Selection of appropriate pain assessment tool for patient use.

❑ Pain relief strategies available:

– the need for basic post-operative analgesia;

– the need for supplementary methods;

– patient choice.

❑ Training requirements.

❑ Equipment needed.

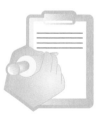

Activity 19.

1. Review and refresh your knowledge by referring to Chapter 4 on pain management.

2. Think about the key issues above and consider:

❑ your own knowledge and skills in relation to pain management;

❑ the patient scenario – identify Teresa's pain management needs following her transfer from intensive care to the surgical post-operative ward.

Additional areas for consideration

Post-operative nausea and vomiting

Post-operative nausea and vomiting (PONV) continues to be a common complication of surgery that can lead to increased recovery time and expanded nursing care (Gan *et al.*, 2003). It has been estimated that approximately 30 per cent of patients recovering from anaesthesia are affected by PONV (Tramer, 2003). Patients say that they would actually prefer to suffer pain than PONV (Van Wiljk and Smallbout, 1990).

Management and treatment of PONV is a complex process that requires the recognition of high-risk patients, the selection of appropriate anaesthetic techniques and knowledge of relieving strategies (Brampton, 2004). In view of this, the Royal College of Anaesthetists (2004) advocate that all patients should receive effective control of pain and PONV and recommend the provision of local guidelines for treatment strategies.

Temperature regulation

During the peri-operative period the surgical patient is often subjected to a number of environmental and physiological changes that can result in the impaired temperature regulation complications of hypothermia and hyperthermia. These complications often occur in the immediate post-operative phase and can be experienced within the post-anaesthetic care environment.

Hypothermia, or a body temperature of below 36°C, often occurs due to the absence of the normal protective shivering reflex resulting from anaesthesia and exposure during surgery. This may result in the patient assuming the temperature of the environment and can lead to difficulties in restoring normothermia post-operatively.

Hyperthermia, or a body temperature of above 38°C, generally occurs because of over-warming. However, the overall condition of the patient needs to be investigated further to see if there is a possibility of sepsis (Young and Sewell, 2004).

Considerations for practice

❑ The anatomy and physiology of temperature regulation.

❑ The monitoring of body temperature.

❑ The use of warming strategies, e.g. blankets, heated intravenous fluids.

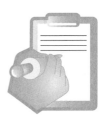

Activity 20.

1. Refresh your knowledge of the anatomy and physiology of temperature regulation.

2. Review the information in Chapter 17 on temperature monitoring and in Chapter 21 on the sepsis care bundle.

Review of key post-operative care issues

The nurse's role within the post-operative period involves managing the care of the post-operative patient through the initiation of both medical and nursing interventions in response to the physiological and psychological effects of both surgery and anaesthesia. This section has explored the key issues required to manage the care and support of the patient in the post-operative period. Issues highlighted include: patient assessment, monitoring and support with reference to the nursing management and interventions required to manage the following body systems: respiratory, cardiovascular and neurological.

Summary

This chapter has taken you on a patient's journey through surgery and has explored the issues involved in the assessment, monitoring and support of a patient requiring both pre- and post-operative care. By reviewing the key areas listed in this chapter, and by referring to the chapter scenario, you will have developed an understanding of the necessary knowledge and competency in the skills required to support a patient from pre-operative assessment to post-operative recovery. Of course, additional support and guidance must be sought if the patient's condition deteriorates or if the patient requires further specialist interventions and treatment.

References

Ang, P., Pagan, A. and Lewis, P. (2002) 'Determining patients' readiness for release from postanesthesia recovery unit'. *Association of Operating Room Nurses*, 76(4): 664–6

Association of Anaesthetists of Great Britain and Ireland (2006) *Consent for Anaesthesia*. London: AAGBI

Bateman, N.T. and Leach, R.M. (1998) 'ABC of oxygen acute oxygen therapy'. *British Medical Journal*, 317: 798–801

Baxter, H. and Chinn, P. (2004), cited in Sheppard, M. and Wright, M. (2006) *Principles and practice of high dependency nursing*. London: Ballière Tindal

Behar, J.M., Gogalniceanu, P. and Bromley L. (2007) 'Anaesthesia: post-operative care'. *Student BMJ*, 15: 138–41

Bothamley, J. and Mardell, A. (2005) 'Preoperative fasting revisited'. *British Journal of Preoperative Nursing*, 15(9): 370–4

Brady, M., Kinn, S. and Stuart, P. (2003) 'Preoperative fasting for adults to prevent perioperative complications (Cochrane Review)'. *Cochrane Library*, Issue 4. Chichester: Wiley

Brampton, W.J. (2004), cited in Royal College of Anaesthetists (2004b) *Raising the standard: a compendium of audit*. London

Briggs, E. (2001) 'Principles of pain assessment in older people', cited in Bird, J. (2005) 'Assessing pain in older people'. *Nursing Standard*, 19(19): 45–52

Casey, G. (2001) 'Oxygen transport and the use of pulse oximetry'. *Nursing Standard*, 15(47): 46–53

Chan Mallory, M., Chan Michael, M. and Chan, E.D. (2003) 'What effect of fingernail polish on pulse oximetry'. *Chest*, 123: 2163–4

Dawson, D. and Shah, S. (2006), cited in Sheppard, M. and Wright, M. (2006) *Principles and practice of high dependency nursing*. London: Ballière Tindal

Department of Health (2001) *Consent – what you have a right to expect: a guide for adults*. London: DoH

Department of Health (2005) *Saving lives: a delivery programme to reduce health care associated infection including MRSA*. London: DoH

Department of Health (2007) *Code of practice for the prevention and control of health care associated infections*. London: DoH

Gallacher, S. (2004) 'Oxygen therapy', cited in Moore, T. and Woodrow, P. (2004) *High dependency nursing care observation, intervention and support*. London: Routledge

Gan, T.J., Meyer, T., Apel, C.C., Chung, F., Davis, P.J., Eubanks, S., Kovac, A. *et al.* (2003) 'Concensus guidelines for managing postoperative nausea and vomiting'. *Anesthesia Analgesia*, 97: 62–71

Garrioch, M. (2004) 'Premedication', cited in Royal College of Anaesthetists (2004) *Raising the standard: a compendium of audit*. London: RCA

Hamilton, H. (2006) 'Complications associated with venous access devices: part one'. *Nursing Standard*, 20(26): 43–50

Hughes, E. (2004) 'Principles of post-operative patient care'. *Nursing Standard*, 19(5): 43–51

Hurley, C. and McAleavy, J. (2006) 'Preoperative assessment and intraoperative care planning'. *Journal of Perioperative Practice*, 16(1): 187–94

James, E. (2004) 'Consent to anaesthesia', cited in Royal College of Anaesthetists (2004a) *Raising the standard: a compendium of audit*. London: RCA

Janke, E., Chalk, V. and Kinley, H. (2002) *Pre-operative assessment: setting a standard through learning*. University of Southampton.

Kitcatt, S. (2003), cited in Hughes, E. (2004) 'Principles of post-operative patient care'. *Nursing Standard*, 19(5): 43–51

Laight, S., Currie, M. and Davies, N. (2006) 'Cardiac care', cited in Sheppard, M. and Wright, M. (2006) *Principles and practice of high dependency nursing*. London: Ballière Tindal

Macintyre, P.E. (2001) 'Safety and efficacy of patient – controlled analgesia'. *British Journal of Anaesthesia*, 87(1): 36–46

National Institute for Clinical Excellence (2002) *Guidance on the use of ultrasound locating devices for placing central venous catheter no. 49*. London: NICE

National Institute for Clinical Excellence (2003) *Guidelines: preoperative tests – the use of routine preoperative tests for surgery*. London: NICE

Nursing and Midwifery Council (2005) *Guidelines for records and record keeping*. London: NMC

Olive, P. (2005) *Cardiac monitoring*. University of Central Lancashire

Pasero, C. (2003) 'Epidural analgesia for postoperative pain: excellent analgesia and improved patient outcomes after major surgery'. *American Journal of Nursing*, 103(10): 62–4

Pasero, C. and McCaffery, M. (2005) 'Authorized and unauthorized use of PCA pumps: clarifying the use of patient-controlled analgesia, in light of recent alerts'. *American Journal of Nursing*, 105(7): 30–2

Pratt, R.J., Pellowe, C.M., Wilson, J.A., Loveday, H.P., Harper, P.J., Jones, S.R.L.J., McDougall, C. and Wilcox, M. .H (2007) 'National evidence-based guidelines for preventing healthcare-associated infections in NHS hospitals in England'. *Journal of Hospital Infection*, 65(Suppl.): S1–S64

Resuscitation Council (2005) 'In-hospital resuscitation'. In *Adult advanced life support*. London: Resuscitation Council (UK)

Royal College of Anaesthetists (2004a) 'Guidance on the provision of anaesthetic services for pre-operative care'. *Guidelines for the provision of anaesthetic services*. London: RCA

Royal College of Anaesthetists (2004b) 'Guidance on the provision of anaesthetic services for post-operative care'. *Guidelines for the provision of anaesthetic services*. London: RCA

Sewell, A. and Young, P. (2003) 'Recovery and post-anaesthetic care'. *Anaesthesia and Intensive Care Medicine*, 4(10): 329–32

Smith, A.F. (2004) 'Preoperative fasting in adults', cited in Royal College of Anaesthetists (2004) *Raising the standard: a compendium of audit*. London: RCA

Smith, G. (2000) *Acute life-threatening events recognition and treatment (ALERT)*. Open Learning Centre, University of Portsmouth

Tramer, M.R. (2003) 'Treatment of postoperative nausea and vomiting'. *British Medical Journal*, 327: 762–3

Van Wijk, M.G.E. and Smallbout, B.A. (1990) 'Postoperative analysis of the patients' view of anaesthesia in a Netherlands teaching hospital'. Cited in Tramer, M.R. (2003) 'Treatment of postoperative nausea and vomiting'. *British Medical Journal*, 327: 762–3

Weetman, C. and Allison, W. (2006) 'Use of epidural analgesia in post-operative pain management'. *Nursing Standard*, 20(44): 54–64

Young, G. and Purdy, R. (2006), cited in Sheppard, M. and Wright, M. (2006) *Principles and practice of high dependency nursing*. London: Ballière Tindal

Chapter 21

SPECIMEN COLLECTION AND INFECTION CONTROL

Sue Quayle

The Nursing and Midwifery Council (2007) has set standards to measure your performance in taking specimens. The Essential Skills Clusters (ESCs) covered are:

Patients/clients can trust a newly registered nurse to:

Section 3	Treat people with dignity and respect them as individuals.
Section 6	Listen and provide information which is clear, accurate and meaningful.
Section 8	Ensure that consent will be sought prior to care or treatment being given and that their rights will be respected.
Section 9[xi]	Perform routine diagnostic tests under supervision.
Section 10[v]	Detect, report and respond appropriately to signs of deterioration and or improvement.
Section 22	Maintain effective standard infection control precautions.

Introduction

The purpose of this chapter is to introduce you to the practice of taking specimens. Taking specimens is an important and common part of nursing. This chapter will cover urinalysis using a reagent strip, mid-stream and catheter specimens of urine. It will also include the taking of sputum and stool specimens. This chapter begins with a brief introduction to infection control that applies to all procedures in this book, as well as to the procedures in this chapter.

Infection control

It is very important that standard infection control precautions are a priority with all procedures in this book. Health care associated infections (HCAIs) cost the National Health Service about £1 billion a year and cause at least 5000 deaths (National Patient Safety Agency, 2004). While the economic cost is high, the emotional cost to patients and their families and friends cannot be counted. It is vital that the risk of the spread of infection is reduced as much as possible. The NMC Skills

Cluster Section 22 states that it is important to use effective hand hygiene and the appropriate standard infection control precautions when caring for all patient/clients. Standard infection control precautions mean treating all blood and body fluids as a risk, whether or not any infection is known to be present.

The maintenance of infection control involves following national and local guidelines. *The Health Act: code of practice for the prevention and control of hospital acquired infections* (DoH, 2006b) states that all NHS bodies must have policies in place for standard infection control precautions. It is therefore important that you check your own Trust's infection control policy. Induction and training programmes should also be in place for all staff (DoH, 2006).

The Department of Health has set specific targets for the reduction in the rate of infection within hospitals. They have linked the evidence base for clinical processes with simple methods to ensure that quality health care is delivered (DoH, 2006).

Standard infection control precautions

The standard infection control precautions are summarised in Table 1.

Food hygiene	Staff hygiene	Asepsis	Personal protective equipment
Hand hygiene	Decontamination of equipment	Safe disposal of waste	Body fluid spillage
Safe management of linen	Safe use of sharps	Specimen handling	

Table 1
Standard infection control precautions

Hand hygiene

Hand washing by health care staff is vitally important in the control of infection (DoH, 2003). The Department of Health has set out very clear guidelines for washing hands in an effective manner. These are as follows.

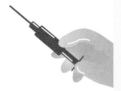

1. Staff should always clean their hands before and after each care activity using the correct hand hygiene procedure.

2. Hands should be wet first under running water.

3. Hand wash solution is then applied (see Figure 1):

   – using hand wash solution clean the hands palm to palm;

   – right palm over left dorsum and left palm over right dorsum;

   – interlace palm to palm with fingers;

   – interlock backs of fingers to opposing palms;

   – rub right thumb with left thumb, rub left fingers in right palm and vice versa.

4. Rinse thoroughly.

5. Dry hands thoroughly.

Figure 1
Hand washing
procedure

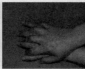

Hand rubs

Evidence has shown that many members of staff find that:

❑ they are too busy to wash their hands properly;

❑ there are not enough sinks in the ward area;

❑ there may not be enough hand rubs; or

❑ they may suffer skin problems from the soaps.

As a result of this most Trusts supply staff with their own hand rubs that they can carry around with them. Hand rubs may also be placed on beds or lockers. These are alcohol based. Alcohol rub may be used if the hands are socially clean as the alcohol reduces the microbial count on clean hands (National Patient Safety Agency, 2004). It is important that you find out which microbes may be reduced by the hand gel supplied to your Trust as the gel may not be effective against some organisms. There is much research in this area and, as a nurse, it is important that you check on a regular basis for any new evidence that may be published. Figure 2 shows the routines for hand washing and for using a hand rub.

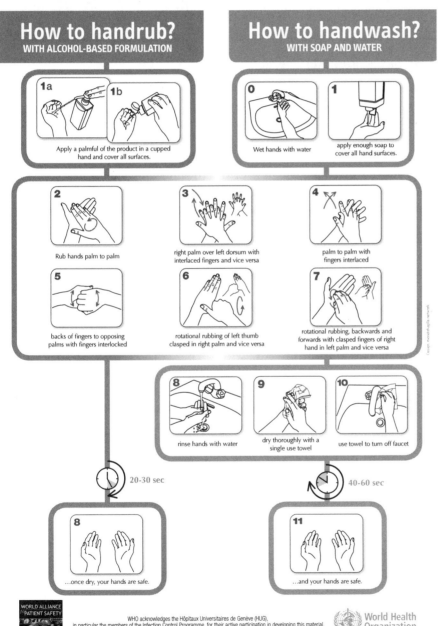

Figure 2 Hand washing and using hand rubs (reproduced with permission from the World Health Organisation).

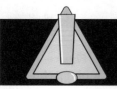

With any patient who has Clostridium Difficile, hands should be washed with soap and water before and after contact with each patient. Disposable gloves and apron should always be worn when handling body fluids.

Areas missed when washing hands

It is very easy to miss out areas when washing your hands. When assessing hand washing techniques I find that one of the most common areas missed are the cuticles. Even with a lot of scrubbing this is still a problem area. When wearing false nails bacteria can harbour very easily by the nail bed. For this reason, false nails should not be worn. Other areas easily missed are the base of the thumbs and the back of the hands. In addition, it is important to ensure that the wrists are clean. For this reason wrist watches should not be worn.

Personal protective equipment (PPE)

If you are at risk of exposure to blood or body fluids it is important that you wear personal protective equipment. This includes gloves, aprons, masks, goggles or visors. Gloves and aprons should be single-use items (Department of Health, 2006b) as this reduces the risk of cross-infection. They will also need to be properly disposed of after use. This means that you will need to find out about the correct way to dispose of contaminated waste in your clinical area.

Gloves

When you have been wearing gloves it is important to wash your hands after you take them off. Bacteria can contaminate the hands through small defects in the gloves or during glove removal (Boyce, 2002, cited in Flores, 2006).

Aprons

While hand hygiene is recognised as the most important factor for the prevention of cross-infection, contact transfer of bacteria from uniforms is also a problem (RCN, online 2007). Plastic aprons must be worn when assisting patients with toileting, bathing or with any activities that may result in the dispersal of pathogens. Plastic aprons should also be worn with procedures causing the splashing of blood or bodily fluids (RCN, online 2007).

Personal hygiene

The Royal College of Nursing (RCN) has developed the 'Wipe It Out' campaign. This gives guidelines on personal hygiene, which involves wearing a clean uniform daily, avoiding wearing a uniform outside the clinical area, not wearing jewellery and wrist watches, keeping nails short and polish free, and wearing hair neat and tidy off the collar.

Safe disposal of sharps

When taking some specimens, such as a catheter specimen of urine, sharps will be used. There will also be many other occasions in your nursing career when you will use sharps. The Department of Health has created specific guidelines on the safe disposal of sharps:

❑ A sharps container should be available at the point of use.

❑ Whoever uses the sharps must dispose of the sharps themselves.

❑ Staff should not remove the needle from the syringe before disposing of them in the sharps container.

❑ Needles should never be re-sheathed.

❑ Sharps should never be passed from hand to hand.

❑ Sharps containers should not be overfilled.

(Department of Health, 2006b)

A clean and safe technique

Aseptic technique, or aseptic non-touch technique (ANTT), should be used when taking some specimens. Non-touch technique involves the identification of key parts of the equipment that must remain uncontaminated. For example, this could be between the tip of a syringe and the needle. If you are unable to do the procedure without touching key parts then a dressing pack should be used. If you are able to do the procedure without touching the key parts as in, for example, a catheter specimen of urine, then gloves should be worn. It is important to check your local Trust policy, as wards with patients who are immunosuppressed or have immature immune systems may require *sterile* gloves to be used.

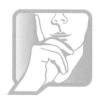

Reflection

Look at the clinical area you are currently working in and consider the ways in which you might possibly contaminate a patient with bacteria from another patient or from yourself. Then consider how you would prevent this from happening.

Specimen collection

Returning to the patient in the scenario, we find that, 24 hours following admission to the surgical ward, Teresa complains of feeling generally unwell. On closer examination Teresa is hot to touch, clammy and perspiring and has a body temperature of 38°C. In view of these findings routine specimens for urine, sputum and stool are requested.

Sepsis

Sepsis is a common problem and is often not recognised until too late. This is due partly to the growing use of invasive procedures as well as to the increasing numbers of patients who are at high risk of infection like, for example, those on chemotherapy, the elderly and those living with HIV infection. The 'Surviving Sepsis' campaign has been organised to improve the management, diagnosis and treatment of sepsis. For more details, see the website at **www.survivingsepsis.org**. Guidelines have been developed to ensure that diagnosis and, therefore, the management and treatment of sepsis is prompt.

Sepsis screening tools

Many hospitals have developed the use of the severe sepsis screening tool. A patient may be suspected of having an infection if they have:

❏ a temperature of 38.3°C or over, or less than 35°C;

❏ a heart rate of over 90 beats per minute;

❏ a respiratory rate of over 20 a minute;

❏ a systolic blood pressure of under 90 mm/hg;

❏ chills, rigors or headache with neck stiffness;

❏ a high white blood cell count.

The doctor will want to determine if there is an infection present and where this infection may be coming from. Therefore, specimens will need to be taken. Cultures may also determine antibiotic sensitivity.

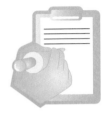

Activity 1.

Review sepsis, its disease process, recognition and appropriate interventions.

Taking specimens

When taking specimens it is important to remember a few basics. Any specimen must be labelled correctly. This usually means it is labelled with:

❏ the patient's name;

❏ the date of birth;

❏ the hospital number;

❏ the ward and/or doctor;

❏ the date of collection; and

❏ often the time of collection is required as well, especially if it is a repeated specimen.

The specimen needs to be accompanied by a request form that has the following information written on it:

❏ a name;

❏ date of birth;

❏ hospital number;

❏ ward and/or doctor;

❑ often a diagnosis or list of symptoms;

❑ date of collection and often the time as well.

All writing on the form should be legible and accompanied by a signature if required.

When collecting specimens it is very important to think of the principles of infection control. This means ensuring that:

❑ there is no contamination to the outside of the container or on the request forms;

❑ specimens are sent to the laboratory as quickly as possible;

❑ gloves and aprons should be worn as appropriate and discarded in the appropriate bins;

❑ hands should be washed before and after each specimen collection;

❑ any sharps used are disposed of immediately at the point of contact into the correct container.

Once specimens have been taken it is important to document this. Any abnormalities must be noted and, if required, reported to the doctor. Once the results are available check them, report any abnormalities and document them.

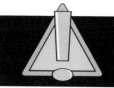

I have seen many specimens thrown away because they have not been labelled and it is impossible to identify them. Also, labelling them with the wrong patient's details is extremely dangerous.

Consent

Consent should be sought before taking any specimens. Information about what is being taken, the reasons why and the way it will be done should be given to the patient in a clear accurate and meaningful way. It is also important to respect the patient's privacy and dignity throughout the process of specimen collection. Many people find it embarrassing to have someone handle specimens taken from them. This should be taken into account with all specimen collection and the patient's dignity maintained at all times.

Urine

Urine is the waste product produced by the kidneys. It is often tested as it gives us an indication of the physical status of the patient. By testing the urine it is possible to detect diseases such as diabetes, liver disease, kidney disease, billiary disease, bleeding from the urinary tract, infections, problems causing high protein levels such as heart failure and hypertension (both in the pregnant person and the non-pregnant). It can also show the presence of malignant tumours. Testing the urine can give a baseline observation and can also be used as a monitoring tool.

Urinalysis is the testing of the physical characteristics and composition of freshly voided urine. Obtaining a urinalysis is a good time to assess the urine to see if it is cloudy or clear, to see if it has an offensive smell and to see what colour it is. Reagent strips should be available and these test for:

❑ leukocytes;

❑ nitrates;

❑ protein;

❑ glucose;

❑ ketones;

❑ uribilinogen;

❑ bilirubin;

❑ blood;

❑ pH.

Urinalysis

Hands should be washed before and after a urinalysis. Gloves and an apron should be worn. Eight simple steps can be used.

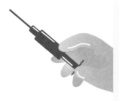

Urinalysis

1. Wash hands, put on gloves and an apron.

2. Use fresh, room temperature urine.

3. Using a reagent strip, dip it into the urine for about one second so that all the areas are moistened.

4. Wipe the edge of the strip on the container to remove excess urine.

5. Take care to avoid urine running from square to square.

6. Wait 60 seconds (depending on the brand of strip) and compare the reaction colours with the colours on the test label. After 120 seconds (depending on the brand of strip), test the colour against the leukocyte label.

7. Dispose of gloves and apron and wash hands.

8. Document and report findings.

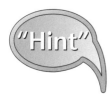

"Hint"

To prevent urine running from one square to another, which may give a false result, try and hold the reagent strip at an angle.

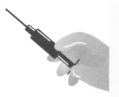

Midstream specimen of urine

A midstream specimen of urine is collected to send to the laboratory for testing for micro-organisms. If micro-organisms are detected the laboratory will also determine which antibiotics the organisms are sensitive to.

1. The patient is encouraged to go to the toilet with a specimen container and some clean wipes.

2. A woman should be encouraged to wipe from front to back (clean to dirty) before passing a small amount of urine.

3. The container is then held underneath the flow of urine and the specimen collected. It does not take much imagination to realise that one needs to be quite dexterous to accomplish this task!

4. If the patient is able to control their flow of urine this makes it easier.

5. It is very easy to contaminate the outside of the pot with this procedure so care must be taken and gloves worn when touching the container.

6. Hands should be washed before and afterwards.

A catheter specimen of urine

Urinary catheterisation is the insertion of a special tube into the bladder. Patients may be catheterised for many reasons. As the bladder is a sterile area catheterisation and any washing out, urine sampling and removal is done as an aseptic procedure as the risk of infection is very high. It is important to ensure that there is no potential for infection to reach the bladder. Catheterisation should therefore only be done by trained and competent staff using strictly aseptic techniques (Department of Health, 2003).

Specimens of urine may be taken from the catheter tubing and sent to the laboratory for testing. As the specimen is taken from the tubing it is important that there is no risk of contamination to the tubing that may then enter the bladder. The specimen must be taken from a fresh sample of urine coming down the tube, not from the clamp at the bottom of the bag where it may have been sitting for a while. Remember that many people will find having a catheter embarrassing and would not like friends or relatives to see it. It is important to maintain their dignity and privacy.

A catheter specimen of urine

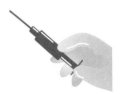

1. Wash hands and put on gloves and an apron.

2. Ensure that there is sufficient urine in the catheter tubing. If there is not enough urine in the tube, clamp the tubing below the access port until there is sufficient.

3. Clean the access point to the catheter with a 70 per cent isopropyl alcohol swab or other appropriate cleaning material.

4. Take a sterile needle and syringe. Use the aseptic non-touch technique to connect the needle onto the end of the syringe.

5. Insert the needle into the access point at a 45° angle to prevent the needle going straight through the tubing and withdraw the required amount of urine. (Some tubing may provide an access point which does not require a needle.)

6. Any sharps used will need to be disposed of immediately in the sharps container.

7. Re-clean the access point with a 70 per cent isopropyl alcohol swab or other appropriate cleaning material.

8. Place the urine into a sterile container. Be careful to do this gently to avoid splashing or spillage.

9. Send to the laboratory with the appropriate documentation.

10. Document the action taken in the patient's notes and record any abnormalities.

11. Remove gloves and apron. Wash hands.

(Procedure adapted from Dougherty and Lister, 2004, p.341.)

Taking a stool specimen

While the thought of taking a stool sample may seem pretty awful, taking and analysing a patient's stool specimen can give a good indication as to the health of the patient. It can show things such as blood, fats, bacteria, virus and even parasites which may be living in the gut. Remember that it is important to be sensitive to the patient's needs at this time.

Stool specimen

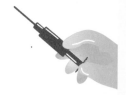

1. Hands should be washed and gloves and an apron worn before handling any faecal specimens.

2. The patient will need to defecate in a clean container of some sort.

3. The specimen may be tested for occult blood (FOBs) on the ward using occult blood testing packs. To do this it is best to follow the manufacturer's instructions.

4. Otherwise, the stool is sent to the laboratory for testing with the appropriate documentation.

5. Gloves and apron should be removed and disposed of correctly. Hands should be washed afterwards.

> *If you are using a bed pan it is important not to contaminate the stool with urine, menstrual product or toilet paper.*

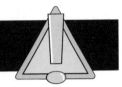

Taking a sputum sample

Sputum is produced by the lungs, usually in response to infection, and it should not be confused with saliva. Testing sputum can reveal infection and can help to identify which antibiotics can be given to the patient.

Sputum sample

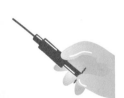

1. Encourage the patient to sit up, if possible, and to breathe deeply.

2. The patient should be encouraged to cough up any secretions. If you find it difficult to obtain a sputum sample, a physiotherapist is proficient in this and may be able to offer you some assistance.

3. Ensure that the patient coughs directly into the sputum container.

4. To prevent the spread of infection, cover the container as quickly as possible.

5. Note the colour and amount of sputum, and whether it has come from the nose, sinuses or chest. Document this in the patient's notes.

6. Send the sample to the laboratory with the appropriate documentation.

7. Wear gloves when touching the container. Hands should be washed afterwards.

Scenario review

Teresa starts to feel better quite quickly and the rest of her recovery remains quite uneventful. Routine screening of her specimens was inconclusive, with no abnormalities detected (NAD). Ten days following admission to the assessment unit, Teresa was discharged home.

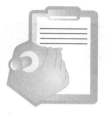

Activity 2.

Review and refresh your knowledge of and skills for the specimen collections required and identify those factors that will aid in diagnosis.

Summary

In this chapter you have seen the importance of specimen collection. You should have a sound knowledge of how to take:

❏ a urinalysis;

❏ a midstream specimen of urine;

❏ a catheter specimen of urine;

❏ a stool specimen;

❏ a sputum specimen.

You will have learnt the importance of obtaining a specimen correctly and of ensuring that the correct documentation accompanies it. You will have learnt to report any abnormalities and document these accurately. You will also have seen the importance of following infection control procedures to prevent contamination to yourself and also cross-contamination to other patients and staff.

References

Department of Health (2003) *Winning ways: working together to reduce health care associated infection in England.* London: HMSO

Department of Health (2006a) *Essential steps to safe clean care.* Online at: **www.dh.gov.uk/en/Publicationsandstatistics/Publications/PublicationsPolicyAnd Guidance/DH_4136212** (last accessed 22 May 2007)

Department of Health (2006b) *The Health Act: code of practice for the prevention and control of health care associated infections.* London: HMSO

Flores, A. (2006) 'Appropriate glove use in the prevention of cross infection'. *Nursing Standard*, 21(5): 45–8

Kozier, B., Erb, G., Berman, A. and Snyder, S. (2002) *Kozier and Erb's techniques in clinical nursing: basic to intermediate skills.* Englewood Cliffs, NJ: Pearson/Prentice Hall

National Patient Safety Agency (2004) *Ready, steady, go! The full guide to implementing the CleanYourHands campaign in your trust.* Online at: **www.npsa.nhs.uk**

Royal Marsden Hospital (2004) *Manual of clinical nursing procedures*, 6th edn. Oxford: Blackwell

Websites

www.rcn.org.uk – Royal College of Nursing (last accessed 22 May 2007)

www.survivingsepsis.org – the 'Surviving Sepsis' campaign is an initiative of the European Society of Intensive Care Medicine, the International Sepsis Forum and the Society of Critical Care Medicine

Appendix: Essential Skills Clusters (ESCs) for Pre-registration Nursing Programmes

This document should be read in association with NMC Circular 07/2007 that provides supporting information.

The term patient/client is used throughout and includes service users and, where appropriate, significant others (including parents/carers).

This document has been reproduced here with permission from the Nursing and Midwifery Council.

Key:

❑ **Standard** (e.g. 3, 4b, 7d, 8f) relates to respective outcomes and proficiencies within the *Standards of proficiency for pre-registration nursing education* (NMC, 2004). See Annexe 3 for codes.

❑ **Code** (e.g. 1.1, 1.2, 1.3, 7.1) relates to the *Code of professional conduct: standards for conduct, performance and ethics* (NMC, 2004).

❑ *** Items requiring numerical assessment (9, 27, 28, 29, 31, 32, 33, 36, 38).**

❑ **Items requiring specific assessment (25 and 42).**

Summative health-related numerical assessments are required to test skills identified (*) within the ESCs that encompass baseline assessment and calculations associated with medicines, nutrition, fluids and other areas requiring the use of numbers relevant to the field of practice:

❑ For entry to the branch, programme providers will use the ESCs to inform the nature and content of the assessment, including whether to assess through simulation. They will determine their own pass mark and number of attempts.

❑ For entry to the register, programme providers will use the ESCs to inform the nature and content of numerical assessment in the branch programme where a 100% pass mark is required and all assessment must take place in the practice setting. The number of attempts is to be determined by the education provider.

Care, Compassion and Communication

Patients/clients can trust a newly registered nurse to:	For entry to branch	For entry to the register
1 Provide care based on the highest standards, knowledge and competence.	i. Demonstrates the underpinning values of the NMC code of professional conduct: standards for conduct, performance and ethics ii. Works within limitations of the role and recognises own level of competence iii. Promotes a professional image iv. Shows respect for others v. Is able to engage patients/clients and build caring professional relationships vi. Forms appropriate and constructive professional relationships with families and other carers vii. Uses professional support structures to learn from experience and makes appropriate adjustments Standard: 7, 1a, b, c, d, e, f, 2d, 4a, d, 7d, 16d Code: 1.1, 1.2, 13, 7.1	viii. Demonstrates clinical confidence through sound knowledge, skills and understanding relevant to branch ix. Is self-aware and self-confident, knows own limitations and is able to take appropriate action x. Acts as a role model in promoting a professional image xi. Acts as a role model in developing trusting relationships, within professional boundaries xii. Recognises and acts to overcome barriers in developing effective relationships with patients/clients xiii. Initiates, maintains and closes professional relationships with patients/clients and carers xiv. Uses professional support structures to develop self-awareness, challenge own prejudices and enable professional relationships, so that care is delivered without compromise Standard: 7, A1, 2, 3, 4, 5, 6, C4, K1, P3 Code: 1.2, 1.3, 2.3, 6.1
2 Engage them as partners in care. Should they be unable to meet their own needs then the nurse will ensure that these are addressed in accordance with the known wishes of the patient/client or in their best interests.	i. Actively involves the patient/client in their assessment and care planning ii. Determines patient/client preferences to maximise comfort & dignity iii. Actively encourages patient/client to be involved in, and/or ensures they are supported in own care/self-care iv. Supports patient/client to identify their goals	vii. Is sensitive to patient/client needs, choice and capability and appropriately incorporates this into planned care viii. Supports access to independent advocacy ix. Recognises situations and acts appropriately when patient/client choice may compromise safety x. Uses strategies to manage situations where the patients'/clients' wishes conflict with planned care

	v. Assesses patient's/client's level of capability for self-care	xi. Acts to ensure that patients/clients who are unable to meet their activities of living have these addressed in a sensitive and dignified manner and a record is kept in relation how these needs are met, e.g. bathing, elimination, care of the skin, nails, hair, eyes, teeth and mouth
	vi. Provides care (or makes provisions) for those who are unable to maintain own personal care (e.g. mouth care, elimination, bathing, care of skin, cleaning teeth, hair washing, cleaning eyes and cleaning and cutting nails)	xii. Works confidently, collaboratively and in partnership with patients/clients, their families and other carers to ensure that needs are met in care planning and delivery, including strategies for self-care and peer support
		xiii. Helps the patient/client to identify and use their strengths to achieve their goals and aspirations
	Standard: 7a, b, c, 8f	Standard: C3, D1, E1, G1, 2, 3,
	Code: 2.1, 4.1, 4.2	Code: 2.1, 3.1, 3.2, 4.4
3 Treat them with dignity and respect them as individuals.	i. Takes a person-centred approach to care	vii. Acts professionally to ensure that personal judgements, prejudices, values, attitudes and beliefs do not compromise the care provided
	ii. Demonstrates respect for diversity and individual patient/client preference, regardless of personal view	viii. Is proactive in promoting and maintaining dignity
	iii. Applies the concept of dignity	ix. Challenges situations/others when patient/client dignity may be compromised
	iv. Delivers care with dignity making appropriate use of the environment, self, skills and attitude	x. Uses appropriate strategies to encourage and promote patient/client choice
	v. Identifies factors that influence and maintain patient/client dignity	Standard: C4, E3, J1
	vi. Acts in a way that demonstrates respect for others promoting and valuing differences	Code: 1.4, 2.1, 2.2
	Standard: 3, 4b, 7d, 8f, 9	
	Code: 2.2, 2.3, 2.4	

Care, Compassion and Communication

Patients/clients can trust a newly registered nurse to:	For entry to branch	For entry to the register
4 Care for them in an environment and manner that is culturally competent and free from discrimination, harassment and exploitation.	i. Demonstrates an understanding of how culture, religion, spiritual beliefs, gender and sexuality can impact on illness and disability	iv. Delivers care that is culturally competent and free from discrimination, harassment and exploitation
	ii. Respects people's rights	v. Upholds patients'/clients' legal rights and speaks out when these are at risk of being compromised
	iii. Adopts a principled approach to care underpinned by the *NMC code of professional conduct: standards for conduct, performance and ethics*	vi. Takes into account differing cultural traditions, beliefs, UK legal frameworks and professional ethics when planning care
		vii. Is proactive in promoting care environments that are culturally sensitive and free from discrimination, harassment and exploitation
	Standard: 1e, 2d, e, 3a, 9	viii. Manages challenging situations effectively
	Code: 2.3, 2.4, 2.5, 3.1, 3.2	Standard: B1, 4, C1, 2, 3, 4, K2, 3, 4
		Code: 2.1, 2.2, 3.2, 8.1
5 Provide care that is delivered in a warm, sensitive and compassionate way.	i. Is attentive and acts with kindness and sensitivity	vi. Anticipates how the patient/client might feel in a given situation and responds with kindness and empathy to provide physical and emotional comfort
	ii. Takes into account a patient's/client's physical and emotional responses when carrying out care	vii. Makes appropriate use of touch
	iii. Delivers care in a manner that is interpreted by the patient/client as warm, sensitive, kind and compassionate	viii. Listens to, watches for, and responds to verbal and non-verbal cues
	iv. Delivers care that addresses both physical and emotional needs and preferences	ix. Delivers care that recognises need and provides both practical and emotional support
	v. Evaluates ways in which own interactions affect relationships to ensure that they do not impact inappropriately on others	x. Has insight into own values and how these may impact on patient/client interactions

Care, Compassion and Communication	For entry to branch	For entry to the register
Patients/clients can trust a newly registered nurse to:		
6 Listen, and provide information that is clear, accurate and meaningful at a level at which the patient/client can understand.	i. Communicates effectively both orally and in writing, so that the meaning is always clear	vii. Consistently shows ability to communicate safely and effectively with patients/clients providing guidance for juniors
	ii. Uses strategies to enhance communication and remove barriers to effective communication	viii. Communicates effectively and sensitively in different settings, using a range of methods and styles
	iii. Records information accurately and clearly on the basis of observation and communication	ix. Provides accurate and comprehensive written and verbal reports based on best available evidence
	iv. Always seeks to confirm understanding	x. Acts to reduce and challenge barriers to effective communication and understanding
	v. Responds in a way that confirms what the patient/client is communicating	xi. Is proactive and creative in enhancing communication and understanding
	vi. Effectively communicates the patient's/client's stated needs/wishes to other professionals	xii. Where appropriate uses the skills of active listening, questioning, paraphrasing and reflection to support a therapeutic intervention
Standard: 3b, c, 4b, d	Standard: 4a, c, 6b, 7c, d, 9, 10c	xiii. Uses appropriate and relevant communication skills to deal with difficult and challenging circumstances (e.g. responding to emergencies, unexpected occurrences, saying 'no', dealing with complaints, resolving disputes, de-escalating aggression, conveying 'unwelcome news')
Code: 1.4, 2.3, 7.1	Code: 2.1, 4.3, 4.4	Standard: C4, D1, E1, 2, F1, 3, G3, H4, J1, K2, M1, N1, 2, Q2, 3
		Code: 2.2, 3.2, 4.3, 4.4, 6.1

xi. Recognises circumstances that trigger personal negative responses and takes action to prevent this compromising of care

xii. Recognises and responds to emotional discomfort/distress in self and others

xiii. Through reflection and evaluation demonstrates commitment to personal and professional development

Standard: A2, B5, C3, 4, D1, D1, E2, H4, P2, 3

Code: 2.3, 2.5, 6.1

Care, Compassion and Communication

Patients/clients can trust a newly registered nurse to:	For entry to branch	For entry to the register
7 Protect and treat as confidential all information relating to themselves and their care.	i. Applies the principles of confidentiality	v. Acts professionally and appropriately in situations where there may be limits to confidentiality (e.g. public interest, protection from harm)
	ii. Protects and treats information as confidential except where sharing information is required for the purposes of safeguarding and/or public protection	vi. Recognises the significance of information and who does/does not need to know
	iii. Applies the principles of data protection	vii. Acts appropriately in sharing information to enable and enhance care (carers, MDT and across agency boundaries)
	iv. Distinguishes between information that is relevant to care planning and information that is not	viii. Works within the legal frameworks for data protection (e.g. access to and storage of records)
		ix. Acts within the law when confidence has to be broken
	Standard: 1e, 2a, b, d	Standard: A4, B1, 2, 3, 4, D2, G1, K2, 3, 4, M1, 2, 3, P4
	Code: 3.1, 3.2, 5.1, 5.3	Code: 1.2, 3.2, 3.3, 5.1, 5.2, 5.3
8 Ensure that their consent will be sought prior to care or treatment being given and that their rights will be respected.	i. Applies principles of consent in relation to restrictions relating to specific client groups and seeks consent for care	iv. Uses appropriate strategies to enable patients/clients to understand treatments and other interventions in order to give informed consent
	ii. Ensures that the meaning of consent to treatment and care is understood by the patient/client	v. Works within legal frameworks when seeking consent
	iii. Seeks consent prior to sharing confidential information outside of the professional care team (subject to agreed safeguarding protection procedures	vi. Assesses the needs and wishes of carers and / or relatives in relation to information and consent
	Standard: 1e, 2a, b, d	vii. Demonstrates respect for patient/client autonomy and their right to withhold consent in relation to treatment within legal frameworks (safeguarding/protection procedures)
	Code: 3.1, 3.2, 3.3, 5.1, 5.3	Standard: A1, B1, C2, 3, E2, K2, 3, 4, P4
		Code: 3.1, 3.2, 5.3, 5.4

Organisational Aspects of Care

Patients/clients can trust a newly registered nurse to:	For entry to branch	For entry to the register
9 Make a holistic and systematic assessment of their needs and develop a comprehensive plan of nursing care that is in their best interests and which promotes their health and well-being and minimises the risk of harm.	i. Contributes to the assessment of physical, emotional, psychological, social, cultural and spiritual needs, including risk factors by identifying, recording, sharing and responding to clear indicators and signs	xiii. Makes a holistic and systematic assessment of physical, emotional, psychological, social, cultural and spiritual needs, including risk, and creates a comprehensive plan of nursing care in partnership with the patient/client, carer, family or friends
	ii. Accurately undertakes and records a baseline assessment of weight, height, temperature, pulse, respiration and blood pressure *	xiv. Takes responsibility for assessment and planning of care delivery
	iii. Contributes to the planning of safe and effective care by recording and sharing information based on the assessment	xv. Applies evidence to practice
	iv. Where relevant, applies knowledge of age and condition-related anatomy, physiology and development when interacting with patients/clients	xvi. Works within the context of a multi-professional team to enhance the care of patients/clients
	v. Understands the benefits of a healthy lifestyle and the potential risks involved with various lifestyles or behaviours	xvii. Promotes health and well-being through teaching patients/clients and carers about their condition and treatment
	vi. Recognises indicators of unhealthy lifestyles	xviii. Uses a range of techniques to discuss treatment options with patients/clients
	vii. Contributes to care based on an understanding of how illness and disability impact on patients/clients and carers at different stages	xix. Enables patients/clients to take an active role in making choices concerning their care
	viii. Makes constructive and appropriate relationships with patients/clients and their carers	xx. Discusses sensitive issues and provides appropriate advice and guidance, e.g. contraception, substance misuse, impact of lifestyle on health
	ix. Measures and documents vital signs under supervision and responds appropriately to findings outside the normal range *	xxi. Refers to specialists when required
	x. When faced with sudden deterioration in patients'/clients' physical or psychological condition or emergency situations (e.g. abnormal vital signs,patient/client collapse, cardiac arrest, self harm, extremely challenging behaviour, attempted suicide) responds appropriately by seeking assistance from a senoir colleague	xxii. Acts appropriately when faced with sudden deterioration in patients'/clients' physical or psychological condition or emergency situations (e.g. abnormal vital signs, patient/client collapse, cardiac arrest, self-harm, extremely challenging behaviour, attempted suicide)
	xi. Performs routine, diagnostic tests (e.g. urinalysis) under supervision as part of assessment process (near patient/client testing)	xxiii. Measures, documents and interprets vital signs and acts appropriately on findings
	xii. Collects and interprets data, under supervision, related to the assessment and planning of care from a variety of sources	xxiv. Performs routine diagnostic tests(e.g. urinalysis) relevant to the area of work and acts appropriately on findings
		xxv. Works within a public health framework to groups
	Standard: 1c, 4d, 6a, c, 7a, c, 8b, c, f, 8, 10c, 11a, b, c	Standard: A3, 4, 6, C3, 4, E1, 2, 3, 4, F2, 3, G3, H1, 2, 5, 6, J1, 2, K1, 2, 3, 4, M1, 2, 3, Q1, 2, 3
	Code: 2.1, 2.3, 2.4, 3.1, 3.2, 6.1	Code: 1.2, 1.4, 2.1, 2.4, 3.1, 4.3, 4.4, 6.5, 8.1

Organisational Aspects of Care Patients/clients can trust a newly registered nurse to:	For entry to branch	For entry to the register
10 Deliver and evaluate care against the comprehensive assessment and care plan.	i. Works collaboratively with patients/clients and their carers enabling them to take an active role in the delivery and evaluation of their care	vi. Provides safe and effective care in the context of patients'/clients' age, condition and developmental stage
	ii. Works within the limitations of own knowledge and skills to question and provide safe and holistic care for patient/client group	vii. Prioritises the needs of groups of patients/clients and individuals in order to deliver care effectively and efficiently
	iii. Prepares patients/clients for clinical interventions as per local policy	viii. Detects, records and reports deterioration/improvement and takes appropriate action
	iv. Actively seeks to extend knowledge and skills using a variety of methods in order to enhance care delivery	ix. Implements strategies for evaluating the effect of interventions, taking account of the patients'/clients'/carers' interpretation of physical, emotional and behavioural changes.
	v. Detects, records, reports and responds appropriately to signs of deterioration and/or improvement	x. Reviews and makes adjustments to the care plan in response to evaluation, communicating these changes to colleagues
	Standard: 7a, c, 10a, 16a, b, c	Standard: A4, E2, 3, F3, G1, 3, J1, 2, L1, M3
	Code: 2.1, 4.3, 6.1, 6.3	Code: 2.1, 4.3, 6.1
11 Act to safeguard children and adults requiring support and protection.	i. Acts within legal frameworks and local policies in relation to the protection of vulnerable adults and children	v. Recognises and responds appropriately when people are vulnerable, at risk or in need of support and protection
	ii. Shares information with colleagues and seeks advice from appropriate sources where there is a concern or uncertainty	vi. Shares information safely with colleagues and across agency boundaries for the protection of individuals/the public
	iii. Documents concerns and information about patients/clients which may be significant	vii. Makes effective referrals to safeguard and protect children and adults requiring support and protection
	iv. Uses support systems to recognise, manage and deal with own emotions	viii. Works collaboratively with other agencies to develop, implement and monitor strategies to safeguard and protect vulnerable individuals and groups
	Standard: 2e, 8f, 9, 10c, 11a, b, 12a, c	ix. Supports patients/clients in asserting their human rights

	For entry to branch	For entry to the register
	Code: 1.5, 5.4, 8.1, 8.2	x. Challenges practices which do not safeguard those requiring support and protection Standard: A2, 5, B2, 4, C2, E2, K4, L2, 4, 5, M2, O1 Code: 1.5, 3.9, 3.10, 5.4, 8.1

Organisational Aspects of Care

Patients/clients can trust a newly registered nurse to:	For entry to branch	For entry to the register
12 Respond appropriately to feedback from patients/clients, the public and a wide range of sources as a vehicle for learning and development.	i. Responds appropriately to compliments and comments ii. Responds appropriately when patients/clients want to complain, providing assistance and support iii. Uses supervision and other forms of reflective learning to make effective use of feedback iv. Takes feedback from colleagues, managers and other departments seriously and shares the messages and learning with other members of the team Standard: 10b, 11c, 13c Code: 1.2, 3.1, 4.3	v. Shares complaints, compliments and comments with the team in order to improve care vi. Responds appropriately and effectively to feedback vii. Supports patients/clients who wish to complain viii. As an individual and team member, actively seeks and learns from feedback to enhance care and own professional development ix. Works within legal frameworks and local policies to deal with complaints, compliments and concerns Standard: A4, 6, B1, 4, C2, D1, E2, H3, K2, 4, L5, M3, P1, 3, 4 Code: 1.5, 4.3, 6.1
13 Promote continuity when their care is to be transferred to another service or person.	i. Assists in preparing patients/clients and carers for transfer/transition through effective dialogue and the provision of accurate information ii. Reports issues and patients'/clients' concerns regarding the transfer/transition iii. Assists in the preparation of records and reports to facilitate safe and effective transfer Standard: 7d, 8f, 10b Code: 2.1, 4.3, 4.4, 6.1	iv. Works with colleagues in other services to ensure safe and effective transition between services v. Prepares patients/clients and their carers for the transition/transfer between services vi. Works in partnership with the patient/client to develop strategies for smooth transfer/transition and evaluates the outcome Standard: D1, 2, E2, F1, 2, 3, G3, H4, J1, 2, M1, 2, 3 Code: 2.1, 4.3, 5.1

Organisational Aspects of Care

Patients/clients can trust a newly registered nurse to:	For entry to branch	For entry to the register
14 Be confident in their own role within the multidisciplinary/multiagency team and to inspire confidence in others.	i. Works within the *NMC code of professional conduct: standards for conduct, performance and ethics*	vi. Appropriately consults and explores solutions and ideas with others to enhance care
	ii. Supports and assists others appropriately	vii. Appropriately challenges the practice of self and others across the multi-professional team
	iii. Values others' roles and responsibilities within the team and interacts appropriately	viii. Takes appropriate role within the team
	iv. Reflects on own practice and discusses issues with other members of the team to enhance learning	ix. Acts as an effective role model in decision-making, taking action and supporting more junior staff
	v. Communicates with colleagues verbally (face-to-face and by telephone) and in writing and electronically in a way that the meaning is clear, and checks that the communication has been fully understood	x. Works inter-professionally as a means of achieving optimum outcomes for patients/clients
	Standard: 1a, e, 4a, c, 6b, 7c, 10c, 13a, c	Standard: A4, 5, D4, G3, H6, K4, L2, 5, M1, 2, 3, N1, 2, 3, O4
	Code: 1.1, 4.1, 4.2, 4.3, 6.1	Code: 4.3, 4.4, 4.5, 8.1
15 Safely delegate care to others and to respond appropriately when a task is delegated to them.	i. Accepts delegated tasks and elements of care based on knowledge, skill and limitations of role	ii. Works within the requirements in the *NMC code of professional conduct: standards for conduct, performance a and ethics* in delegating care and when care is delegated to them
		iii. Takes responsibility and accountability when delegating care to others
	Standard: 1c, 8b, 11a, c	iv. Prepares, supports and supervises those to whom care has been delegated
	Code: 1.3, 1.4, 4.5, 4.6, 6.3	v. Recognises and addresses deficits in knowledge and/or skill in self and takes appropriate action
		Standard: A1, N1, 2, 3
		Code: 1.3, 4.6, 6.4

16 Safely lead, co-ordinate and manage care.	i. Inspires confidence and provides clear direction to others
	ii. Takes decisions and is able to answer for these decisions when required
	iii. Bases decisions on evidence and uses experience to guide decision-making
	iv. Acts as a positive role model for junior staff
	v. Manages time effectively
	vi. Negotiates with others in relation to balancing competing/conflicting priorities
	Standard: A4, D1, G1, 3, H1, 2, 6, I1, K1, 2, M2, N3
	Code: 1.3, 6.5
17 Work safely under pressure.	i. Contributes as a team member
	vi. Demonstrates good time management
	ii. Demonstrates professional commitment by working flexibly to meet service needs to enable quality care to be delivered
	vii. Prioritises own workload and manages the competing/conflicting priorities of the caseload, ward or department
	iii. Recognises when situations are becoming unsafe and reports appropriately
	viii. Appropriately reports concerns regarding staffing/skill mix
	iv. Understands and applies the importance of rest for effective practice
	ix. Recognises stress in others and provides appropriate support or guidance
	v. Uses supervision as a means of developing strategies for managing own stress and for working safely and effectively
	x. Enables others to identify and manage their stress
	Standard: 2e, 13c, 16d
	Standard: A6, B4, D1, G1, 3, I1, K1, 2, 3, 4, L2, 3, 4, 5, M2, N1, 2, 3,
	Code: 1.4, 4.1, 4.2, 4.3
	Code: 1.3, 6.4, 6.5, 8.1, 8.2

481

Organisational Aspects of Care Patients/clients can trust a newly registered nurse to:	For entry to branch	For entry to the register
18 Identify and safely manage risk in relation to the patient/client, the environment, self and others.	i. Under supervision, works within clinical governance frameworks and contributes to promote safety and positive risk-taking	vii. Reflects on and learns from patient safety incidents as individual and team member and contributes to team learning
	ii. Reports patient/client safety incidents to senior colleagues	viii. Participates in clinical audit to improve patient/client care
	iii. Under supervision assesses risk within current sphere of knowledge and competence	ix. Assesses and implements measures to manage, reduce or remove risk that could be detrimental to patients/clients, self and others
	iv. Follows instructions and takes appropriate action to minimise risk	x. Assesses, evaluates and interprets risk indicators and balances risks against benefits, taking account of the level of risk the patient/client, or others are prepared to take
	v. Under supervision works within legal frameworks for protecting self and others	xi. Works within legal frameworks to promote safety and positive risk-taking
	vi. Knows and accepts own responsibilities and takes appropriate action	xii. Works within policies to protect self and others
	Standard: 2e, 16a, b	xiii. Takes steps not to cross professional boundaries and put self or colleagues at risk
	Code: 1.5, 8.1, 8.2, 8.3	Standard: A4, 5, B1, 3, 4, D1, 2, E4, F1, 2, 3, H1, 2, 3, 4, 5, 6, K3, 4, L2, 3, 4, 5, M1, 3
		Code: 2.2, 2.3, 3.1, 3.2, 8.1, 8.2, 8.3
19 Work to resolve conflict and maintain a safe environment.	i. Recognises signs of aggression and responds appropriately to keep self and others safe	iii. Selects and applies appropriate strategies and techniques for defusing, disengaging and managing actual and potential violence and aggression
	ii. Assists others or obtains assistance when help is required	Standard: B4, D1, 2, F2, J2, K2, 3, L2, 5, O4, Q3
	Standard: 4c, e, 8f	Code: 1.4, 2.2, 2.3
	Code: 1.4, 2.3	

Organisational Aspects of Care

Patients/clients can trust a newly registered nurse to:	For entry to branch	For entry to the register
20 Select and manage medical devices safely.	i. Safely uses and disposes of medical devices under supervision	ii. Works within legal frameworks and applies evidence-based practice in the safe selection and use of medical devices
	Standard: 1g, 2a, c, d, e, 5c, 8f	iii. Safely uses and maintains a range of medical devices appropriate to the area of work, including ensuring regular servicing, maintenance and calibration
	Code: 1.5, 6.1	iv. Keeps appropriate records in relation to the use and maintenance of medical devices and the decontamination processes required as per local and national guidelines
		v. Explains the devices to patients/clients and/or carers and checks understanding
		Standard: E3, L1, 4, 5, P3
		Code: 1.5, 2.1, 6.1

Infection Prevention and Control

Patients/clients can trust a newly registered nurse to:	For entry to branch	For entry to the register
21 Be confident in using health promotion strategies, identifying infection risks and taking effective measures to prevent and control infection in accordance with local and national policy.	i. Participates in assessing and planning care appropriate to the patients'/clients' risk of infection	vi. Works within *NMC code of professional conduct: standards for conduct, performance and ethics* to meet responsibilities for prevention and control of infection
	ii. Participates in completing care documentation and evaluation of interventions to prevent and control infection	vii. Plans, delivers and documents care that demonstrates effective risk assessment, infection prevention and control
	iii. Aware of the role of the Infection Control Team and Infection Control Nurse Specialist, and local guidelines for referral	viii. Identifies, recognises and refers to the appropriate clinical expert
	iv. Recognises potential signs of infection and reports to relevant senior member of staff	ix. Explains risks to patients/clients, relatives, carers and colleagues
	v. Discusses the benefits of health promotion in the prevention and control of infection for improving and maintaining the health of the population	x. Recognises infection risk and reports and acts in situations where there is need for health promotion/protection
	Standard: 8f, 9, 11a, 13a	Standard: A1, 6, E2, 4, F3, H4, L1, 2, 4, 5, O1
	Code: 2.1, 2.2, 4.3, 4.4, 6.1	Code: 1.2, 2.1, 4.4, 6.3

Infection Prevention and Control

Patients/clients can trust a newly registered nurse to:	For entry to branch	For entry to the register
22 Maintain effective Standard Infection Control Precautions for every patient/client.	i. Applies knowledge of transmission routes in describing, recognising and reporting situations where there is a need for Standard Infection Control Precautions	viii. Initiates and maintains appropriate measures to prevent and control infection according to route of transmission of micro-organism, in order to protect patients/clients, members of the public and other staff
	ii. Demonstrates effective hand hygiene and the appropriate use of Standard Infection Control Precautions when caring for all patients/clients	ix. Applies legislation that relates to the management of specific infection risk at a local and national level
	iii. Follows local and national guidelines for Standard Infection Control Precautions	x. Adheres to infection prevention and control policies/procedures at all times and ensures colleagues also work according to good practice guidelines
	v. Participates in the cleaning of multi-use equipment between each patient/client	xi. Challenges the practice of other care workers who put themselves and / or others at risk of infection
	v. Uses multi-use patient/client equipment and follows the appropriate cleaning/disinfecting/decontamination protocol	Standard: A5, B1, H1, 2, 6, K3, L2, N3, Q2
	vi. Safely uses and disposes of, or decontaminates, items in accordance with local policy and manufacturers' guidance and instructions	Code: 6.1, 6.2, 8.1, 8.2
	vii. Adheres to requirements for cleaning, disinfecting, decontaminating of 'shared' nursing equipment (including single patient/client but multiuse equipment) before and after every use as appropriate, according to recognised risk, in accordance with manufacturers' and organisational policies	
	Standard: 2a, d, e, 5c, 8b, c, d	
	Code: 1.4, 4.5, 6.1, 6.5	

23 Provide effective care for patients/clients who have an infectious disease including, where required, the use of standard isolation techniques.	i. Safely delivers care under supervision to patients/clients who require to be nursed in isolation or in protective isolation settings	v. Recognises and acts upon the need to refer to specialist advisors as appropriate
	ii. Takes appropriate actions should exposure to infection occur, e.g. chicken pox, diarrhoea and vomiting, needle stick injury	vi. Assesses the needs of the infectious patient/client or cohort and applies appropriate isolation
	iii. Applies knowledge of an 'exposure prone procedure' and takes appropriate precautions/actions	vii. Ensures that patients/clients, relatives, carers and colleagues are aware of and adhere to local policies in relation to isolation and infection control procedures
	iv. If has a blood-borne virus, consults with occupational health before carrying out exposure-prone procedures	viii. Identifies suitable alternatives when isolation facilities are unavailable
	Standard: 1f, 2d, 4a, c, e, 5a, b, 8a, c, 9, 10c, 12a, b, c, 16a, b, c, d	Standard: A3, 4, B1, E4, G1, 2, 3, H2, J1, L2, 5
	Code: 1.2, 2.3, 7.1	Code: 2.1, 2.2, 6.1, 6.3
24 Fully comply with hygiene, uniform and dress codes in order to limit, prevent and control infection.	i. Adheres to local policy and national guidelines on dress code for prevention and control of infection (including: footwear, hair, piercings and nails)	iv. Acts as a role model to others and ensures colleagues work within local policy
	ii. Maintains a high standard of personal hygiene	Standard: A5, N3, Q2, 3
	iii. Wears appropriate clothing for the care delivered	Code: 1.2
	Standard: 1f, g, 8c, 9, 12a, b, c, 16a, b, c, d	
	Code: 4.3, 6.1	
25 Safely apply the principles of asepsis when performing invasive procedures and be competent in aseptic technique.	i. Demonstrates understanding of the principles of wound care, healing and asepsis	iv. Applies a range of appropriate measures to prevent infection including application of safe and effective aseptic technique relevant to branch
	ii. Safely performs basic wound care using clean and aseptic techniques **through simulation**	v. Safely performs wound care/dressings, applying non-touch and/or aseptic techniques related to Branch and task being performed
	iii. Assists in providing accurate information to patients/clients on the management of a device, site or wound to prevent and control infection and to promote healing	vi. Able to communicate potential risks to junior colleagues and advise patients/clients on management of their device, site or wound to prevent and control infection and to promote healing

Infection Prevention and Control

Patients/clients can trust a newly registered nurse to:	For entry to branch	For entry to the register
26 Act to reduce risk when handling waste (including sharps), contaminated linen and when dealing with spillages of blood and body fluids.	i. Adheres to the requirements of the Health and Safety at Work Act and infection control policies regarding the safe disposal of all waste, soiled linen, blood and/or other body fluids and disposing of 'sharps' Standard: 4a, 6b, 7c, 10c Code: 2.1, 6.1	iii. Manages hazardous waste and spillages in accordance with local health and safety policies Standard: H2, 3, 4, 6, K1, 2, N3, O4, P2, 3, Q1, 2, 3 Code: 1.2, 1.4, 2.1, 4.3, 6.1
	ii. Acts to address potential risks within a timely manner Standard: 2e, 12a, b, c Code: 1.5, 8.1, 8.2	Standard: L1, 2, 3, 5, O3 Code: 6.1, 8.1, 8.2

Nutrition and Fluid Management

Patients/clients can trust a newly registered nurse to:	For entry to branch	For entry to the register
27 Provide assistance with selecting a diet through which they will receive adequate nutritional and fluid intake.	i. Under supervision supports patients/clients to make healthy food and fluid choices	vi. Uses knowledge of dietary and other factors contributing to ill health, obesity, weight loss, poor fluid intake and poor nutrition to inform practice
	ii. Accurately monitors dietary and fluid intake and completes relevant documentation *	vii. Supports patients/clients to make appropriate choices/changes to eating patterns, taking account of dietary preferences (including religious and cultural requirements) and special diets needed for health reasons
	iii. Supports patients/clients who need to adhere to specific dietary and fluid regimens	viii. Refers to specialist member of the multidisciplinary team for additional/specialist advice
	iv. Provides assistance as required (e.g. use of beakers, bottles, adapted cutlery, plates, positioning, etc.)	ix. Discusses with patients/clients how diet can improve health and the risks associated with not eating appropriately
	v. Identifies and reports patients/clients who are unable to or have difficulty in eating or drinking so that they achieve adequate nutrition and fluid intake Standard: 1c, 2e, 5b, c, 6a, 7a, b, 8b, c, f, 9, 10c, 11c, 16a, c, Code: 2.1, 3.1, 3.2, 4.4, 6.1	x. Provides advice and support to mothers who are breast feeding where relevant to branch
		xi. Provides support and advice to carers when there are feeding difficulties Standard: A6, C1, 2, 3, 4, E1, 2, 3, 4, H5, J1, O2, P3, Q1, 2 Code: 1.4, 2.1, 2.2, 2.4, 3.1, 4.3, 6.1, 6.3

28 Assess and monitor nutritional status and formulate an effective care plan.	i. Takes and records accurate measurements of weight, height / length, body mass index and other appropriate measures of nutritional status *	v. Makes a comprehensive assessment of patients'/clients' needs in relation to nutrition identifying, documenting and communicating level of risk *
	ii. Assesses baseline nutritional requirements for healthy person (related to age, mobility, etc.)	vi. Seeks specialist advice as required in order to formulate an appropriate care plan
	iii. Contributes to formulating a care plan through assessment of dietary preferences, including local availability of foods and cooking facilities	vii. Provides information to patient/client and carers
	iv. Reports to other members of the team when agreed plan is not achieved	viii. Monitors and records progress against the plan
	Standard: 5b, c, d, 7a, b, 8a, b, f, 9, 10a, b, 11a, b,	ix. Discusses progress/changes in the patients'/clients' condition with the multidisciplinary team
		x. Reports malnutrition/worsening nutritional status as an adverse event and initiates appropriate action
	Code: 4.2, 4.5, 6.3,	Standard: A3, 4, F1, 2, 3, G2, H3, 4, 5, M2, 3, O2
		Code: 2.1, 4.3, 4.4, 6.3, 8.1
29 Assess and monitor fluid status and formulate an effective care plan.	i. Applies knowledge of fluid requirements needed for health and during illness/recovery so that appropriate fluids can be provided	v. Uses negotiating and other skills to encourage patients/clients who might be reluctant to drink to take adequate fluids
	ii. Accurately monitors and records fluid intake and output *	vi. Identifies signs of dehydration and acts to correct these *
	iii. Recognises and reports reasons for poor fluid intake and output	vii. Works collaboratively with multidisciplinary team to ensure an adequate fluid intake and output
	iv. Reports to other members of the team when fluid intake and output falls below requirements	Standard: A3, 4, D1, 2, J1, M2, 3, O2
	Standard: 3a, b, c, 4c, e, 6a, d, 7a, c, d, 9, 10c, d, 11c, 16c,	Code: 4.1, 4.2, 4.3, 4.4, 6.1
	Code: 2.1, 4.3, 4.4,	

Nutrition and Fluid Management

Patients/clients can trust a newly registered nurse to:	For entry to branch	For entry to the register
30 Provide an environment conducive to eating and drinking.	**In residential care settings:** i. Follows local procedures in relation to mealtimes (e.g. protected mealtimes, indicators of patients who need additional support) ii. Ensures that patients/clients are ready for the meal (i.e. in appropriate location, position, offered opportunity to wash hands, offered appropriate assistance) iii. Reports to appropriate person if a patient/client is unable to eat at the mealtime (e.g. is away from the unit, unwell, etc.) iv. Follows food hygiene procedures Standard: 2e, 8a, d, f, 9,10a, c, 12b, Code: 1.5, 2.2, 6.1, 6.3, 8.1	v. Challenges others who do not follow procedures vi. Ensures appropriate assistance and support is available to enable patients/clients to eat vii. Makes provision for replacement meals for those patients/clients unable to eat at the usual time viii. Ensures that appropriate food and fluids are available as required by the patients/clients Standard: A5, B5, I1, K4, M1, N1, 2, 3, O4, P3, Q3 Code: 1.3, 1.4, 4.3, 4.5, 4.6, 6.4, 8.1, 8.2, 8.4
31 Ensure that those unable to take food by mouth receive adequate nutrition.	i. Recognises, responds appropriately and reports patients who have difficulty eating and/or swallowing ii. Adheres to a plan of care that provides adequate nutrition and hydration when eating or swallowing is difficult Standard: 6a, b, c, d, 7a, b, Code: 1.2, 2.1, 4.2	iii. Takes action to ensure that, where there are problems with eating and swallowing, nutritional status is not compromised iv. Where relevant to branch, administers enteral feeds safely and maintains equipment in accordance with local policy * v. Where relevant to branch safely inserts, maintains and uses nasogastric, PEG and other feeding devices Standard: A6, B1, 4, 5, H1, 2, 3, 4, K1, 2, 3, 4, L1, O2. Code: 1.4, 6.1, 6.2, 8.1,

Nutrition and Fluid Management

Patients/clients can trust a newly registered nurse to:	For entry to branch	For entry to the register
32 Safely administer fluids when fluids cannot be taken independently.		**Where relevant to branch:** i. Understands and applies the knowledge that intravenous fluids are prescribed and works within local administration of medicines policy ii. Monitors and assesses patients/clients receiving intravenous fluids * iii. Documents progress against prescription and markers of hydration * iv. Monitors infusion site for signs of abnormality, reports and documents any such signs Standard: G2, J1, 2, L2, O2 Code: 4.3, 4.3, 6.1, 6.2, 6.5

Medicines Management

Patients/clients can trust a newly registered nurse to:	For entry to branch	For entry to the register	Indicative content
33 Correctly and safely undertake medicine[2] calculations.	i. Is competent in basic medicines calculations* Standard: 15a, 16a Code: 6.1	ii. Accurately calculates medicines frequently encountered within branch * Standard: O2, P4 Code: 6.1	Numeracy skills, drug calculations required to administer medicines safely via appropriate routes in branch including specific requirements for children and other groups.
34 Work within the legal and ethical framework that underpins safe and effective medicines management.	i. Demonstrates understanding of legal/ethical frameworks relating to safe administration of medicines in practice	ii. Applies legislation in practice to safe and effective ordering, receiving, storing administering and disposal of medicines and drugs, including controlled drugs in both primary and secondary care settings	Law, consent, confidentiality, ethics, accountability. Responsibilities under law, application of medicines legislation to practice, including use of controlled drugs, exemption orders in relation to Patient Group Directions (PGD).[3]

[1] Medicines management is 'The clinical cost-effective and safe use of medicines to ensure patients get maximum benefit from the medicines they need while at the same time minimising potential harm.'

[2] A medicinal product is: 'Any substance or combination of substances presented for treating or preventing disease in human beings or in animals. Any substance or combination of substances which may be administered to human beings or animals with a view to making a medical diagnosis or to restoring, correcting or modifying physiological functions in human beings or animals is likewise considered a medicinal product' (Council Directive 65/65/EEC).

[3] The law states that only registered nurses may supply and administer a PGD. This cannot be delegated to any other person, including students.

Medicines Management

Patients/clients can trust a newly registered nurse to:	For entry to branch	For entry to the register	Indicative content
	Standard: 2d, 9, 12b, 16a Code: 1.5, 6.1	Standard: A5, 6, B1 Code: 1.5, 6.1, 6.2	Regulatory requirements: NMC guidance for the administration of medicines and NMC code of professional conduct: standards for conduct, performance and ethics, statutory requirements in relation to Mental Health and Children and Young People and Medicines. National Service Frameworks and other country specific guidance.
35 Work as part of a team to offer a range of treatment options of which medicines may form a part.	i. Demonstrates awareness of a range of commonly recognised approaches to managing symptoms, e.g. relaxation, distraction, lifestyle advice	iii. Works confidently as part of the team to develop treatment options and choices	Health promotion, lifestyle advice, over-the-counter medicines, self-administration of medicines and other therapies.
	ii. Discusses referral options	iv. Questions, critically appraises and uses evidence to support an argument in determining when medicines may or may not be an appropriate choice of treatment	Observation and assessment. Effect of medicines and other treatment options, including distraction, positioning, complementary therapies, etc.
	Standard: 8f, 9,16a Code: 6.1	Standard: A4, D1, G3, H1, 3, 6, K4, L2, 4, M1, 2, 3 Code: 4.2, 8.1, 8.2	
36 Ensure safe and effective practice through comprehensive knowledge of medicines, their actions, risks and benefits.	i. Uses knowledge of commonly administered medicines in order to act promptly in cases where side effects and adverse reactions occur	ii. Applies knowledge of basic pharmacology, how medicines act and interact in the systems of the body, and their therapeutic action related to branch practice	Related anatomy and physiology. Drug pathways, how medicines act.
	Standard: 16a	iii. Safely manages drug administration and monitors effects. *	Pharmaco-therapeutics – what are therapeutic actions of certain medicines Risks versus benefits of medication.
	Code: 6.1	iv. Safely manages anaphylaxis	Pharmacokinetics and how doses are determined by dynamics/systems in body.
		v. Reports adverse incidents and near misses	Role and function of bodies that regulate and ensure the safety and effectiveness of medicines.

	For entry to branch	For entry to the register	Indicative content
		Standard: F2, 3, J2, O2, P4	Knowledge on management of 'adverse drug events', adverse drug reactions, prescribing and administration errors and the potential repercussions for patient safety.
		Code: 6.1, 6.4	
Medicines Management			
Patients/clients can trust a newly registered nurse to:			
37 Order, receive, store and dispose of medicines safely in any setting (including controlled drugs).	i. Demonstrates ability to safely store medicines under supervision	ii. Orders, receives, stores and disposes of medicines safely in relation to branch (including controlled drugs)	Managing medicines in in-patient or primary care settings, e.g. schools and homes.
	Standard: 2d, 12b	Standard: B1, L3, 5	Legislation that underpins practice, related to a wide range of medicines including controlled drugs, infusions, oxygen, etc.
	Code: 1.5, 6.1	Code: 1.5, 6.1, 6.2	Suitable conditions for storage, managing out-of-date stock, safe handling medication, managing discrepancies in stock, omissions.
			www.dh.gsi.gov.uk – see *Safer management of controlled drugs*
38 Administer medicines safely in a timely manner, including controlled drugs.	i. Uses prescription charts correctly and maintains accurate records	iv. Safely and effectively administers medicines via routes and methods commonly used within the branch and maintains accurate records *	Patient/client involvement, fear and anxiety, importance of non-verbal and verbal communication.
	ii. Utilises and safely disposes of equipment needed to draw up/administer medication (e.g. needles, syringes, gloves)	Standard: A1, G2, H4, L1, O2	Use of prescription charts including how to prepare, read and interpret them and record administration and non-administration. Use of patient/client drug record cards for controlled drugs.
	iii. Administers medication safely under direct supervision, including orally and by injection in simulation and/or in practice	Code: 4.4, 6.1	Preparing and administering medication in differing environments, hygiene, infection control, compliance aids, safe transport and disposal of medicines and and equipment.
	Standard: 1c, d, 8f, 10d, 12b, 15a		Safety, checking patient/client identity, last dose, allergies, anaphylaxis, polypharmacy, monitoring of effect and record-keeping.

Medicines Management

Patients/clients can trust a newly registered nurse to:	For entry to branch	For entry to the register	Indicative content
	Code: 4.4, 6.3		Where and how to report contra-indications, side effects, adverse reactions.
			Skills needed to administer safely via various means, e.g. oral, topical, by infusion, injection, syringe driver and pumps, e.g. in relation to branch.
			Aware of own limitations and when to refer on.
			Legal requirements, mechanisms for supply, sale and administration of medication, self-administration.

Medicines Management

Patients/clients can trust a newly registered nurse to:	For entry to branch	For entry to the register	Indicative content
39 Keep and maintain accurate records within a multidisciplinary framework and as part of a team.	i. Demonstrates awareness of the roles and responsibilities within the MDT for medicines management, including how and in what ways information is shared	ii. Effectively keep records of medication administered and omitted, including controlled drugs	Links to legislation, use of controlled drugs, *NMC code of professional conduct: standards for conduct, performance and ethics*, in relation to confidentiality, consent and record-keeping.
	Standard: 5d, 9, 13a, b, c	Standard: A1, B1, G2, O2	Use of electronic records.
	Code: 4.2, 4.3	Code: 4.4	
40 Work in partnership with patient/clients and carers in relation to concordance and managing their medicines.	i. Under supervision involves patient/client and carers in administration/self-administration of medicines.	ii. Works with patients/clients, parents and carers to provide clear and accurate information	Cultural, religious, linguistic and ethical beliefs, issues and sensitivities around medication.
	Standard: 4c, 7c, d, 9	iii. Gives clear instruction, explanation before checking understanding relating to use of medicines and treatment options	Ethical issues relating to compliance and covert administration of medicines.
	Code: 2.1, 2.2	iv. Assesses the patients'/clients' ability to safely self-administer their medicines	Self-administration, patient/client assessment explanation and monitoring.

Learning outcome	Competency	Competency	Notes / resources
			Concordance.
		v. Assists patients/clients to make safe and informed choices about their medicines Standard: C3, 4, E1, 2, 3, G2, 3, H3, J1 Code: 4.2, 4.3	Meeting needs of specific groups including self-administration, e.g. the mentally ill, learning disabled, children and elderly.
41 Use and evaluate up-to-date information on medicines management and work within national and local policies.	i. Accesses commonly used evidence-based sources relating to the safe and effective management of medicines Standard: 2d, 9, 12b Code: 1.5, 6.1	ii. Works within national and local policies relevant to the branch Standard: B4, E1, 2, H5 Code: 1.5, 2.1, 5.4	Evidence-based practice, identification of resources, the 'expert' patient/client. Using sources of information, national and local policies, clinical governance, formularies, e.g. British National Formulary and the Children's British National Formulary.
42 Demonstrate understanding and knowledge to supply and administer via a Patient Group Direction (PGD).[1]	i. Demonstrates knowledge of what a Patient Group Direction is and who can use them Standard: 9, 16a, b, 13c Code: 6.1	ii. **Through simulation and course work** demonstrates knowledge and application of the principles required for safe and effective supply and administration via a Patient Group Direction including an understanding of role and accountability iii. **Through simulation and course work** demonstrates how to supply and administer via a Patient Group Direction Standard: H4, P4 Code: 6.1	National Prescribing Centre Competency Framework **www.npc.co.uk.**

[1] The law states that only registered nurses may supply and administer a PGD. This cannot be delegated to any other person, including students.

List of abbreviations

A&E	Accident and Emergency Department
AAGBI	Association of Anaesthetists of Great Britain and Ireland
ABCDE	Airway, Breathing, Circulation, Disability, Exposure
ACLS	advanced cardiac life support
ADD	Assessment of Discomfort in Dementia Protocol
AED	automatic external defibrillator
ALERT	Acute Life-threatening Events Recognition and Treatment
ANTT	aseptic non-touch technique
AVPU	Alert, Voice, Pain, Unconscious
BAOT/COT	British Association/College of Occupational Therapists
BAPEN	British Association for Parenteral and Enteral Nutrition
BBV	blood-borne virus
BMA	British Medical Association
BMI	body mass index
bpm	beats per minute
BRASS	Blaylock Risk Assessment Screening Score
BUN	blood urea nitrogen
BVM	bag, valve and mask device
CDCP	Centers for Disease Control and Prevention
COPD	chronic obstructive pulmonary disease
CPR	cardio-pulmonary resuscitation
CRCU	Critical Resus Care Unit
CSM	Committee on Safety of Medicines
CSP	Chartered Society of Physiotherapy
CT	computerised tomography

CVA	cerebral vascular accident
CVP	central venous pressure
DoH	Department of Health
DNAR	do not attempt resuscitation
DS-DAT	Discomfort Scale – Dementia of the Alzheimer's Type
ECRI	Emergency Care Research Institute
EDTA	ethyline diamine tetra-acetic acid
EMD	electromechanical dissociation
EPINet	Exposure Prevention Information Network
EPUAP	European Pressure Ulcer Advisory Panel
ER	emergency room
ESC	Essential Skills Cluster
EWS	Early Warning Score
FBC	full blood count
F_IO_2	fraction of inspired oxygen
FOB	[test] for occult blood
GCS	Glasgow Coma Scale
GI	gastrointestinal
GSCC	General Social Care Council
GSL	general sale list [medicine]
GTN	glyceryl trinitrate
HASAWA	Health and Safety at Work Act 1974
HCAI	health care associated infection
HIV/AIDS	human immunosuppressive virus/acquired immune deficiency syndrome
HMSO	Her Majesty's Stationery Office
HO	house officer
HSE	Health and Safety Executive

IHCD	Institute of Health and Care Development
IDDM	insulin-dependent diabetes mellitus
INS	Intravenous Nurses Society
IV	intravenous
LMA	laryngeal mask airway
MCA	Medicines Control Agency
MDA	Medical Devices Agency
MDI	metered dose inhaler
MDT	multidisciplinary team
MEWS	Modified Early Warning Score
MHOR	Manual Handling Operations Regulations 1992 (as amended 2002)
MHRA	Medicines and Healthcare Products Regulatory Agency
MRSA	methicillin resistant Staphylococcus aureus
MSD	musculoskeletal disorder
MUST	Malnutrition Universal Screening Tool
NAD	no abnormalities detected
NBPA	North British Pain Association
NG	nasogastric
NHO	National Hospice Organisation
NHS	National Health Service
NICE	National Institute for Health and Clinical Excellence
NMC	Nursing and Midwifery Council
NNP	night nurse practitioner
NPSA	National Patient Safety Agency
NSAID	non-steroidal anti-inflammatory drug
PAINAD	Pain Assessment in Advanced Dementia Scale

PCA	patient-controlled analgesia
PEA	pulseless electrical activity
PEARL	pupils equal and reacting to light
PEG	percutaneous endoscopic gastrostomy
PGD	Patient Group Direction
POM	prescription only medicine
PONV	post-operative nausea and vomiting
POTTS	Physiological Observation Track and Trigger System
PPE	personal protective equipment
RCGP	Royal College of General Practitioners
RCN	Royal College of Nursing
RCPCH	Royal College of Paediatrics and Child Health
RPS	Royal Pharmaceutical Society of Great Britain
SALT	speech and language therapist
SAP	Single Assessment Process
SHO	senior house officer
SIGN	Scottish Intercollegiate Guidelines Network
SOAD	second opinion approved doctor
TENS	transcutaneous electrical nerve stimulation
TM	traditional medicine
TPN	total parenteral nutrition
TPR	temperature, pulse and respirations
UKCC	United Kingdom Central Council for Nursing, Midwifery and Health Visiting
UTI	urinary tract infection
VF	ventricular fibrillation
VT	ventricular tachycardia
WHO	World Health Organisation

Glossary

Adjuvants Substances that, when added to a medicine, speed or improve its action.

Aetiology The area of medical science that deals with the causes of disease.

Agonist drug A drug that binds to a receptor on the plasma membrane of a cell and initiates a change in the function of the cell. A drug that is an agonist has attraction to bind to a given receptor and will activate the receptor and subsequently lead to a change in the function of the cell.

Anaphylactic reaction Anaphylaxis is a severe and rapid systemic allergic reaction to a trigger substance, called an allergen. Minute amounts of allergens may cause a life-threatening anaphylactic reaction. Anaphylaxis may occur after ingestion, inhalation, skin contact or injection of a trigger substance. The most severe type of anaphylaxis – anaphylactic shock – will usually result in death if untreated.

Antagonist drugs Bind to a receptor site but will not cause any change in the function of the receptor or the cell. They will effectively block the receptor, thus preventing the agonist compound from having any effect on the cell.

Anthropometrical measurements A non-invasive way of scientifically measuring an individual's body composition including body weight and height, upper arm, chest and head circumference, in order to assess physiological development and nutritional status.

Apraxia Defined as the inability to make voluntary movements, despite being able to demonstrate normal muscle function.

Arrhythmias Variations from the normal rhythm of the heart beat (sinus rhythm).

Aspiration pneumonia A term used to describe the inhalation (aspiration) of a substance, commonly food, drink, gastric acid or vomit, leading to lung damage or a respiratory infection such as pneumonia. If the infection is insufficiently treated it can become life-threatening, leading to respiratory failure.

Asystole Absence of a heart beat, coupled with absence of cardiac electrical activity.

Auscultation A term used to refer to the action of listening to internal organs, usually with the aid of a stethoscope.

Bacteraemia A condition in which bacteria are present in the bloodstream.

Body mass index (BMI) Also known as the Quetelet Index, is a calculation used to determine body weight in relation to height and whether an individual's body weight is within the expected range (value) for their height. A BMI value of less than 19 indicates that a person is underweight, the normal range is 20–25 and anything greater than 26 is considered overweight or obese. The calculation is based on weight in kilograms divided by height in metres squared:

$$BMI = \frac{Weight\ (kg)}{Height\ (m^2)}$$

Cardiac arrest Refers to cessation of the pumping mechanism of the heart. It is a major emergency but can be reversed using life support techniques.

Colloids A concentrated substance, containing larger insoluble particles that do not pass easily through a semi-permeable membrane. These are used in clinical practice as plasma expanders to boost blood volume and blood pressure.

Crystalloids An aqueous substance containing water-soluble molecules that enable them to pass freely through a semi-permeable membrane.

Detrusor hyperreflexia A term used solely in reference to those individuals who have a clearly defined neurologic disease causing involuntary bladder contractions. Examples of neurologic disease states that can lead to detrusor hyperreflexia are stroke, Parkinson's disease, multiple sclerosis and Alzheimer's disease.

Diastolic pressure The resting period in the cardiac cycle is known as diastole. The pressure exerted on the arterial walls during diastole is known as the diastolic pressure. It is represented by the lower value of a blood pressure reading.

Dietician A health care professional who specialises in the study of food, diet and nutrition. Dieticians plan and manage diet and dietary advice for patients with special dietary requirements. They form part of the wider multidisciplinary team.

Dysarthria A weakness or incoordination of the muscles controlling speech. This may result in slurred or weak speech patterns. It is common following stroke.

Dysphagia A difficulty with, or inability to, swallow.

Dysphasia A speech disorder in which there is an impairment of speech and of comprehension of speech.

Dyspnoea Difficulty in breathing. For example, a breathless patient may be described as dyspnoeic.

Dysrhythmia An abnormal heart rhythm.

Erythema Diffuse or patchy redness of skin, blanching on pressure, due to congestion of cutaneous capillaries.

Extravasation Escape of fluid from the vessel that is meant to contain it. This can apply to the swelling around an intravenous infusion cannula that occurs when the vein collapses.

Fistula A channel originating from a cavity (such as the bowel) to another cavity (such as the bladder) or the skin surface, which should not be there.

Gallipot A container for solutions, ointments or medicines, usually made from plastic.

Haematemesis Vomiting blood.

Homeostasis Maintenance of a stable, internal environment. Physiological processes work together to maintain homeostasis which is the basis for what we call 'health'.

Hyperglycaemia Excess sugar (glucose) in the blood. It is usually associated with diabetes mellitus.

Hypertension Abnormally high blood pressure.

Hyperthermia Abnormally high body temperature. Also known as pyrexia or fever.

Hypotension Abnormally low blood pressure.

Hypothermia Abnormally low body temperature, below 35°C.

Hypovolaemia A reduced circulating blood volume. This may be caused by bleeding, sweating, vomiting or diarrhoea.

Ischaemia A condition characterised by a lack of blood supply to an area of the body. This may be due to blockage of blood vessels, such as the coronary arteries, leading to angina or a heart attack

Korotkoff sounds The sounds that are listened for when taking a blood pressure reading using a non-invasive technique. They are named after Dr Nikolai Korotkoff, a Russian physician who described them in 1905.

Micturition The act of passing or voiding urine.

Necrosis This term refers to tissue death as a result of ischaemia or a disease process.

Nociceptors Sensory receptors that respond only after a high level of stimuli, enough to hurt the individual. When they are activated they can generate a reflex and pain.

Occult blood Blood in the stool that is not visible but can be detected by simple laboratory tests.

Oedema An abnormal accumulation of fluid beneath the skin, or in one (or more) of the body cavities.

Oliguria An abnormally low excretion of urine. This may be a characteristic of renal impairment.

Osteomyelitis Inflammation of the bone marrow, usually due to infection.

Palpation Examination by pressing on the surface of the body to feel the organs or tissues underneath.

Parenteral nutrition A method of feeding that bypasses the gastrointestinal tract and administers a slow infusion of nutrients directly into the veins. Total parental nutrition (TPN) provides the sole source of nutrients to a patient.

Pharmacodynamics The study of the action of drugs on the human body and the way in which a drug works.

Pharmacokinetics The study of the action of drugs in the body and the way in which the body metabolises a drug.

Phlebitis Inflammation of a vein, often due to the presence of an intravenous cannula.

Postural hypotension An abnormal drop in blood pressure on standing up.

Pulseless electrical activity (PEA) Previously known as electro-mechanical dissociation (EMD). This may occur during cardiac arrest. The pumping mechanism of the heart stops, despite normal cardiac electrical activity being present.

Pyrexia Abnormally high body temperature.

Receiver A container for fluid or equipment. These are usually disposable, but you may come across stainless steel 'kidney dishes', which are examples of receivers.

Receptive aphasia Also known as Wernicke's aphasia: loss of the power of speech, characterised by fluent but meaningless speech and severe impairment of the ability to understand spoken or written words.

Septicaemia Infection (usually bacterial) of the blood. May also be termed as 'blood poisoning'.

Speech and language therapist (SALT) A health care professional who specialises in the assessment and management of communication problems and swallowing difficulties in patients following a stroke.

Steret™ A disposable, alcohol impregnated swab.

Sterile field An area, covered by a sterile sheet, which serves as a clean space when performing an aseptic procedure.

Stridor An abnormal inspiratory noise caused by narrowing of the upper airway, particularly the larynx.

Systolic pressure Contraction of the heart is referred to as systole. The pressure exerted on the walls of arteries during this contraction is known as the systolic pressure. It is represented by the upper value in a blood pressure reading.

Tachycardia Rapid pulse (greater than 100 beats per minute).

Thrombo-embolism Part of a blood clot that becomes detached and occludes another blood vessel further up the vascular tree.

Turgor Being or becoming swollen or engorged.

Vasoconstriction Narrowing of blood vessels.

Vasodilatation Widening of blood vessels.

Vasovagal reflex Sudden slowing of the heart rate due to the action of the vagus nerve. This may lead to a temporary loss in consciousness (a common cause of fainting). It may be caused by shock, acute pain, fear or stress.

Ventricular fibrillation (VF) An arrhythmia of the ventricles that is characterised by uncoordinated electrical activity and a cessation of the pumping mechanism of the heart. It is a common cause of cardiac arrest and may be reversed by defibrillation.

Ventricular tachycardia (VT) An arrhythmia that originates in the lower chambers of the heart, usually to a rate of 150–200 beats per minute; it may result in fainting, low blood pressure, shock or even sudden death; it is a common and often lethal complication of myocardial infarction (heart attack).

Index